Psychological Evaluations in Immigration Cases:

Theory, Practice, and Ethical Considerations

Ana Maria Gamez
California Baptist University, USA

IGI Global
Scientific Publishing
Publishing Tomorrow's Research Today

Vice President of Editorial	Melissa Wagner
Director of Acquisitions	Mikaela Felty
Director of Book Development	Jocelynn Hessler
Production Manager	Mike Brehm
Cover Design	Phillip Shickler

Published in the United States of America by
IGI Global Scientific Publishing
701 East Chocolate Avenue
Hershey, PA, 17033, USA
Tel: 717-533-8845
Fax: 717-533-7115
Website: https://www.igi-global.com E-mail: cust@igi-global.com

Library of Congress Cataloging-in-Publication Data

Names: Gamez, Ana M. editor
Title: Psychological and medical evaluations in immigration cases : theory, practice, and ethical considerations / edited by Ana Gamez.
Description: Hershey, PA : IGI Global Scientific Publishing, [2025] | Includes bibliographical references and index. | Summary: "This book aims to offer a thorough overview of the cultural, psychological, medical, and legal aspects inherent in immigration cases. It provides theoretical and practical insights into the crucial aspects of psychological and medical evaluations in immigration cases"-- Provided by publisher.
Identifiers: LCCN 2024061598 (print) | LCCN 2024061599 (ebook) | ISBN 9798369379448 hardcover | ISBN 9798369379455 paperback | ISBN 9798369379462 ebook
Subjects: LCSH: Emigration and immigration--Psychological aspects--Case studies | Immigrants--Psychology--Case studies | Immigrants--Medical examinations--Case studies
Classification: LCC JV6013 .P767 2025 (print) | LCC JV6013 (ebook) | DDC 362.89/912--dc23/eng/20250313
LC record available at https://lccn.loc.gov/2024061598
LC ebook record available at https://lccn.loc.gov/2024061599

British Cataloguing in Publication Data
A Cataloguing in Publication record for this book is available from the British Library.

Table of Contents

Detailed Table of Contents

The Latino immigrant population in the US plays a major role in society. The US Census Bureau (2022) reports that a substantial number of Spanish speaking individuals report having limited English proficiency (LEP). Furthermore, LEP patients report language barriers as the greatest challenge to receiving healthcare service which may negatively impact their treatment and may lead to negative health outcomes. This chapter provides a brief overview of the Latino immigrant population, the challenges they experience, both societally and personally, as they navigate the immigration process in the US. Specifically, this chapter addresses the concerns and issues related to administering psychological evaluations for the LEP individuals. We expound upon the various challenges that may arise in the interaction between the LEP client and the provider. Clinical implications and recommendations are suggested for the assessor for mitigating communication and cultural disparities for this population.

The United States is often noted as the land of immigrants. Despite this national and international nomenclature, crimes against immigrants have received less empirical examination in comparison to crimes against U.S. citizens. This disparity is an issue since this gap in the literature can potentially obscure and minimize policy and practice. It can be surmised that diminished responses to crime victims, especially violent crimes, is an issue and the inability to consider potential barriers and other contextual factors associated with language and cultural barriers impedes the effectiveness of the justice system and other social institutions. Therefore, the purpose of this chapter is to explore the importance between immigrants and violent crime.

Care and Connection via Day Labor Centers and Others Like Them: Creating Informal Sources of Critical Support for (Im)Migrants In this chapter, the role of day labor centers, and others like them, is considered as a potential source of critical support for (im)migrant workers. Through an ethnographic study of a particular day labor center alongside recent scholarship, this chapter discusses the core challenges of labor migration, the precariousness of day labor in particular, and how labor centers (and others like them) can offer tangible and emotional support for (im)migrants. Centers like these may expand to offer psychological and social services, medical care, and access to important physical provisions. In so doing, (im)migrants may improve their resiliency, knowing that they have an emotionally and physically supportive space from which to draw strength and resources, and ultimately, improve their chances for positive mental health outcomes as they contribute to their families and communities.

The purpose of this chapter is to equip readers with the understanding of factors that may get in the way of mental health care for immigrants, what may help improve access and use and lastly how to provide culturally relevant mental health care for immigrants. In the first section, this chapter will provide the reader with an understanding of barriers to both access and use of mental health care for immigrants. Further, the chapter will identify facilitators towards improving access and use of mental health care for immigrants. The second half of the chapter will provide recommendations for clinical practice via a five step framework which may be applied in working with immigrants in mental health care settings.

This chapter explores the profound psychological impacts of domestic violence and human trafficking, highlighting their role as pervasive human rights violations. It delves into the psychological effects, including PTSD, depression, and dissociation,

The results indicate that K-Means clustering provided the best balance of accuracy and computational efficiency, offering insights into the psychological profiles of immigrants and their coping mechanisms under stress.

Preface

INTRODUCTION

As the editor of *"Psychological Evaluations in Immigration Cases: Theory, Practice, and Ethical Considerations*," I am proud to present this volume that brings together leading scholars, clinicians, and researchers to explore the theoretical foundations and practical applications of psychological, legal, and human rights in immigration cases. This book is a vital resource for professionals seeking to understand and navigate the nuanced process of psychological evaluations within the context of immigration and university professors teaching immigration psychology.

Our contributors provide peer-reviewed research and share real-world case studies illustrating immigrants' challenges. The chapters offer in-depth discussions on a wide range of issues, including trauma, culture shock, acculturation, psychological testing, and trauma-informed treatment approaches, as well as gang violence, political persecution, human trafficking, family separation, and the psychological impact of detention.

The primary audience for this book includes graduate students, academic researchers, attorneys, psychologists, and policymakers. Whether you are preparing to conduct evaluations, represent clients in legal proceedings, or contribute to academic research and policy development, this textbook offers critical insights and evidence-based strategies for effective, compassionate, and informed work in immigration cases.

I hope this book serves as both a foundational text and a practical guide for those committed to justice and the psychological well-being of immigrant populations.

ORGANIZATION OF THE BOOK

This volume opens with Chapter 1, which provides foundational context for understanding *The Role of Psychological Evaluations in Immigration Proceedings*. Psychological assessments help inform judicial decision-making in emotionally and culturally complex cases. The chapter outlines how these evaluations are often integral to legal processes such as asylum, hardship waivers, and applications under VAWA, U, and T Visas.

Chapter 2 turns our attention to *The Psychological Sequelae of Trauma and Stress as Immigrants Adapt to a New Country*. It unpacks the unique psychological factors inherent in stress, trauma, and mental health disorders such as PTSD and depression frequently found among immigrants. The chapter advocates for trauma-informed clinical practice and emphasizes the need for cultural competence in recognizing and treating these conditions.

In Chapter 3, the focus shifts to *Language Barriers in the Mexican Immigrant Population*, analyzing the role of limited English proficiency in complicating the delivery of psychological services. Drawing from demographic data and clinical experience, the authors offer recommendations for overcoming linguistic and cultural challenges in assessments, ensuring fair and accurate evaluation outcomes.

Chapter 4, titled *The Land of Dreams or Muffled Screams*, examines the intersection of immigration and violent crime in the United States. The authors argue that a lack of empirical attention to crimes against immigrants has policy implications and undermines justice. This chapter highlights cultural and systemic barriers and urges a more inclusive and informed response from institutions serving immigrant populations.

Chapter 5, explores *Care and Connection via Day Labor Centers and Others Like Them: Providing Informal Sources of Critical Support for (Im)Migrants*, through an ethnographic lens. This chapter examines how such informal spaces provide vital emotional, and social support to vulnerable (im)migrant laborers. The discussion illustrates how these community-based networks bolster resilience and fill critical service gaps often left unattended by formal systems.

Chapter 6, *Mental Health Care with Immigrants, Barriers, Facilitators, and Recommendations for Clinical Practice* provides a practical roadmap for clinicians. It details the barriers immigrants face in accessing care and identifies facilitators that can bridge these divides. A five-step framework is presented, equipping practitioners with culturally competent strategies for delivering effective and equitable mental health care.

In Chapter 7, titled *From Trauma to Triumph*, the psychological aftermath of domestic violence and human trafficking is examined through forensic and therapeutic perspectives. The chapter highlights victim resilience and showcases evidence-based interventions like trauma-focused CBT, emphasizing multidisciplinary collaboration to support survivors' mental health and legal needs.

Chapter 8 delves into *Ethical Challenges in Multicultural Social Work with Immigrants*. This chapter critically reflects on the ethical challenges and encourages reflection, cultural humility, and transformative practice to address inequality and promote justice within immigrant-serving systems.

Finally, Chapter 9 presents an innovative approach in *Legal and Psychological Resilience: A Cluster Analysis of Immigrant Populations*. The use of cluster analysis offers new empirical insights into how immigrants cope and adapt, contributing valuable knowledge for both legal and clinical professionals.

CONCLUSION

This collection is designed as both a scholarly resource and a practical guide. It provides tools, frameworks, and real-world insights for professionals at the intersection of immigration and mental health.

Bringing together the diverse chapters in this volume reveals a powerful narrative highlighting the often-overlooked psychological complexities immigrant populations face.

Each chapter enriches our understanding of immigrant experiences and calls attention to the role of the forensic psychologist and other practitioners in immigration proceedings. It also highlights the ethical responsibility of professionals—clinicians, social workers, legal advocates, and researchers—to respond with cultural humility, clinical precision, and unwavering compassion.

The aim is to encourage ethical practice, advocacy, and care that promotes dignity, resilience, and equity for immigrant communities around the globe.

Chapter 1
The Role of Psychological Evaluations in Immigration Proceedings

Ana M. Gamez
https://orcid.org/0000-0003-4523-1470
California Baptist University, USA

Kelsey A. Michaels
California Baptist University, USA

Garrett P. Murrieta
https://orcid.org/0009-0000-4440-7062
California Baptist University, USA

Daniel Abdala
https://orcid.org/0009-0009-6717-9045
California Baptist University, USA

ABSTRACT

Immigrants pursuing changes in their legal status often encounter the complexities and challenges of the U.S. immigration system. This chapter examines the critical role psychological evaluations play in various immigration cases. These assessments are frequently essential for guiding legal decisions, particularly when psychological factors are pivotal. Psychological evaluations are essential in asylum claims, extreme hardship waivers, and evaluations related to asylum and cases involving VAWA, U Visas, and T Visas.

DOI: 10.4018/979-8-3693-7944-8.ch001

INTRODUCTION

The U.S. has the largest immigrant population as compared to any other country, and these numbers are predicted to increase (Moslimani & Passel, 2024; Prabhu & Baranoski, 2012; Tazi et al., 2023). In 2023, approximately 47.8 million immigrants lived in the U.S., an increase of about 1.6 million from the previous year, representing naturalized U.S. Citizens, lawful permanent residents, lawful temporary residents, and unauthorized immigrants (Gramlich & Passel, 2024). Since the 1960s, the number of foreign-born persons living in the U.S. has substantially increased, representing about 14.3% of the U.S. population in 2023 (Moslimani & Passel, 2024). Relocating to the U.S. and adapting to life in a new country can be particularly demanding on an individual's overall well-being. Immigrants seeking changes in legal status soon realize the inherent challenges of navigating the complexity of the U.S. immigration system. The U.S. immigration law poses many challenges for those seeking immigration relief within the U.S. There is a growing demand for qualified mental health professionals in immigration proceedings. Forensic psychologists provide immigration adjudicators with valuable insights regarding an individual's psychological functioning to address legal questions.

Many types of immigration relief exist for immigrants seeking legal status in the U.S. Psychological evaluations for immigration proceedings provide legal decision-makers with critical information regarding the type of relief the applicant seeks. Psychological evaluations are recommended to assess the applicants' psychological traumas, history of symptoms and diagnoses, and current psychological functioning. This chapter will explore different types of immigration relief that often benefit from a psychological expert opinion. These include immigration cases on asylum, cancellation of removal, extreme hardship waivers, Violence Against Women Act (VAWA) cases, U Visas, and T Visas.

THE PSYCHOLOGICAL EVALUATION IN IMMIGRATION CASES

Psychological evaluations in immigration cases are specialized forensic evaluations that should be conducted by licensed professionals practicing within the scope of practice dictated by their license and trained in conducting psychological evaluations in immigration cases. Psychological evaluations allow the trained mental health professional (e.g., Licensed Clinical Psychologist) to conduct a forensic interview that helps answer a psycho-legal question. Psychological evaluations generally use mixed-method forms of data collection and analysis. For example, the forensic interview with the applicant may include record reviews, interviews with family members and spouses, and psychological testing. The psychological evaluation helps provide vital information to the immigration adjudicator or judge.

The psychologist's role in conducting immigration evaluations is to remain neutral and objective (Barber-Rioja et al., 2022). Before beginning the interview, the psychologist must inform the qualifying relative(s) about the process and purpose of the psychological evaluation for their immigration case and advise the interviewee about the psychologist's role during the evaluation (Shibley & Holt, 2022). The psychologist must also clarify their role and the purpose of the evaluation. Educating the applicant that the psychologist is acting as an evaluator, not as a clinician or therapist, is essential. The psychologist should inform the interviewee that they will be asked about different aspects of their life that may be uncomfortable to discuss. Notably, the psychologist must clarify the limits of confidentiality and that any information disclosed during the interview may be included in the final report, which will be shared with the applicant's immigration attorney and the immigration adjudicator (Shibley & Holt, 2022).

Psychological measures, such as symptom-specific assessments, structured clinical interviews, and personality assessment tests, may examine the quality of relationships and tests for malingering of symptoms to answer the referral question (Barber-Rioja et al., 2022; Evans & Hass, 2018; Meyers, 2020; Shibley & Holt, 2022; Weiss & Rosenfeld, 2012). Objective psychological measures should be valid, reliable, and empirically grounded to provide valuable fact-based evidence for immigration adjudicators (Barber-Rioja et al., 2022; Evans & Hass, 2018). An advantage of psychological assessments is that they help to assess and identify current symptoms, the existence of a mental health disorder, or other psychological vulnerabilities. This information can validate immigration claims, such as extreme hardship or fear of persecution (Evans & Hass, 2018).

Many psychological measures are used in assessing applicants going through immigration proceedings. The decision of which assessments to use depends on the forensic evaluator's clinical judgment, scope of practice, training, and competence (Evans & Hass, 2018; Shibley & Holt, 2022). Many of the assessments used in immigration evaluations are self-report measures (Shibley & Holt, 2022). Psychological evaluators must be competent in assessing the psychological tests' appropriateness given the applicant's cultural and linguistic background (Melikyan et al., 2019).

A psychologist or any mental health professional considering this type of work must have the requisite scope of practice, education, training, and experience to conduct these psychological evaluations. Culture, language, acculturation, and language proficiency are among the many factors that must be considered with this diverse population, given that immigrants can come from all over the world. Forensic evaluators must consider whom they are assessing (i.e., language, culture, education), the psychometric properties of the assessment (i.e., standardization, validity, reliability), and the purpose of the assessment (Meyers, 2020; Shibley & Holt, 2022).

ASYLUM

The number of asylum applications in the U.S. has steadily risen from 262,046 in 2022 to 862,638 in 2024 (U.S. Department of Justice, 2024). Many asylum-seekers have experienced unimaginable trauma and violence in their native countries, as well as enduring traumatic experiences along their migration journey. Asylum seekers report having experienced persecution due to political violence, gang violence, war, genocide, gender-based violence, and insurrections. Many of these individuals develop psychiatric symptoms, including anxiety, depression, and posttraumatic stress disorder (Singer et al., 2020). Consequently, the need for forensic mental health professionals in asylum immigration proceedings is growing.

To qualify for asylum eligibility within the U.S., the asylee must meet the definition of a refugee according to Section 101(a)(42) of the Immigration and Nationality Act (INA). Essentially, a refugee is an individual who is outside their country of nationality and is unable or unwilling to return to their country due to persecution or a well-founded fear of persecution based on one of the five protected grounds: race, religion, political opinion, nationality, or membership to a particular social group (Meyers, 2020). Individuals who request protection while outside of the U.S. are considered refugees, whereas asylum applies to individuals already in the U.S. (Rosenberg, 2019).

According to U.S. laws, there are two pathways for asylum-seekers: affirmative asylum processing and defensive asylum processing. Affirmative asylum applies to individuals who have entered the U.S., have applied for asylum within one year, and are not in removal proceedings (Rosenberg, 2019). Individuals seeking affirmative asylum receive a non-adversarial interview with a USCIS officer, who determines whether the applicant should be granted asylum as a matter of discretion (Meyers, 2020). Individuals not granted asylum are placed in removal (deportation) proceedings in immigration court and can file a defensive asylum application (Rosenberg, 2019).

Asylum applicants bear the burden of proof, which can be difficult, as applicants often lack adequate evidence of persecution, such as documentation or witness testimony (Prabhu & Baranoski, 2012). Ultimately, the case will depend heavily on the applicant's testimony, in which they must demonstrate that they have suffered from past persecution or have a well-founded fear of future persecution if forced to return to their home country. Demonstrating a well-found fear of future persecution requires both a subjective and an objective component. The subjective component requires demonstrating a genuine fear of future persecution. The objective component is established by demonstrating that there is a reasonable possibility (i.e., a 10% chance) that they will be targeted for persecution by a government entity or that the government entity cannot or will not protect them from persecution on account of the five protected grounds (NIJC, 2022). Whether the applicant's testimony describes past persecution or a well-founded fear of future persecution, the immigration adjudicator must determine if the applicant's claims are credible. A determination of credibility is based on the totality of the circumstances, as well as relevant factors that include the applicant's demeanor, candor, or responsiveness, the inherent plausibility of the testimony, and any inconsistencies or falsehoods within the written or oral statements provided by the applicant or witnesses (Meyers, 2020). The psychological effects of persecution and violence include depression, anxiety, PTSD, suicidal ideation, sleep difficulties, somatic complaints, difficulty concentrating, fatigue, memory loss, insomnia, and nightmares (McKenzie, 2022; Meyers, 2020). Due to the distressing nature of their experiences, applicants may exhibit emotional numbing, an avoidance or reluctance to discuss their trauma, a flat affect, and difficulty concentrating or recalling details of the traumatic event (Evans & Hass, 2018; Rosenberg, 2019).

Psychological evaluations provide an objective and comprehensive narrative explaining the traumatic event(s), the resulting psychological and cognitive impact of trauma, and how trauma manifests across individual and cultural factors. Evaluations help document the traumatic experiences of asylum-seekers fleeing persecution and provide evidence that adds to the credibility of the asylum claims. Psychological evaluations for asylum cases must include clinical interviews, reliable psychological testing, and collateral evidence. Furthermore, while conducting these evaluations, it is essential for interviewers to be aware of the trauma experienced by asylum seekers and to employ techniques that facilitate a safe and supportive environment for disclosure. These evaluations not only document the applicant's experience in their home country but also explain how trauma can manifest in several ways, further adding to the credibility of their testimony (Evans & Hass, 2018; Rosenberg, 2019).

HARDSHIP CASES

Immigrants seeking to enter or remain in the U.S. must gain permission from the U.S. government. Some individuals may be subject to grounds of inadmissibility or even removability. Inadmissibility applies to individuals prohibited from obtaining a visa and entering the country (Shibley & Holt, 2022). Furthermore, inadmissibility may also apply to those prohibited from adjusting their lawful status within the U.S.

(U.S. Department of Homeland Security, 2024). In contrast, removability refers to individuals no longer permitted to remain in the U.S. (Shibley & Holt, 2022).

The grounds for inadmissibility and removability are outlined in sections §212 and §237 of the Immigration and Nationality Act (INA). Some of the reasons why a noncitizen may be prohibited from entering or remaining in the U.S. include health-related grounds, criminal conduct, national security, immigration violations, prior unlawful presence or removal, failure to provide valid documentation, fraud, and lack of labor certification (Immigration and Nationality Act, 1952; Kolker & Smith, 2024; Meyers, 2020). For most immigrants and their family members, some degree of hardship or adversity is expected in most, if not all, cases involving separation or relocation. Inadmissibility or removal may result in several expected consequences, such as family separation or economic loss (Shibley & Holt, 2022). For some families, family separation or relocation poses a hardship. These hardships are evaluated on a case-by-case basis by the U.S. Department of Immigration. At the same time, while complex, separation or relocation may not always rise to the hardship required for immigration relief.

There are two legal standards of hardship in immigration law as they apply various forms of immigration relief: *extreme hardship* and *exceptional and extremely unusual hardship* (Evans & Hass, 2018; Meyers, 2020; Shibley & Holt, 2022). These two hardship standards are differentiated by the degree of hardship applicants must prove when applying for immigration relief and are evaluated on a case-by-case.

Exceptional & Extremely Unusual Hardship

Exceptional and extremely unusual hardship requires a much higher standard of proof than the less stringent standard of extreme hardship (Donahue, 2018; Shibley & Holt, 2022). The exceptional and extremely unusual standard is much more challenging because the hardship is substantially different or beyond what would generally be expected (Meyers, 2020; Shibley & Holt, 2022). Exceptional and extremely unusual hardship is the required standard of proof for cases concerning removal (deportation) proceedings.

Extreme Hardship

Immigrants can apply for an inadmissibility waiver. Waivers of inadmissibility are referred to as I-601 or I-601A extreme hardship waivers. In general, these waivers seek to waive the reasons for inadmissibility in order to gain permission to enter the U.S. or adjust their status to lawful permanent resident (LPR).

The I-601 waiver, also known as the waiver of grounds of inadmissibility, applies to individual's ineligible for entry and currently outside the U.S. Several grounds of inadmissibility can be waived within the I-601 waiver: health-related grounds, certain criminal conduct, a bar due to prior unlawful presence, immigration fraud, membership in a totalitarian party, and alien smuggling (Meyers, 2020). The I-601A waiver, known as the provisional unlawful presence waiver, is available for individuals unlawfully in the U.S., either because they entered the country without permission or remained in the U.S. longer than permitted (Shibley & Holt, 2022). To be granted either the I-601 or the I-601A, USCIS officials must determine if the applicant meets all regulatory requirements (United States Citizenship and Immigration Services, 2024).

Qualifying Relatives. There are different statutory requirements for each form of immigration relief, which dictate the type of relief an individual can apply for, the standard of hardship an applicant must prove, and whose hardship will be considered. For most hardship waivers, immigration officials focus on the hardship that a family member would experience if the applicant is denied rather than the hardship of the applicant (Donahue, 2018). Within immigration law, these family members are known as qualifying relatives (Donahue, 2018; Meyers, 2020). With hardship waivers, the qualifying relatives are generally limited to spouses, parents, sons, or daughters who are U.S. citizens or lawful permanent residents (Evans & Hass, 2018). Depending on why an individual is seeking immigration relief, the focus of whose hardship will be considered may be more or less limited. For instance, if an individual was deemed inadmissible due to a preexisting 3- or 10-year bar because of a prior unlawful presence, the qualifying relatives are limited only to spouses or parents who are U.S. citizens or lawful permanent residents (United States Citizenship and Immigration Services, 2024).

Separation and Relocation. In considering extreme hardship for qualifying relatives, two potential scenarios must be considered if the applicant were denied entry or prevented from remaining in the country. Separation involves a scenario in which a qualifying relative remains in the U.S., and the applicant remains in their country of citizenship. Conversely, relocation involves a situation in which the qualifying relative relocates to the applicant's country of citizenship (Shibley & Holt, 2022; United States Citizenship and Immigration Services, 2024). Notably, the USCIS Policy Manual explains that applicants must only demonstrate hardship in at least one of these scenarios (Donahue, 2018). These two scenarios act as a guide in establishing extreme hardship, and it is essential to consider two requisite questions: How would separation or relocation impact the qualifying relative's well-being if the applicant were denied admission? Would the consequences of separation or relocation rise to extreme hardship for the qualifying relative(s)?

Extreme Hardship Factors. In establishing extreme hardship, it is crucial to identify factors that impact the qualifying relative(s) beyond what would commonly be expected if the applicant were denied. In other words, do the factors and consequences of denial qualify as extreme, or are they common? Common consequences of inadmissibility or removal do not necessarily warrant a finding of extreme hardship; however, combined with other factors, they may contribute to a finding of extreme hardship (United States Citizenship and Immigration Services, 2024).

The USCIS Policy Manual provides a list of common consequences. It includes family separation, economic loss, difficulties adjusting to life in a new country, inadequate educational opportunities abroad, inferior medical care, and an inability to pursue chosen employment abroad. This list of consequences provides some understanding concerning the factors that USCIS considers common rather than extreme. For many immigrants and their qualifying relatives, these consequences, on a personal level, may present as extreme in that there is a long-lasting and painful impact on the well-being of the family and the immigrant. However, these consequences alone may not be sufficient to meet the standard of extreme hardship. The USCIS Policy Manual also provides information on factors that support the finding of extreme hardship. These categories include family ties, social and cultural impact, economic impact, health conditions and care, and country conditions (Donahue, 2018; Shibley & Holt, 2022; United States Citizenship and Immigration Services, 2024).

Family Ties. The psychological evaluator examines the nature of the qualifying relative's relationship with the applicant and how separation or relocation would adversely impact the relationship. This may include factors such as the qualifying relative's family and community ties within the U.S. and the country of relocation, caregiver responsibilities of any family members within the U.S., the potential impact of caregiver responsibilities due to separation or relocation, prior or current military service, and the nature of their relationship with the applicant (Meyers, 2020; Shibley & Holt, 2022). Other factors to consider may include the qualifying relative's age, length of residence within the U.S., and prior residence in the country of relocation. When considering scenarios where there is a shift in caregiver responsibilities due to separation or relocation, it is vital to consider the social, emotional, and cognitive impact on the qualifying relative's well-being (Shibley & Holt, 2022; United States Citizenship and Immigration Services, 2024).

Social and Cultural Impact. This category acknowledges different social and cultural factors that may impact the applicant and the qualifying relative. For example, social and cultural differences between U.S. laws and social practices in the country of relocation and how this might impact the qualifying relative and the applicant may be considered (Shibley & Holt, 2022). Laws or social practices within the country of relocation and their impact on the qualifying relative due to their affiliation with the U.S. and Western values must also be considered. The psychological evaluation may assess the extent of the qualifying relative's cultural familiarity within the U.S. and the country of relocation, language proficiency, and ability to adapt to another culture within the relocation (Meyers, 2020). Additionally, access to educational and work opportunities is another set of factors that could impact the applicant or the qualifying relative (Meyers, 2020; Shibley & Holt, 2022).

Financial Impact. Financial hardships for the qualifying relative and the applicant factors are also considered. Financial hardship may occur because of an inability to obtain employment in the country of relocation for either the applicant or the qualifying relative (Meyers, 2020; Shibley & Holt, 2022). Other factors may include the cost of care for family members and extraordinary needs, such as special education or care for children (Shibley & Holt, 2022).

Health Conditions and Care. Medical and psychological issues for the qualifying relative are also considered (Meyers, 2020). This will provide context when considering factors such as the availability and quality of medical care in the country of relocation, which may also include the cost and course of treatment (Meyers, 2020; Shibley & Holt, 2022). Other factors within this category that require consideration are the psychological impact on the qualifying relative due to separation or relocation if the applicant is denied. Additionally, the psychologist conducting the evaluation should assess the psychological impact on the qualifying relative due to worrying about the applicant's suffering or how the qualifying relative's preexisting trauma could worsen due to separation or relocation (Shibley & Holt, 2022).

Country Conditions. The conditions of the country they would be relocating to are also factors. For example, is the country experiencing civil unrest, environmental catastrophes, violence, economic sanctions, or political conditions that jeopardize repatriation or result in reasonable fear or harm? Do these conditions indicate that the applicant's country of origin is unsafe or unstable?

Establishing Extreme Hardship. Within immigration law, the applicant bears the burden of proof when applying for an extreme hardship waiver. The applicant must demonstrate that, based on the preponderance of evidence, inadmissibility would more likely than not result in extreme hardship for the qualifying relative (Donahue, 2018; Shibley & Holt, 2022). In proving extreme hardship for qualifying relatives, the applicant must demonstrate that the resulting hardship would transcend what is usually expected if the applicant is prohibited from entering or remaining in the U.S. (Evans & Hass, 2018; Meyers, 2020; Shibley & Holt, 2022).

Psychological Evaluation: Extreme Hardship

The central focus of an extreme hardship evaluation is to collect information about how separation or relocation would impact the qualifying relative(s) if the applicant is denied the hardship waiver. In assessing current or future hardships, the forensic evaluator should address each scenario (separation or relocation) separately (Shibley & Holt, 2022). To answer the referral question for extreme hardship cases, a psychologist will gather relevant background information, conduct the forensic clinical interview, administer psychological assessments, and collect necessary information. A referral question helps guide the type of information a psychologist must gather, assess, and report on when conducting an immigration evaluation (Evans & Hass, 2018; Mercado et al., 2022; Shibley & Holt, 2022). Accordingly, immigration evaluations are tailored explicitly toward answering a legal question.

Simply put, psychologists conducting an immigration evaluation should ask themselves, what will the report aim to answer? In extreme hardship cases, the referral question can be divided into two parts: How would separation or relocation impact the qualifying relative(s)? Would the consequences of separation or relocation affect the qualifying relative beyond what would generally be expected (Shibley & Holt, 2022; Tazi et al., 2023)?

Background Information. An essential aspect of a psychological evaluation for an immigration case involves gathering background information to understand the individual better. Establishing a comprehensive understanding of the interviewee's history may include the following: family history and upbringing, relationship history, quality of relationships with the applicant, children, employment and academic history, immigration history, medical and psychiatric history, substance abuse history, and trauma history (Evans & Hass, 2018; Shibley & Holt, 2022; Walker et al., 2020). Walker et al. recommend using open-ended questions, as it encourages more detailed responses. A thorough background history serves as a blueprint for the types of information the evaluator must collect to develop a comprehensive report for the immigration adjudicator.

It is recommended that evaluators have an explicit written agreement with the applicant's attorney guaranteeing access to the case file (American Psychological Association, 2013; Evans & Hass, 2018). The evaluator must examine the information beyond what was provided by the applicant and their qualifying relative (Barber-Rioja et al., 2022; Evans & Hass, 2018). Collateral and third-party information is often necessary to include in extreme hardship cases. It serves two functions: (a) it corroborates claims made by the qualifying relative or the applicant, particularly claims regarding extreme hardship, and (b) collateral information can provide context for the immigration adjudicator, who is ultimately responsible for interpreting case evidence and deciding the case outcome (Mercado et al., 2022). Therefore, evaluators are encouraged to provide multiple sources of collateral and third-party information, thereby increasing the reliability and objectivity of their final report (Barber-Rioja et al., 2022).

VIOLENCE AGAINST WOMEN ACT (VAWA)

The Violence Against Women Act (VAWA), enacted in 1994, is a response to the many forms of gender-based violence for which women experience the highest rate of victimization (Black et al., 2023; Sacco, 2019). VAWA addresses crimes such as domestic violence, sexual assault, dating violence, and stalking (Sacco, 2019; Seghetti & Bjelopera, 2012). Provisions of VAWA also include special protections for immigrants who are victims of domestic violence and abuse (Black et al., 2023; Sacco, 2019; Seghetti & Bjelopera, 2012; Shibley & Holt, 2022). The Violence Against Women Act provides immigration relief for victims of domestic violence in several ways: (a) Victims can self-petition for deferred action and lawful permanent resident (LPR) status without the cooperation of their abuser, and (b) victims can request cancellation of removal due to domestic violence victimization (Barber-Rioja et al., 2022; Evans & Hass, 2018; Kandel, 2013; Scott et al., 2018; Shibley & Holt, 2022). For immigrants trapped in abusive relationships, VAWA enables victims to pursue both freedom and safety from their abusive spouses, parents, or children.

Immigrants within the U.S., particularly immigrant women, are at an increased risk of experiencing intimate partner violence as compared to the general population (Ingram et al., 2010; Sabri et al., 2018). Thus, the VAWA immigration protections are vital to help ensure the protection of immigrant victims of intimate partner violence (IPV). The study by Sabri and colleagues (2018) analyzed 147,092 intimate partner homicides within the U.S. and found that foreign-born women in the U.S. were more likely to be victims of intimate partner homicide compared to native-born women. This, in part, may be due to several factors that increase the risk of victimization, such as social, institutional, and structural inequalities among immigrant populations (Counts et al., 1999; Erez et al., 2009; Raj & Silverman, 2002; Sabri et al., 2018).

U.S. immigration law provides several forms of domestic violence-based relief, as defined within the Immigration and Nationality Act (Barber-Rioja et al., 2022; Evans & Hass, 2018; Shibley & Holt, 2022). These include the VAWA Self-Petition, the Battered Spouse Waiver, the VAWA Cancellation of Removal, and U Visas (Barber-Rioja et al., 2022; Evans & Hass, 2018; Shibley & Holt, 2022). The eligibility and requirements per each form vary, and therefore, applicants, immigration attorneys, and forensic evaluators must pay close attention to the concepts outlined in each immigration relief form. This includes legal concepts such as good-faith marriage, good moral character, and extreme cruelty. These three concepts represent a set of requirements that applicants must prove when petitioning for domestic violence-based relief.

Psychological Evaluation for VAWA Immigration Petitions

Within VAWA immigration petitions, forensic evaluators are tasked with determining the applicant's psychological functioning about their claim of extreme cruelty. Psychological evaluations involving VAWA immigration petitions must assess the nature and extent of the domestic abuse by examining all available information, conducting a clinical interview with the victim and relevant third parties, and using valid and reliable psychological tests that measure psychological symptoms and the emotional impact of trauma.

Assessing the Impact of Extreme Cruelty. Extreme cruelty evaluations have three objectives: Explore whether the applicant is suffering from trauma, assess the psychological impact of the trauma, and examine whether there is a causal link between the psychological trauma and the abusive behavior that the applicant is claiming (Meyers, 2020). To this end, the psychologist conducting the immigration evaluation must determine the applicant's psychological functioning before, during, and after the abuse (Evans & Hass, 2018). Retrospective reporting on previous functioning helps contextualize the applicant's current psychological functioning. This involves asking the applicant about their ability to contend with day-to-day activities prior to and during the abuse, such as eating and sleeping habits, self-care, work, school, home life, the quality of relationships, recreational activities, satisfaction with life, mood, and ability to manage emotions (Evans & Hass, 2018). Collateral information, including medical records and interviews with family, can help shed light on premorbid psychological functioning.

Using psychological instruments that assess the impact of trauma by assessing the current level of functioning, such as the Trauma Symptom Inventory-2 (TSI-2; Briere, 2010) and the Posttraumatic Stress Disorder Checklist (PCL-5; Blevins et al., 2015), both of which have been validated for use among immigrant populations (Barber-Rioja et al., 2022). Additionally, it is helpful to consider myths about victims of intimate partner violence, such as why the victim waited to leave or seek help. Immigration adjudicators may not fully understand the extent of power behind the abuser's threat, as well as the increased risk of harm or death a victim faces when leaving an abusive relationship.

Therefore, the forensic evaluator should speak to the psychological and emotional control that a domestic abuser can exert over a victim. This can be done by citing literature demonstrating the heightened risk of leaving an abusive relationship. Additionally, the psychologist evaluator may also use risk assessments, such as the Danger Assessment for Immigrant Women (DA-I; Messing et al., 2013), which can provide objective information about the level of danger a victim faces within the abusive relationship (Evans & Hass, 2018; Graham et al., 2019). Ultimately, the psychologist conducting the immigration evaluation must track the applicant's psychological functioning over time.

Extreme Cruelty. Immigrants who have experienced domestic violence will need to demonstrate that they were a victim of battery or extreme cruelty by a spouse, parent, or child who is either a U.S. citizen or a lawful permanent resident (Shibley & Holt, 2022). Notably, claims of extreme cruelty can be substantiated by psychological evaluation (Kandel, 2013). Extreme cruelty is described as a deliberate pattern of abusive behaviors aimed at harming, threatening, and controlling a victim (Barber-Rioja et al., 2022; Evans & Hass, 2018; Kandel, 2013; Shibley & Holt, 2022; Sullivan & Orloff, 2013). Within immigration law, extreme cruelty includes all forms of abuse, such as physical, sexual, psychological, and emotional abuse, as well as immigration-related abuse and economic abuse (Evans & Hass, 2018; Shibley & Holt, 2022; Sullivan & Orloff, 2013).

At face value, some of these abusive actions may not appear to be violent or fit within one of the previously mentioned categories of abuse; however, when considering the intent and the subsequent impact of an abuser's actions, it may become clear that the harmful behavior fits within the overall pattern of abuse. Psychologists conducting these types of evaluations must familiarize themselves with the various forms of abuse within the context of domestic violence and how these abuses specifically impact immigrants. Because extreme cruelty includes many forms of domestic violence, it may be beneficial to examine the different forms of abuse within the framework of coercive control.

Coercive Control. Coercive control is described as a strategic pattern of coercive behaviors designed to isolate, exploit, degrade, intimidate, and punish an individual, all to maintain power and control over the victim (D'Costa, 2023; Evans & Hass, 2018; Shibley & Holt, 2022). The notion of coercive control is a central feature within abusive relationships. When analyzing the nature and extent of abuse within domestic violence, the complexities of an abusive relationship cannot be adequately understood through a single type or instance of abuse. Instead, domestic violence is best described as existing in an insidious framework in which an abuser utilizes a variety of tactics to gain and maintain power and control over their victim. Within this framework, physical violence is a tool, as are other forms of abuse. Consequently, the tools that a coercive controller chooses to employ in an abusive relationship can vary across a multitude of contexts.

To assess extreme cruelty, a psychologist may need to gather information to determine if the abusive behaviors were used as tools of control, the intent behind the abuse, and whether there was a consistent pattern of power and control by the abuser. Coercive control extends beyond a single type of abusive behavior or an isolated incident of abuse; instead, it involves a systematic pattern of abuse involving a combination of physical, sexual, psychological, and economic abuse, as well as other tactics designed to subjugate and undermine victim's autonomy (D'Costa, 2023; Dutton & Goodman, 2005; Meyers, 2020). Abusive tactics lead to a sense of hopelessness and can have long-lasting consequences on the victim's well-being even after the abusive relationship has ended. Several types of abusive behaviors are often identified in VAWA cases. These include the following.

Physical Abuse. Physical abuse, one of the most common forms of abuse, is described as a deliberate act of physical force that typically results in injury, trauma, or death (Evans & Hass, 2018; Shibley & Holt, 2022; Sullivan & Orloff, 2013). Some examples of physical abuse may include physically assaultive behavior, such as punching, kicking, slapping, throwing objects, hair pulling, grabbing, smothering, or choking. However, it may also entail physically restrictive acts, such as blocking exits, forceful imprisonment or confinement, holding or tying someone down, using a weapon to threaten and control, or withholding food or medical care (Meyers, 2020; Sullivan & Orloff, 2013). Recurrent threats of physical violence towards a person are considered to be a form of physical abuse (Shibley & Holt, 2022). It has long been established that domestic abusers often threaten or harm children and pets as a way of controlling intimate partner victims (Blaney et al., 2020; L. Walker, 1984).

Sexual Abuse. Sexual abuse can be understood through a range of nonconsensual sexual behaviors inflicted on another person. It may include forced sexual acts that were either attempted or completed, sexual coercion, reproductive coercion, sexual exploitation or forced prostitution, and harassment or stalking with sexual implications (Evans et al., 2018; Meyers, 2020; Shibley & Holt, 2022; Walker et al., 2020). Forced sexual acts may include attempted or completed nonconsensual sex (vaginal, oral, or anal), molestation, touching, groping, incest, or marital rape (Evans et al., 2018; Meyers, 2020; Shibley & Holt, 2022; Walker et al., 2020). The cultural and legal perspectives of marital rape vary from country to country. Many countries have yet to criminalize marital rape, and in fact, marital rape was not criminalized in the U.S. until the mid-1970s (Bennice & Resick, 2003; Yllö & Torres, 2016). Accepting attitudes and beliefs regarding marital rape may be reflective of traditional gender roles within a marriage, reinforcing the notion of a 'wifely duty' or the idea that a wife is the property of her husband (Bennice & Resick, 2003).

Bearing this in mind, forensic evaluators must consider how a victim's perceptions of sexual abuse will vary across cultures.

Psychological Abuse. Psychological aggression is another type of abuse that may include emotional and verbally abusive behaviors involving manipulative tactics intended to intimidate, harm, and control a person (Evans & Hass, 2018; Leemis et al., 2022; Meyers, 2020; Shibley & Holt, 2022; Sullivan & Orloff, 2013). Psychological abuse aims to distort and undermine a victim's sense of self-worth, trust, and safety. Common forms of psychological abuse include, but are not limited to constant criticism, shaming, verbal attacks, isolating the victim from their social support system, emotional neglect, guilt-tripping, monitoring the victim's behaviors, threats and intimidation, gaslighting, as well as control and manipulation of a victim's thoughts, behaviors, and sense of reality (Evans & Hass, 2018; Shibley & Holt, 2022; Sullivan & Orloff, 2013). Immigration-related psychological abuse may consist of demeaning or derogatory comments about a person's ethnicity, intelligence, cultural values, physical appearance, or ability to work within the U.S. (Evans & Hass, 2018; Meyers, 2020). Immigrants experiencing psychological abuse may feel increasingly isolated from their friends, family, and community support systems due to the rules and regulations that the abuser implemented. Gaslighting and withholding information about the victim's immigration status is also common (Evans & Hass, 2018; Sullivan & Orloff, 2013).

Financial Abuse. Financial abuse is another form of harmful behavior in which an abuser restricts, exploits, and controls a person's economic resources and financial independence (Evans & Hass, 2018; Meyers, 2020; Shibley & Holt, 2022; Sullivan & Orloff, 2013). The goal of economic abuse is to create a situation in which the victim is financially dependent on the abuser, thereby creating a power imbalance within the relationship (Evans & Hass, 2018). Common ways in which immigrants experience economic abuse include restricting employment or education, forcing them to work without obtaining a work permit, forcing them to work multiple jobs, sabotaging current employment by harassing a victim at work, withholding money or resources, limiting their access to transportation or childcare, confiscating their earnings or salary, and coercing financial decisions in which the victim incurs debt or takes out a loan (Evans & Hass, 2018; Meyers, 2020; Shibley & Holt, 2022; Sullivan & Orloff, 2013).

Legal Status Manipulation; "Immigration Abuse". In this form of abuse, the abuser uses the victim's immigration status as a tool to manipulate and control them (Evans & Hass, 2018; Huang, 2022; Shibley & Holt, 2022; Sullivan & Orloff, 2013). This is accomplished by exploiting the victim's legal vulnerabilities, fear of deportation, and unfamiliarity with the U.S. legal system. This form of abuse is especially damaging for immigrants who are experiencing domestic violence, such that it strongly influences a victim's willingness to contact social services or law enforcement due to fear of legal repercussions (Huang, 2022).

Common examples of immigration-related abuse include the following (Gray, 2024; Huang, 2022; Sullivan & Orloff, 2013):

1. Threatening deportation if the victim attempts to leave or seek help,
2. Withholding or threatening to withhold paperwork or sponsorship necessary for securing immigration status,
3. Deliberately failing to file immigration paperwork that would legalize the victim's immigration status,
4. Prohibiting access to or destroying essential documents (e.g., passports, birth certificates),
5. Providing misleading information about the victim's legal rights,
6. Threatening to take custody of children and have the victim deported,
7. Exploiting a victim's undocumented immigration status, thereby preventing them from leaving or seeking help.

Immigration-related abuse is particularly effective at creating a significant power imbalance within a relationship by which the victim is dependent on the abuser for legal stability, subsequently trapping the victim in an abusive relationship.

Good Faith Marriage and Good Moral Character

Both the VAWA Self-Petition and the Battered Spouse Waiver require evidence of a good-faith marriage, such that victims of spousal abuse entered the marriage in good faith (Evans & Hass, 2018; National Immigration Women's Advocacy Project, 2015), meaning that the marriage was not entered into to avoid immigration laws (Meyers, 2020; Sullivan & Orloff, 2013). Similarly, proof of good moral character is required for VAWA Self-Petitions and VAWA Cancellation of Removal, but it is not a requirement for the Battered Spouse Waiver (National Immigration Women's Advocacy Project, 2015; Shibley & Holt, 2022).

The concept of good moral character is not expressly defined in the Immigration and Nationality Act; rather, it is understood by evaluating an individual's actions and conduct, which may or may not violate the moral standards of the community in which they live (Meyers, 2020). A finding of good moral character is determined at the discretion of the immigration adjudicator. It is based on the facts and circumstances of a case, which may include both favorable and unfavorable factors. Factors demonstrating good moral character, or the lack thereof, include the following: history of criminal convictions and offenses that have led to permanent or conditional bars, probation compliance, history of drug and alcohol addiction, applicant credibility, law-abiding behavior, employment history, education, volunteer work, family ties, community involvement, and the stability of different relationships (Evans & Hass, 2018; Meyers, 2020).

Assessing good moral character involves reviewing relevant documents, conducting interviews, collecting collateral information from third parties, and administering psychological assessments, such as risk and personality assessments (Barber-Rioja et al., 2022; Evans & Hass, 2018; Meyers, 2020). It is helpful to consider other contributing factors that would have impaired an individual's decision-making abilities, such as a history of psychiatric or neurological disorders, intoxication, adverse childhood experiences, trauma-related behaviors, coercion, peer pressure, developmental immaturity, level of education, financial hardship, and homelessness (Barber-Rioja et al., 2022). Ultimately, the evaluator is tasked with providing an objective and neutral opinion regarding the causal link between the applicant's claims of domestic violence and their past behaviors.

NONIMMIGRANT VISA FOR VICTIMS OF CRIME (U VISA)

The U visa is another type of victim-based relief for immigrants who have suffered substantial mental or physical abuse because of criminal activity that took place within the U.S. Due to the alarming statistics regarding the frequency of crimes committed against immigrants in the U.S., Congress developed the U visa to protect victims of certain crimes by providing several forms of immigration relief for individuals who have: (1) suffered substantial mental or physical abuse due to criminal activity, (2) who have information regarding the crime or criminal activity, and (3) have assisted or are willing to assist law enforcement or government officials in the detection, investigation, or prosecution of a qualifying criminal activity committed against the victim (Orloff et al., 2013).

The benefits provided by the U visa are intended to promote trust and facilitate cooperation with law enforcement officials without fearing deportation or retaliation for reporting crimes, especially among immigrants who are undocumented. Ultimately, the U visa strengthens the justice system's effectiveness in combatting criminal activity, thus promoting the community's safety. If approved, the U visa offers several benefits for victims directly or indirectly impacted by crime. These benefits include (1) temporary immigration status for up to four years, thereby shielding recipients from removal; (2) certain family members of the victim may also qualify for temporary immigration status; (3) work authorization; and (4) victims may also be eligible for lawful permanent resident status (Hass et al., 2014; Shibley & Holt, 2022).

Qualifying Crimes for the U Visa

Within immigration law, Congress has provided an extensive list of qualifying crimes that fulfill the eligibility requirements for the U visa. These qualifying crimes include abduction, abusive sexual contact, hostage, blackmail, domestic violence, extortion, false imprisonment, female genital mutilation, felonious assault, fraud in foreign labor contracting, incest, involuntary servitude, kidnapping, manslaughter, murder, obstruction of justice, peonage, perjury, prostitution, rape, sexual assault, sexual exploitation, slave trade, stalking, torture, trafficking, witness tampering, unlawful criminal restraint, and other related crimes (Orloff et al., 2013). Qualifying crimes may also include attempts, conspiracy, or solicitation to commit any of the abovementioned crimes.

Willingness to Cooperate with Law Enforcement

The U visa requires that an applicant demonstrate a willingness to assist or cooperate with law enforcement or other government officials in the detection, investigation, prosecution, conviction, or sentencing of the qualifying criminal activity (Orloff et al., 2013). A victim's desire and intention to help can be hindered by several external factors that are out of their control, and subsequently, there are reasonable justifications for non-cooperation. Reasonable factors contributing to a victim's refusal to cooperate include continued abuse and threats perpetrated against the victim and their family, coercion, controlling behaviors by the abuser, fear of being subjected to ostracism or discrimination within their community, preexisting conditions (e.g., mental or physical disabilities), lack of transportation, severe economic hardship, history traumatic experiences, fear of deportation or other legal ramifications, language barriers, and lack of trust with law enforcement due to problematic incident responses in the past (Evans & Hass, 2018; Hass et al., 2014).

Substantial Mental Abuse

When applying for a U visa, an applicant must demonstrate that they suffered substantial mental or physical abuse because of the qualifying criminal activity. For the forensic evaluator, the concept of substantial mental or physical abuse is the primary focus of the psychological evaluation for U visa cases. Mental or physical abuse refers to harm or trauma that affects the victim's physical person or impairs the victim's emotional or psychological soundness (Barber-Rioja et al., 2022; Orloff et al., 2013). Title 8 of the Code of Federal Regulations §214.14(b)(1) states that a determination of whether the abuse is substantial depends on several factors: the nature of the injury, the severity of the abusive conduct, the severity of the harm suffered, the duration of the abuse, and the extent of severe or permanent harm to the victim's appearance, health, or physical or mental soundness, including the worsening of any preexisting conditions (U.S. N.A.R.A., 2021). In weighing these factors, immigration adjudicators consider each factor individually and cumulatively. Based on the credible evidence standard under the Violence Against Women Act, U visa applicants are permitted to present evidence demonstrating that they suffered substantial mental or physical abuse (Orloff et al., 2013). Keeping this in mind, forensic evaluators can provide immigration adjudicators with an objective and neutral report oriented toward answering the referral question.

VICTIMS OF HUMAN TRAFFICKING AND VIOLENCE (T VISA)

As a part of the Victims of Trafficking and Violence Protection Act of 2000 (2000), Congress also enacted the Trafficking Victims Protection Act (TVPA) in response to the emergent problem of human trafficking across the U.S. (Carlson, 2023). The TVPA serves a dual purpose: to provide protection and immigration relief for victims of trafficking, as well as combat human trafficking by encouraging cooperation between law enforcement and trafficking victims (Shibley & Holt, 2022). In passing the TVPA, Congress created the T nonimmigrant status for victims of human trafficking, commonly referred to as the T visa. This visa enables victims of human trafficking and their qualifying family members to remain in the U.S. for up to four years if they assist law enforcement during the investigation or prosecution of human trafficking (Novak et al., 2021). Additional benefits include employment authorization, access to federal benefits and services, and the opportunity to apply for lawful permanent resident status within the U.S. after three years (Carlson, 2023; Sloan, 2018).

To qualify for a T visa, an immigrant is required to demonstrate that they:

1. Have been a victim of a severe form of trafficking (sex or labor trafficking) through the use of force, fraud, or coercion.
2. Are physically present in the U.S. (or its territories) on account of trafficking.
3. Cooperate with any reasonable request from law enforcement to assist with the investigation or prosecution of human trafficking or qualify for an exception due to age or trauma suffered.
4. Would suffer extreme hardship involving unusual and severe harm upon removal from the U.S.
5. Are admissible to the U.S. or qualify for a waiver of any applicable grounds of inadmissibility.

The exploitative and depraved nature of human trafficking involves a range of abusive behaviors over an extended period. Traffickers utilize a variety of methods to exploit and control their victims: fraud, coercion, force, and isolation. These methods may include acts of physical or sexual violence, threats designed to intimidate and control, economic abuse, exploitation of victim vulnerabilities, deception, psychological manipulation, monitoring of victim behaviors, isolation, imprisonment, and the deprivation of fundamental human rights. The long-lasting psychological consequences of human trafficking are profound. Their sense of self and autonomy have eroded away, and their perceptions of themselves and others have been severely distorted. Trafficking victims may also experience a great deal of shame, self-blame, anger, and feelings of naivety as a result of being forced, coerced, or deceived by the perpetrator (Evans & Hass, 2018; Pascual-Leone et al., 2017). Hypervigilance permeates their everyday life, and victims have learned to mistrust others and themselves. Consequently, victims of human trafficking are at high risk of developing PTSD, somatic symptoms, depression, anxiety, dissociation and memory problems, and substance use disorders (Hopper & Hidalgo, 2006; Pascual-Leone et al., 2017).

UTILITY OF PSYCHOLOGICAL EVALUATIONS

Psychological evaluations in immigration cases help document applicants' experiences of victimization, such as those of trafficked victims. They also may provide insight into the abusive dynamics of force, fraud, and coercion by traffickers. Victims of trafficking must also provide evidence demonstrating how they would suffer extreme hardship involving unusual and severe harm if removed from the U.S. For T visas, the finding of extreme hardship is directly related to the individual's experience of being trafficked. Psychological evaluations not only assess the nature and severity of the trauma suffered by a trafficked victim but also examine the potential harm that would be experienced by the applicant upon removal (Shibley & Holt, 2022). For instance, if a victim was forced to return to their home country, would they have access to adequate medical or psychological care? Would they experience persecution or ostracism because of their victimization? Or would they be at risk of being re-victimized due to unstable and dangerous conditions in their country of origin? As such, psychological evaluations play a decisive role in providing psychological evidence for the adjudicator during the decision-making process. Ultimately, an adjudicator's decision may have far-reaching consequences for both the immigrant and their family, as well as law enforcement efforts in combatting human trafficking more broadly.

Due to the expansive nature of the statutory provisions for U visas, the scope of the psychological evaluation may be extensive depending on the facts and circumstances of each case. Like VAWA immigration petitions, there are several types of abuse that forensic evaluators can assess in U visa psychological evaluations, which include physical, sexual, psychological, economic, and immigration abuse, as well as negligence (Evans & Hass, 2018). Additionally, considering the wide range of qualifying criminal activities for U visas, applicants may have experienced multiple victimizations after entering the U.S. The type of abuse and the impact of the abuse will vary across each category of criminal activity. For example, a victim of sexual assault will likely have experienced a different type of abuse compared to someone who was blackmailed, not to mention the differences in how each victim was affected.

The purpose of the psychological evaluation for U visa cases is to address the referral question: To what degree has the applicant suffered, mentally or physically, and how is that impairment related to the qualifying criminal activity? It is not, however, for the forensic evaluator to decide whether the mental or physical harm is substantial. Forensic evaluations must examine the applicant's level of functioning before, during, and after the crime to assess the connection between the qualifying criminal activity and subsequent suffering (Shibley & Holt, 2022). This helps illustrate the developmental trajectory of symptoms and document the worsening of preexisting conditions. The forensic evaluator needs to explore how the crime changed the victim. Much like other psychological assessments for immigration proceedings, conducting a psychological evaluation for U visa cases should include a multimethod approach, which consists of clinical interviews, psychological tests, collateral sources of information, and a review of records when available. In such cases, reviewing medical records and conducting psychological testing (e.g., mental status evaluation or neuropsychological) may help compare prior and current functioning. There are several preexisting conditions to consider when assessing a U visa applicant, such as a prior history of abuse and other traumatic experiences, a history of mental health disorders, and current exposures to stressful environmental factors (Evans & Hass, 2018).

The psychological evaluation may provide helpful insight regarding the victim's efforts and intentions to cooperate with the criminal justice process, including past, present, and future helpfulness. The victim's experience with law enforcement, including any reasonable justifications for non-cooperation, should be documented. Questions should be aimed at understanding the victim's role and overall experience within the criminal justice process. Asking whether they called the police, if charges were brought against the perpetrator, how they were treated by law enforcement, whether they were informed of their legal rights, whether a language translator was provided for them, if they participated in or were asked to participate in investigative interviews, and whether they were asked to testify or provide a deposition. The psychologist evaluating the applicant should explore and document any barriers contributing to non-cooperation, such as threats, coercion, or controlling behaviors by the perpetrator or other individuals attempting to suppress the victim's willingness to cooperate.

SUMMARY

This chapter reviewed the types of immigration reliefs and the use of psychological evaluations in these proceedings. The chapter highlights the critical role that forensic psychologists play in assisting the court to navigate complex immigration cases. The chapter delved into the role that psychological evaluation has in (1) asylum cases where individuals reported fear of persecution in their home country and psychological trauma, (2) extreme hardship situations if deported, (3) extreme hardship waiver cases, (4) the role that psychologists play in assessing cases involving violence against women (VAWA), victims of serious crimes (U Visas), and victims of human trafficking (T Visas). The chapter serves as a practical guide for psychologists conducting these evaluations and provides recommendations for effectively conducting psychological evaluations involving immigrant populations.

REFERENCES

American Psychological Association. (2013). Specialty guidelines for forensic psychology. *The American Psychologist*, *68*(1), 7–19. DOI: 10.1037/a0029889 PMID: 23025747

Barber-Rioja, V., Akinsulure-Smith, A. M., & Vendzules, S. (2022). *Mental health evaluations in immigration court: A guide for mental health and legal professionals*. NYU Press., DOI: 10.18574/nyu/9781479802623.001.0001

Bennice, J. A., & Resick, P. A. (2003). Marital rape: History, research, and practice. *Trauma, Violence & Abuse*, *4*(3), 228–246. DOI: 10.1177/1524838003004003003 PMID: 14697124

Black, A., Valerio, M., & Blasdell, R. (2023). United States Violence Against Women Act (VAWA). In Shackelford, T. K. (Ed.), *Encyclopedia of Domestic Violence* (pp. 1–10). Springer International Publishing., DOI: 10.1007/978-3-030-85493-5_1684-1

Blaney, N., Randour, M. L., & Blink, C. (2020). Advances in understanding and addressing the link between pet abuse and intimate partner violence. In Geffner, R., White, J. W., Hamberger, L. K., Rosenbaum, A., Vaughan-Eden, V., & Vieth, V. I. (Eds.), *Handbook of Interpersonal Violence and Abuse Across the Lifespan* (pp. 1–22). Springer International Publishing., DOI: 10.1007/978-3-319-62122-7_286-1

Blevins, C. A., Weathers, F. W., Davis, M. T., Witte, T. K., & Domino, J. L. (2015). The posttraumatic stress disorder checklist for DSM-5 (PCL-5): Development and initial psychometric evaluation. *Journal of Traumatic Stress*, *28*(6), 489–498. DOI: 10.1002/jts.22059 PMID: 26606250

Briere, J. (2010). *Trauma symptom inventory* (2nd ed.). Psychological Assessment Resources., TSI-2. DOI: 10.1002/9780470479216.corpsy1010

Carlson, W. C. (2023). Implementation challenges of T Visa eligibility for human trafficking survivors: A role for social work. *Social Work*, *68*(3), 222–229. DOI: 10.1093/sw/swad017 PMID: 37164622

Counts, D. A., Brown, J. K., & Campbell, J. (Eds.). (1999). *To have and to hit: Cultural perspectives on wife beating*. University of Illinois Press.

D'Costa, M. (2023). Coercive control. In Shackelford, T. K. (Ed.), *Encyclopedia of Domestic Violence* (pp. 1–9). Springer International Publishing., DOI: 10.1007/978-3-030-85493-5_278-1

Donahue, M. (2018). *UNDERSTANDING EXTREME HARDSHIP IN WAIVERS | JANUARY 2018*.

Dutton, M. A., & Goodman, L. A. (2005). Coercion in intimate partner violence: Toward a new conceptualization. *Sex Roles*, *52*(11–12), 743–756. DOI: 10.1007/s11199-005-4196-6

Erez, E., Adelman, M., & Gregory, C. (2009). Intersections of immigration and domestic violence: Voices of battered immigrant women. *Feminist Criminology*, *4*(1), 32–56. DOI: 10.1177/1557085108325413

Evans, B., & Hass, G. (2018). *Forensic psychological assessment in immigration court: A guidebook for evidence-based and ethical practice*. Routledge., DOI: 10.4324/9781315621197

Graham, L. M., Messing, J. T., & Campbell, J. (2019). The danger assessment: An instrument for the prevention of intimate partner homicide. In Geffner, R., White, J. W., Hamberger, L. K., Rosenbaum, A., Vaughan-Eden, V., & Vieth, V. I. (Eds.), *Handbook of Interpersonal Violence and Abuse Across the Lifespan* (pp. 1–21). Springer International Publishing., DOI: 10.1007/978-3-319-62122-7_145-1

Gramlich, J., & Passel, J. (2024, September 27). U.S. immigrant population in 2023 saw largest increase in more than 20 years. *Pew Research Center*. https://www.pewresearch.org/short-reads/2024/09/27/u-s-immigrant-population-in-2023-saw-largest-increase-in-more-than-20-years/

Gray, A. D. (2024). Domestic violence against immigrant women and children in the United States. In Shackelford, T. K. (Ed.), *Encyclopedia of Domestic Violence* (pp. 1–13). Springer International Publishing., DOI: 10.1007/978-3-030-85493-5_426-1

Hass, G., Yang, E., Monahan, K., Orloff, L., & Anver, B. (2014). Barriers and successes in U visas for immigrant victims: The experiences of legal assistance for victims grantees. *Arts Social Sci J S*, *1*, 2.

Hopper, E., & Hidalgo, J. (2006). Invisible chains: Psychological coercion of human trafficking victims. *Intercultural Human Rights Law Review*, *1*, 185–209.

Huang, G. (2022). How domestic violence impacts immigrant victims. In Geffner, R., White, J. W., Hamberger, L. K., Rosenbaum, A., Vaughan-Eden, V., & Vieth, V. I. (Eds.), *Handbook of Interpersonal Violence and Abuse Across the Lifespan* (pp. 2629–2653). Springer International Publishing., DOI: 10.1007/978-3-319-89999-2_163

Immigration and Nationality Act. (1952). 8 U.S.C. § 1182. Https://www.govinfo.gov/content/pkg/COMPS-1376/pdf/COMPS-1376.pdf

Ingram, M., McClelland, D. J., Martin, J., Caballero, M. F., Mayorga, M. T., & Gillespie, K. (2010). Experiences of immigrant women who self-petition under the Violence Against Women Act. *Violence Against Women, 16*(8), 858–880. DOI: 10.1177/1077801210376889 PMID: 20679184

Kandel, W. A. (2013). *Immigration provisions of the Violence Against Women Act.* VAWA.

Kolker, A. F., & Smith, H. R. (2024). *Immigration: Grounds of inadmissibility.*

Leemis, R. W., Friar, N., Khatiwada, S., Chen, M. S., Kresnow, M., Smith, S. G., Caslin, S., & Basile, K. C. (2022). *The National Intimate Partner and Sexual Violence Survey: 2016/2017 report on intimate partner violence.* https://stacks.cdc.gov/view/cdc/124646#moretextPAmods.subject_name

McKenzie, K. C. (Ed.). (2022). *Asylum medicine: A clinician's guide.* Springer International Publishing., DOI: 10.1007/978-3-030-81580-6

Melikyan, Z. A., Agranovich, A. V., & Puente, A. E. (2019). 19—Fairness in psychological testing. In Goldstein, G., Allen, D. N., & DeLuca, J. (Eds.), *Handbook of Psychological Assessment* (4th ed., pp. 551–572). Academic Press., DOI: 10.1016/B978-0-12-802203-0.00018-3

Mercado, A., Antuña, C., Bailey, C., Garcini, L., Hass, G., Henderson, C., Koslofsky, S., Morales, F., & Venta, A. (2022). Professional guidelines for psychological evaluations in immigration proceedings. *Journal of Latina/o Psychology, 10*(4), 253–276. Advance online publication. DOI: 10.1037/lat0000209

Messing, J. T., Amanor-Boadu, Y., Cavanaugh, C. E., Glass, N. E., & Campbell, J. C. (2013). Culturally competent intimate partner violence risk assessment: Adapting the danger assessment for immigrant women. *Social Work Research, 37*(3), 263–275. DOI: 10.1093/swr/svt019

Meyers, R. S. (2020). *Conducting psychological assessments for U.S. immigration cases.* Springer International Publishing., DOI: 10.1007/978-3-030-49868-9

Moslimani, M., & Passel, J. (2024, September 27). *What the data says about immigrants in the U.S.* Pew Research Center. https://www.pewresearch.org/short-reads/2024/09/27/key-findings-about-us-immigrants/

National Immigration Women's Advocacy Project. (2015). *Comparing forms of immigration relief for immigrant victims of crime.* Author. Retrieved from http://niwaplibrary.wcl.American.edu/pubs/imm-relief-forms-comparison

NIJC. (2022). *NIJC procedural manual for asylum representation*. National Immigrant Justice Center. https://immigrantjustice.org/for-attorneys/legal-resources/file/nijc-procedural-manual-asylum-representation-pdf

Novak, E. A., Kulig, T. C., & Doña-Reveco, C. (2021). *Human trafficking and the T visa process: Insights from legal representatives working with victims from Latin America*. OLLAS Reports., DOI: 10.32873/uno.dc.ollas.1016

Orloff, L., Angel, C., & Robinson, S. (2013). *Empowering survivors: Legal rights of immigrant victims of sexual assault*.

Pascual-Leone, A., Kim, J., & Morrison, O.-P. (2017). Working with Victims of human trafficking. *Journal of Contemporary Psychotherapy*, *47*(1), 51–59. DOI: 10.1007/s10879-016-9338-3

Prabhu, M., & Baranoski, M. (2012). Forensic mental health professionals in the immigration process. *The Psychiatric Clinics of North America*, *35*(4), 929–946. DOI: 10.1016/j.psc.2012.08.012 PMID: 23107571

Raj, A., & Silverman, J. (2002). Violence against immigrant women: The roles of culture, context, and legal immigrant status on intimate partner violence. *Violence Against Women*, *8*(3), 367–398. DOI: 10.1177/10778010222183107

Rosenberg, J. (2019). Why are you seeking refuge? Conducting evaluations of Central American asylum seekers. *Journal of Human Rights and Social Work*, *4*(4), 229–237. DOI: 10.1007/s41134-019-00097-x

Sabri, B., Campbell, J. C., & Messing, J. T. (2018). Intimate partner homicides in the United States, 2003-2013: A comparison of immigrants and nonimmigrant victims. *Journal of Interpersonal Violence*, *36*(9–10), 4735–4757. DOI: 10.1177/0886260518792249 PMID: 30095027

Sacco, L. N. (2019). *The Violence Against Women Act (VAWA): Historical overview, funding, and reauthorization*.

Scott, M., Weaver, S., & Kamimura, A. (2018). Experiences of immigrant women who applied for Violence Against Women Act (VAWA) Self- petition in the United States: Analysis of legal affidavits. *Diversity and Equality in Health and Care*, *15*(4). Advance online publication. DOI: 10.21767/2049-5471.100168

Seghetti, L. M., & Bjelopera, J. P. (2012). The Violence Against Women Act: Overview, legislation, and federal funding. *Congressional Research Service*, *10*, 1–35.

Shibley, M. G., & Holt, M. (2022). *Conducting immigration evaluations: A practical guide for mental health professionals*. Routledge. https://api.taylorfrancis.com/content/books/mono/download?identifierName=doi&identifierValue=10.4324/9781003139973&type=googlepdf

Singer, E., Eswarappa, M., Kaur, K., & Baranowski, K. A. (2020). Addressing the need for forensic psychological evaluations of asylum seekers: The potential role of the general practitioner. *Psychiatry Research*, *284*(112752), 112752. Advance online publication. DOI: 10.1016/j.psychres.2020.112752 PMID: 32000095

Sloan, M. (2018). *T visas protect victims of human trafficking and strengthen community relationships.*

Sullivan, K., & Orloff, L. (2013). *BREAKING BARRIERS: A COMPLETE GUIDE TO LEGAL RIGHTS AND RESOURCES FOR BATTERED IMMIGRANTS.*

Tazi, K. Y., Rogers, R., & Chang, Y.-T. (2023). Forensic evaluations for immigration courts: A critical commentary on legal and ethical considerations. *Psychological Injury and Law*, *16*(4), 303–319. DOI: 10.1007/s12207-023-09489-x

United States Citizenship and Immigration Services. (2024). *USCIS policy manual.* U.S. Citizenship and Immigration Services. Https://www.uscis.gov/policy-manual

U.S. Department of Homeland Security. (2024). *Application for waiver of grounds of inadmissibility.* USCIS. https://www.uscis.gov/i-601

U.S. Department of Justice. (2024). *Adjudication statistics: Total asylum applications*. U.S. Department of Justice, Executive Office for Immigration Review. https://www.justice.gov/eoir/media/1344871/dl?inline

U.S. N.A.R.A. (2021). *Alien victims of certain qualifying criminal activity. 8 C.F.R. §214.14.* United States: National Archives and Records Administration (US NARA): Office of the Federal Register. https://www.govinfo.gov/app/details/CFR-2021-title8-vol1/CFR-2021-title8-vol1-sec214-14

Victims of Trafficking and Violence Protection Act of 2000, 22 U.S.C. § 7101 (2000). https://www.govinfo.gov/content/pkg/PLAW-106publ386/pdf/PLAW-106publ386.pdf

Walker, L. (1984). *The battered women syndrome*. Springer.

Walker, L. E., Shapiro, D., & Akl, S. (2020). *Introduction to forensic psychology: Clinical and social psychological perspectives*. Springer International Publishing., DOI: 10.1007/978-3-030-44470-9

Weiss, R. A., & Rosenfeld, B. (2012). Navigating cross-cultural issues in forensic assessment: Recommendations for practice. *Professional Psychology, Research and Practice*, *43*(3), 234–240. DOI: 10.1037/a0025850

Yllö, K., & Torres, M. G. (2016). *Marital rape: Consent, marriage, and social change in global context (Eds).* Oxford University Press.

Chapter 2 The Psychological Sequelae of Trauma and Stress as Immigrants Adapt to a New Country

Ana M. Gamez
https://orcid.org/0000-0003-4523-1470
California Baptist University, USA

Dylan Lacson
California Baptist University, USA

Kelsy A. Michaels
California Baptist University, USA

Jerrondralyn K. Beltran
California Baptist University, USA

ABSTRACT

This chapter explores the unique and often complex experience of immigrants' stress and trauma as they seek to adjust to a new country. The chapter examines the psychological impact of migration and adaptation, along with the challenges faced during and after relocation to a new country. It delves into the common mental health conditions that often accompany the immigrant experience, such as anxiety, depression, PTSD, and acculturative stress. It further explores how these conditions can present differently across cultures and in the context of the immigrant experience, emphasizing the importance of cultural competence in clinical practice. Understanding the psychological aspects of trauma and other mental health

DOI: 10.4018/979-8-3693-7944-8.ch002

conditions and symptoms presented by many immigrants is necessary to be able to document the case adequately.

INTRODUCTION

Approximately 281 million people worldwide have migrated from their home countries to pursue a better life abroad; many have fled from war, poverty, and persecution (McAuliffe & Triandafyllidou, 2021; Perreira & Ornelas, 2013). The psychological effects of immigration and acculturation are an increasingly urgent area of concern for researchers and mental health professionals alike as the number of immigrants worldwide continues to grow rapidly. The drastic shift in cultural environment requires immigrants to adjust their lifestyles, attitudes, and behaviors in ways that enable them to thrive in the new country. This urgent need to conform may cause crises among immigrants, who, in addition to being separated from family and loved ones and possibly forgoing their original cultural identities, are pressured to integrate into the social norms of a new country or risk being ostracized, discriminated against, or even deported (Breslau, 2011; Garcini et al., 2023; Zhou et al., 2019). The hardships of acculturation and separation from one's familiar lifestyle in their country of origin introduce several other stressors that may lead to even more traumatic experiences, the effects of which tend to span across several generations among immigrants.

Complex trauma resulting from exposure to war, displacement, and resettlement can be challenging to assess for healthcare providers with limited experience and training, which may result in the misunderstanding and misinterpretation of symptoms (Murray et al., 2010; Sundvall et al., 2015). Therefore, evaluators conducting immigration evaluations must not only be adequately trained to conduct evaluations for immigration proceedings, but also be culturally competent. Mental health providers should be trained and equipped to provide trauma-informed care to adequately support the needs of immigrants, as many present with trauma histories (Vukcevic et al., 2016). Difficulties in fully understanding the mental status of immigrants can severely hinder assessment outcomes, as evaluators may resort to relying on their generalized understandings and assumptions about the migrant's cultural factors.

The purpose of this chapter is to examine the role of stress and trauma in the psychological well-being and adaptation of immigrants as they navigate the complexities of settling in a new country. While the emphasis will primarily be on the experiences of immigrants in the United States, the chapter draws from several studies accounting the collective experiences of immigrants worldwide, as their experiences with stress and trauma remain consistent, regardless of their original or host countries. Immigration is multifaceted, involving the physical relocation to the new country and a profound emotional, physical, social, and cultural impact on the individual and family system. The process of adaptation to a new environment can be overwhelming and amplified by stress and trauma experienced in the home country, during the journey or travel, and post-arrival to the host country.

IMMIGRANT STRESS AND ADAPTATION

Stress is a complex, multifaceted process wherein an environmental factor, otherwise known as a stressor, triggers a significant physical, psychological, and behavioral response that can overwhelm the system and consequently, the individual must cope and adapt to changes in their environment (Bustamante et al., 2017; Vélez-Coto et al., 2021). Among immigrants, migration is an inherently stressful process that introduces many difficulties, risks, and stress factors that increase the likelihood of exposure to traumatic events (Sangalang et al., 2019). Prior research has associated migration with several unique stressors that primarily occur because of acculturation and adaptation to a new host country, leading to negative consequences in mental health among immigrants (Lechner, 2007). These consequences include psychological distress, depressive symptoms, anxiety, and general pessimism about the future; several studies have found that migrant populations tend to be especially vulnerable to physical and mental health issues that are worsened by the lack of a reliable social support network, and feelings of isolation and confusion (Coffman & Norton, 2010). Contributing factors include language barriers, feelings of loss of one's cultural identity, and separation from family; all of these are further exacerbated when combined with the lack of education or familiarity with a foreign country's health care system. Barriers to mental health treatment make it difficult to receive adequate physical and mental care, thus, medical conditions such as depression, anxiety and trauma may be overlooked and go untreated (Zhou et al., 2019).

Adaptation is often dynamic, as individuals must continuously change their thoughts, behaviors, feelings, and physiological mechanisms to adjust to a new, foreign, and unfamiliar environment (Costa et al., 2003). This constant need for change and adaptation for immigrants may be overwhelming and negatively affect their psychological well-being including, increasing the likelihood of psychological deterioration and engaging in high-risk behaviors (Bisson & Sakhuja, 2006). Researchers have identified five sources of immigrant stress in Latina women, including a lack of English proficiency, the lack of legal immigration status, workplace disadvantages, separation from family and home country, and cultural dissonance (Sternberg et al., 2016).

ACCULTURATION PROCESS

The acculturation process primarily involves four dimensions (Figure 1; Berry, 1997). The first dimension is integration, in which immigrants are expected to maintain elements of their original culture while acquiring aspects of the host country's current culture. The extent to which an immigrant must integrate and acquire the new culture largely depends on the host population's tolerance for cultural diversity, as well as the levels of prejudice, racism, ethnocentrism, and discrimination. The second dimension is assimilation, wherein the migrant forgoes their original cultural identity to fully acquire the traits of the host population's culture in order to be further accepted. The third dimension, separation, occurs when an individual refuses to adjust to the cultural norms of the new country, as they prefer only to uphold their original culture. The fourth and final dimension is marginalization, wherein the individual is unable to maintain their original cultural identity while also being unable to identify with the new culture, resulting in feelings of anxiety, loss of identity, and alienation from both groups. According to Berry (1997), stressors resulting from these four dimensions tend to occur when there is a wider gap and a more significant difference between the immigrant's original culture and the host population's culture, as this would necessitate the need for extensive cultural relearning and possibly lead to repeated conflict and adaptive difficulties.

Figure 1. The acculturation process (Berry, 1997)

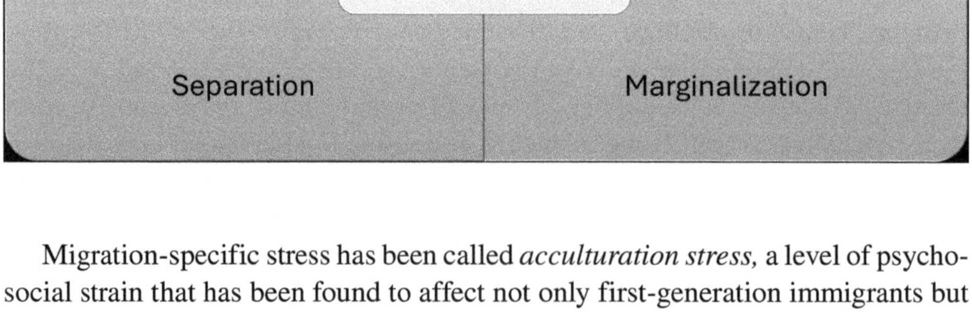

Migration-specific stress has been called *acculturation stress,* a level of psychosocial strain that has been found to affect not only first-generation immigrants but their descendants as well, as the persistent challenge to adapt and integrate with a new culture may span across multiple generations (Arbona et al., 2010). Immigrants tend to experience unique stressors resulting from acculturation, wherein many change and adjust aspects of their livelihoods, such as culture, language, ethnic identity, attitudes and beliefs, values, social behaviors and relations, diets, artistic expression, and communication (LeMaster et al., 2018).

A meta-analysis by Bustamante et al. (2017) identified chronicity as a critical characteristic of migration-related stress. The Chronicity refers to the many stressors that are ongoing and which become a major part of an immigrant's life (e.g., living conditions, difficulty finding secure employment due to legal status, victimization and social factors). According to these authors, other sources of migration-related stress include feelings of alienation and insecurity, impoverished social conditions, exploitation, poor housing conditions, drastic changes in language and culture, loneliness, and the broad everyday struggles to survive. They compare moving away from one's home country to mourning and loss, as migration often requires separation from what is safe and familiar: family and loved ones, native language and culture, local geography, and social status. According to these authors, post-migration stressors include PTSD risk factors, such as poor social environments that foster weak social integration and loneliness, poor access to mental health services, socioeconomic instabilities, difficulties in communication, and detention. The excessive mourning and overwhelming feelings of loss following leaving one's home country are associated with the risk of exhibiting depressive, anxiety, and somatic symptoms (Atxotegui, 2000). Researchers have found that some Latino immigrants in the USA mourn the separation from their family, have difficulty learning a new language, experience difficulty adjusting to the new culture, and may experience employment and living condition challenges (Mehta et al., 2002; Simich, 2006).

Immigrants must learn to adjust to the stressors of acculturation such as gender roles, intergenerational differences, communication difficulties, changing of roles within the family, and negotiation of loyalty towards one's culture of origin and the new country's culture (Bustamante et al., 2017). A study by Portes (2001) found generational conflict common among migrant families. The conflict was attributed to an acculturational gap between parents and their children, as migrant children adapted their behavior to the host country's culture at a more rapid rate than the parents. These disagreements or tension between migrant parents and their children, specifically in the areas of relationships, marriage, gender roles, and career choices, are common as immigrant parents try to hold on to more traditional attitudes and beliefs of their culture. Familial cultural differences pose additional stress on the children of immigrant families who may feel forced to take on more independent, self-reliant roles due to either being unable to rely on their parents for providing sound advice and help, or due to the parents' need for translation, education, and cultural navigation from their children (Melander & Shmulyar Gréen, 2023).

Figure 2. The acculturation process (Grove & Torbiörn, 1985)

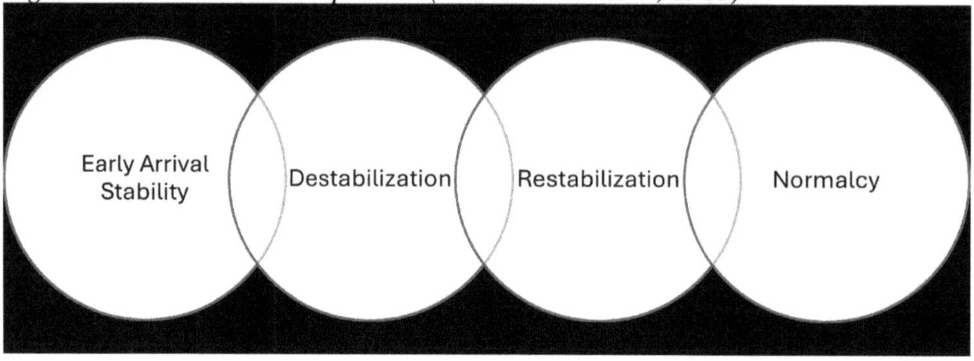

Grove and Torbiörn (1985) developed a four-staged longitudinal model to explore the effects of pre- and post-migration stressors on immigrants' psychological symptoms and behaviors as they resettle in their new host country. The first stage, early arrival stability, occurs immediately upon arrival, wherein migrants are made aware of the host country's cultural expectations and must adjust their behaviors accordingly. The second stage, destabilization, then occurs when migrants are faced with the dilemma of balancing their commitment to their original cultures and the host population's culture; some may prefer only to interact and be surrounded by people from the same culture of origin while remaining hostile to the host culture, while other migrants may prefer to fully assimilate to the new culture. Afterward, the re-stabilization stage occurs when migrants remain open to progressively exploring the new culture and gradually adjusting to their livelihoods, culminating in the fourth and final stage; the return to everyday life.

In reality, this smooth transition into normalization in a foreign land and culture is often complicated and inaccessible for migrants, leading to a further divide between migrants who can acculturate and those who cannot (LeMaster et al., 2018). This inability to acculturate and adapt to the new country may result in a chronic state of stress and feeling overwhelmed, leading to psychological decompensation (Gonsalves, 1992). Migration often puts significant strain on social networks and support systems. Cultural adaptation involves learning the new country's social norms, values, and expectations. Thus, becoming socially integrated into the new environment may seem necessary for the family system, as fitting in and adopting roles and mainstream expectations within the family could serve as a survival strategy (Kroening & Dawson-Hahn, 2019).

An immigrant's post-migration experience, however, is plagued by many fears (see Figure 3), including the fear of failure, fear of deportation, fear of an inability to communicate and be understood due to language barriers, fear of not fitting in, fear of law enforcement and the fear of death (Gamez, 2024). The fear of deportation is by far one of the most significant fears, which creates an overall feeling of uncertainty about the immigrant's status and future in the country they immigrated to. The constant fear of deportation increases the likelihood of immigrants developing symptoms of depression, anxiety, stress, and somatic symptoms.

The fear of deportation extends beyond the fear of detainment and separation from their families; it impacts immigrants' willingness to pursue employment opportunities, education, and healthcare (Arbona et al., 2010; Bailey & Widener, 2022). Furthermore, this fear inadvertently puts immigrants at an increased risk for exploitation and victimization and presents a barrier against integrating into society. Similarly, other fears, such as the fear of failure, fear of encountering law enforcement, and fear of death, have a powerful psychological impact on the individual, mainly when they have experienced traumatic events prior to migration, during their journey, or in the new country; these heightened fears often cause anxiety, frustration, as well as helplessness and other adverse psychological effects (Chong & Chong, 2023).

Figure 3. Common fears among immigrants (Gamez, 2024)

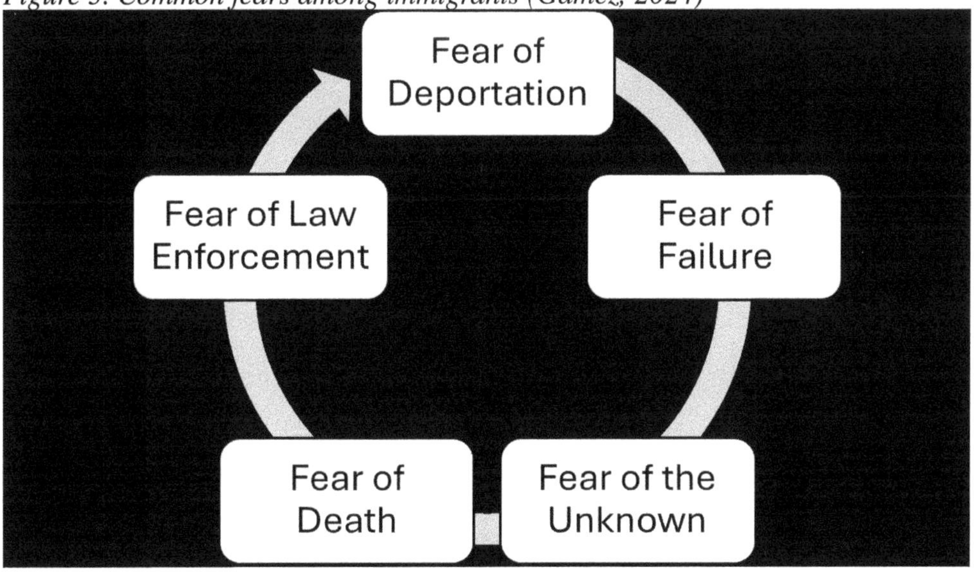

CULTURAL CONSIDERATIONS AND TRAUMA

Culture has a profound impact on our thoughts, emotions, and behaviors. Thus, culture cannot be set aside when considering psychological trauma. This is particularly important when examining the cultural variation of symptoms among immigrant populations experiencing trauma and other mental illnesses, as culture influences how we interpret and respond to psychological symptoms and disorders. Culture not only influences our internal processes, but it also shapes how we interact with individuals from other cultural backgrounds. An individual's cultural identity may be central to understanding why they have endured traumatic experiences. For instance, the ethnicity, sexual orientation, or gender identity of an individual may elicit profound consequences on their well-being within some areas of the world, as they may experience persecution and ostracism due to their cultural identity.

Furthermore, cultural attitudes can shape how mental health practitioners assess and interpret the causes of psychological distress and symptomology among diverse immigrant populations. Subsequently, these cultural attitudes may affect the final diagnosis. Psychologists must demonstrate multicultural competency and humility when working with diverse populations. This section will discuss multicultural factors, the impact of culture on mental health, and how trauma is experienced, expressed, and explained across cultures.

Multicultural Factors

Trauma affects people in different ways due to a range of individual differences. Integrating a multicultural approach is vital in understanding individual differences within the context of mental health, as there is a dynamic intersectionality of individual factors. These factors may include cultural identity, race, ethnicity, gender, age, sexual orientation, gender identity, religion, language, disability, or socioeconomic status (Barber-Rioja et al., 2022; Zangeneh & Al-Krenawi, 2019). The intersection of these factors provides context for how people experience, understand, and convey the psychological symptoms associated with trauma and mental illness. Consider, for example, how a Zulu woman in South Africa experiences, interprets and responds to an armed robbery compared to that of a white South African male. Though this example involves two individuals from South Africa, their experience, understanding, and response to the traumatic event will likely differ. It is important for psychologists working with diverse populations to assess these multicultural differences and how they affect mental health.

There are a variety of cross-cultural assessment models designed to assess cultural information and how this influences mental health, however, the most widely accepted cultural assessment tool is the Cultural Formational Interview (CFI) provided by the *Diagnostic and Statistical Manual of Mental Disorders* (5th ed., text rev.; DSM-5-TR; American Psychiatric Association, 2022). The CFI is a culturally sensitive assessment that offers a comprehensive approach to understanding the influence of cultural factors on an individual's mental health by examining five dimensions: (1) cultural identity of the individual, (2) cultural concepts of distress, (3) psychosocial stressors and cultural features of vulnerability and resilience, (4) cultural features of the relationship between the individual and the clinician, and (5) overall cultural assessment (American Psychiatric Association, 2022a). The CFI provides a culturally informed framework for identifying cultural characteristics and assessing how individuals interpret and respond to their mental health issues.

Impact of Culture on Psychological Distress

Across cultures, individuals endorse varying cultural concepts of distress, which refers to how people experience, interpret, and convey psychological suffering, behavioral problems, or unpleasant thoughts and emotions (American Psychiatric Association, 2022; Barber-Rioja et al., 2022). Within the DSM-5-TR, cultural concepts of distress include cultural idioms, cultural explanations, and cultural syndromes (American Psychiatric Association, 2022). Cultural idioms refer to the way distress is commonly expressed through linguistic terms or phrases that may not include specific symptoms or syndromes. Cultural explanations or perceived causes of distress are described as labels, attributions, or features that are explained through culturally recognized etiology of symptoms, illness, or distress. Cultural syndromes refer to symptoms and attributions that often occur within cultural groups, communities, and contexts that are locally recognized as coherent patterns of experience (American Psychiatric Association, 2022).

The term ‘depression’ can be used to describe all three cultural concepts of distress. For instance, depression can describe a syndrome (e.g., major depressive disorder), it can be used to describe an idiom of distress (e.g., “I feel depressed”), and it can be used to explain the symptoms or illness (e.g., feeling sad, hopeless, and fatigued because of depression). While these cultural concepts of distress set the foundation for identifying the cultural variation of mental and emotional distress within immigrant populations, other cultural phenomena must be considered in order to understand how people experience, express, and explain symptoms associated with trauma and other forms of psychological suffering.

Experience of Trauma Across Cultures

The nature of the traumatic event itself and how people experience traumatic events vary across cultures. Objectively, there are different types of traumatic experiences (e.g., natural disasters, warfare, terrorism, domestic violence, etc.), which can vary both in frequency and duration. For example, consider the paradox between someone from a country where war and violence are a constant part of everyday life compared to that of an individual who has never experienced widespread conflict. The frequency and duration of armed conflict may influence an individual's perception regarding the severity of the traumatic experience. With that in mind, the resulting trauma is not simply dependent on the objective nature of a traumatic experience. The experience of trauma is also subjective, and therefore, a multicultural approach is necessary in order to understand how people perceive and assign meaning to traumatic events.

Consider how culture is defined, such that it refers to an array of values, norms, concepts, and practices learned and shared by a community through multiple generations (American Psychiatric Association, 2022; Barber-Rioja et al., 2022). Culture comprises language, religion, spirituality, customs and rituals, family structures, and political, economic, and legal systems (Barber-Rioja et al., 2022). Take, for example, how laws and cultural norms in different countries influence a victim's perception of a traumatic experience, such as marital violence. In many countries throughout the world (e.g., China, El Salvador, Afghanistan, Nigeria, and India), marital rape is not criminalized, and therefore a victim's perception of the traumatic experience may vary depending on their cultural identity and worldview (Evans & Hass, 2018; Shibley & Holt, 2022).

Expression of Trauma Across Cultures

Not only does culture influence how we experience traumatic events, but also how we express our emotions, our distress, and the psychological symptoms associated with trauma and other mental illnesses. The manner and extent of self-disclosure are, in part, culturally mediated. For instance, topics about mental health, such as alcoholism or thoughts of suicide, may be regarded as taboo among certain cultures, consequently leading to avoidance and a lack of self-disclosure (Barber Rioja & Rosenfeld, 2018). This example points to how cultural stigmas impact individuals' willingness to self-disclose. Within collectivist societies, individuals might refrain from disclosing negative aspects of their lives due to cultural stigmas about mental health, as it could reflect poorly on their families (Barber Rioja & Rosenfeld, 2018).

The extent and how individuals disclose traumatic experiences also depends on the language used to discuss trauma. Language not only shapes how we think, feel, and perceive, but it also influences how and what we share, such that it can be used to modulate emotions (Evans & Hass, 2018; Shibley & Holt, 2022). This is based on the notion that the use of one's native language is associated with emotional content, whereas the use of a second language is associated more with rational or intellectual content (Bond & Lai, 2001; Shibley & Holt, 2022). For example, when discussing embarrassing topics compared to comfortable topics, bilingual participants spoke more in their second language than in their primary language (Bond & Lai, 2001). This demonstrates how language is used as a protective tool in order to avoid conversations with emotionally charged material.

Emotional expression and symptomology also vary among cultures. This is particularly relevant concerning specific diagnoses, such as depression, posttraumatic stress disorder, anxiety, and schizophrenia (Barber-Rioja et al., 2022). Many cultures value emotional restrain more than emotional expressiveness, and consequently, a stoic and even-keeled emotional expression may be misinterpreted as callous, anhedonia, or as a flat affect (Barber-Rioja et al., 2022; Qureshi & Eiroa-Orosa, 2013). Additionally, among cultures that value emotional restraint, individuals who have experienced trauma may express emotional or mental health symptoms through somatic complaints, such as headaches, back pain, gastrointestinal difficulties, or fatigue (Benuto et al., 2020). Ultimately, individuals from culturally diverse backgrounds each have their normative ways of expressing their emotions, distress, and psychological symptomology.

Explanation of Trauma Across Cultures

How psychological suffering and distress are explained varies considerably across cultures. This not only affects how people interpret the causes of mental illness but also how people respond to and treat mental illness. In many cultures, it is commonly believed that psychiatric symptoms are caused by supernatural or spiritual forces, which may be the result of witchcraft, disrespecting spirits or Gods, family or relationship conflict, financial problems, alcohol abuse, violation of social norms, or envy (Subu et al., 2022; Subudhi, 2014; Zangeneh & Al-Krenawi, 2019). For mental health professionals who rely on the biomedical approach for explaining the causes of mental illness, it is crucial to understand that the issue is not about which explanation is correct. Instead, it is about acknowledging the different types of explanations that may emerge when dealing with culturally diverse populations and how these beliefs affect an individual's interpretation and response to trauma and mental illness (Schouler-Ocak, 2015).

THE PSYCHOLOGICAL SEQUELAE OF TRAUMA AMONG IMMIGRANT POPULATIONS

Stressors have been found to increase the risk of physical and mental health problems in Latino immigrants (Kouyoumdjian et al., 2003; Vargas-Willis & Cervantes, 1987). Immigrants are at a disproportionately high risk of experiencing traumatic events before and during resettlement (Alegría et al., 2017; Crouch et al., 2000; McLaughlin et al., 2013). Prior to migration, immigrants may be exposed to the traumas of war, poverty, and hunger, which influence their decision to leave their home countries. Travel itself may present traumatic experiences in the form of violence, forced labor, detention, inhumane treatment, and lack of access to essential services. Lastly, upon arriving in their host countries, migrants may experience trauma in the form of prejudice and discrimination, lack of access to primary care, financial struggles, impoverished living conditions, and the broad stresses of acculturation, which may increase the risk of mental illnesses such as depression, anxiety, and PTSD (Bhugra & Becker, 2005).

Posttraumatic Stress Disorder

Trauma is defined as an event or a series of events that are physically or emotionally harmful or potentially life-threatening that tend to have chronic adverse effects on a person's physical, mental, social, or emotional well-being (Miller et al., 2019). Severe trauma that exceeds a person's ability to cope can lead to the development of posttraumatic stress disorder (PTSD). PTSD is a chronic impairment disorder that is common among individuals who have witnessed or experienced a traumatic event or have been exposed to extreme stressors (Miao et al., 2018). According to the American Psychiatric Association (2022), it is the only psychiatric disorder that requires the occurrence of an external traumatic event prior to the emergence of its symptoms and diagnosis. This may include direct exposure to the traumatic event, witnessing a person who had experienced the trauma firsthand, or learning of a tragic event that a close relative or friend had been exposed to (Hyland et al., 2018). The disorder can cause significant disturbance and impairment in daily functioning.

Research has identified several factors that contribute to the duration and severity of PTSD symptoms. A study in South Africa found that PTSD symptoms were most severe among those who had witnessed the traumatic events firsthand, whereas a European study found that experiences involving physical and sexual violence and living through war were associated with the longer duration of symptoms compared to other types of trauma (Atwoli et al., 2013, 2015).

In the United States alone, immigrants, mainly from Hispanic communities, are at a higher risk of witnessing or exposure to racial discrimination, urban violence, abuse by law enforcement, forced removal from families, detention, and the threat of deportation (De Arellano et al., 2018; Perreira & Ornelas, 2013). These post-migration stressors are not specific to immigrants in the USA and have been found in other countries. For instance, one study conducted in Finland examined the impact of pre and post-migration factors on Somali refugee mental health outcomes and found that higher levels of both pre- and post-migration stressors were associated with higher levels of PTSD symptoms (Mölsä et al., 2017). These pre- and post-migration factors associated with higher levels of PTSD symptoms included higher levels of war trauma, childhood adversity, shorter duration in Finland, non-permanent legal status, and more severe and frequent discrimination (Mölsä et al., 2017). Prior research suggests that experiencing multiple traumatic events, such as repeated abuse during childhood and adolescence, can lead to more severe symptoms of mental illness and poorer cognitive functioning compared to those who have experienced a single traumatic event (Lewis et al., 2021).

Research indicates that PTSD is disproportionally prevalent among immigrants, with estimates ranging as high as 47%, as opposed to the general, non-immigrant population, which is estimated to be around 3% (Bisson et al., 2015; Lindert et al., 2009). However, the prevalence of PTSD tends to decrease over generations, as the risk of third-generation migrants developing PTSD is estimated to be more similar to the general population (Guardia et al., 2017). This has been attributed to first-generation immigrants being directly exposed to the stressors and traumas of moving and resettling (Cohodes et al., 2021). When compared to voluntary migrants, refugees are much more likely to meet the criteria for PTSD due to a collectively increased exposure to traumatic events, such as violence, war, and political persecution, which often act as primary motivators for migration (Rasmussen et al., 2012). Risk factors for developing PTSD include peri- and posttraumatic components, which pertain to an individual's living conditions prior to and after the traumatic event (Carlson et al., 2016). In the context of immigration, migrants are often exposed to possible stressors and traumatic events due to their collective experiences in their home countries, during the process of migration, and their experiences of resettlement and acculturation in the new host country (Bas-Sarmiento et al., 2017).

The prevalence of traumatic events and exposure to risk factors for PTSD widely vary between countries that both import and export migrants (Atwoli et al., 2015). A study by Trabsa et al. (2023) examined the prevalence of traumatic experiences and PTSD among non-refugee immigrants in Spain, most of whom had emigrated from Northern Africa or South America. The participants consisted of immigrant patients and Spain-born patients who had previously been diagnosed with non-substance-induced psychotic disorders, such as nonspecific psychosis and schizophrenia, the symptoms and real-life consequences of which are notably more severe when paired with a diagnosis of PTSD (Fan et al., 2008). The researchers found that 31% of psychotic, non-refugee immigrants met the diagnostic criteria for PTSD, whereas only 7.1% of native-born psychotic participants had met the criteria. Furthermore, immigrants were more likely to report experiences of childhood trauma and other violent, life-threatening traumatic events compared to native-born individuals.

Furthermore, the types of trauma immigrants are exposed to may be unique to a specific country. The meta-analysis by Atwoli et al. (2015) compared the prevalence of PTSD among immigrants from a diverse array of countries and found that immigrants from low-income countries were more likely to be exposed to trauma than immigrants from high-income countries. Other studies have found a high correlation between witnessing trauma and experiencing PTSD among South African immigrants. These findings have been attributed to the long history of socio-political oppression and criminal violence in South Africa, which are commonplace in South Africa (Kaminer et al., 2008).

This differs from higher-income countries such as Japan, Spain, Italy, and Northern Ireland, wherein more personal, isolated traumatic experiences such as sexual and physical violence or the unexpected death of a loved one were more prominent risk factors for PTSD. Immigrants who have higher fluency in the host country's language are more likely to experience worse PTSD outcomes. This may be due to the increased pressure from higher societal expectations both within their communities and in the host country (Chu et al., 2013). Considering the vastly complex and often unpredictable distribution of risk factors worldwide, researchers must take historical context and personal experiences into account when assessing the experiences of immigrants with PTSD (Bustamante et al., 2017).

Anxiety Disorders

The prevalence of anxiety disorders among U.S. immigrants varies, with newly arrived immigrants reportedly being less likely to experience anxiety compared to US-born individuals, with the exception of immigrants from Puerto Rico and Mexico, both of whom were found to be at a greater risk for anxiety disorders (Szaflarski et al., 2017). Anxiety disorders are collectively the most common type of mental illness; they are characterized by excessive fear and avoidance of potential threats, to the extent that it has become persistent and impairing to everyday functioning (Penninx et al., 2021). Often, anxiety is caused by the anticipation of future threats, whether real or imagined, as the anticipation and avoidance of said threat tend to be disproportionate to the actual threat. There are several risk factors commonly associated with anxiety, such as genetic and environmental factors, and it is often comorbid with other mental disorders, such as depression and somatic disorders, which are known to increase the severity of symptoms and the difficulty of treatment (Munir & Takov, 2024). Immigrants are at risk of developing depression and somatic disorders, namely major depressive disorder and psychological distress (García-Sierra et al., 2020; Osooli et al., 2023).

Szaflarski et al. (2017) attributed the lower prevalence of anxiety among newly arrived immigrants to the possibility that the individuals who successfully migrated were more likely to have better physical and mental health than those left behind in their home countries, as this resilience and stability would be necessary for the selection process and for traveling to the U.S., in a phenomenon they call the "healthy immigrant effect." They also suggest that immigrants, upon recent arrival to the U.S., are in a generally better state of mind and mental health compared to their U.S.-born counterparts and are more likely to exhibit symptoms of mental health problems as their stay in the foreign land lengthens. For instance, Mexican immigrants in the U.S. are more likely to suffer from anxiety than Mexico-born individuals living in Mexico, possibly due to the experiences of living away from home, assimilating into the American culture, exposure to political and economic disenfranchisement, and being victims of discrimination (Breslau, 2011). Similarly, Szaflarski et al. (2017) found that immigrants from Asian or Pacific Islander and Hispanic or Latino backgrounds tend to accumulate symptoms of anxiety at a more rapid pace compared to immigrants from other backgrounds, implying a greater need for mental health services and support systems for these populations in the future.

The risk of anxiety likely varies according to the unique and specific conditions found in their new host countries, such as population sizes, nutrition, and access to health services and support systems. The prevalence of anxiety among African and Syrian migrants in Morocco was associated with several risk factors including diabetes, refugee status, overcrowding at home, and low monthly income (Essayagh et al., 2023). Another influencing factor would be the difference in experiences between generations of immigrants, as studies have found that while first-generation immigrants in the U.S. were less likely to be diagnosed with anxiety disorders, mood disorders, and depression, compared to US-born individuals, second-generation immigrants had an increased prevalence of mental health diagnoses (Salas-Wright et al., 2014). This has been a consistent finding worldwide; a cross-sectional survey conducted by Pignon et al. (2018) compared the prevalence of anxiety disorders among three generations of immigrants in comparison to the native French population. Contrary to the findings in the United States, Pignon and colleagues found that migration was associated with a higher prevalence of anxiety disorders and psychiatric comorbidities among all three generations of immigrants in France. However, much like previous American studies, Pignon and colleagues discovered that the prevalence of anxiety disorders increased across generations, with third-generation migrants being significantly more likely to experience anxiety than first-generation migrants.

Some researchers have attributed the increase in anxiety to the ongoing disproportionate amount of second-generation immigrants living in disadvantaged conditions in terms of income and education status, as well as the possible intergenerational differences in exposure to adverse childhood experiences and the common stressors and traumas experienced by immigrant families (Salas-Wright et al., 2014). The age at which immigrants are first exposed to these stressors and adverse living conditions may contribute to the likelihood of them developing anxiety later on, as adverse childhood experiences have been found to increase the risk of anxiety and depression (Elmore & Crouch, 2020). This is supported by the finding that people who migrated to the U.S. as children below the age of 13 tend to have higher rates of anxiety disorders compared to those who migrated during or after adolescence (Breslau et al., 2009).

Depression

Depression is a mood disorder characterized by persistent feelings of sadness, lack of interest, irritability, and physical symptoms that can interfere with daily functioning (American Psychiatric Association, 2022; Rintell et al., 2021). Depression may affect a person physically as they may feel fatigued, experience changes in appetite or sleep, difficulty concentrating, and feelings of hopelessness or guilt. Mood changes, behaviors, and cognition affect daily functioning and increase the risk of several chronic and acute physical health conditions, as well as other mental illnesses.

A depressive disorder may be caused by several factors or triggers, such as stressful events, drastic and unexpected changes in lifestyle, and feelings of loneliness and isolation, all of which are commonly experienced by immigrants (Bennik et al., 2013; Lee et al., 2020; Richter-Levin & Xu, 2018). Traumatic experiences have also been found to increase the risk of depression (Wang et al., 2023). Previous studies have shown that most patients who have experienced depressive episodes have reported traumatic experiences such as adverse childhood experiences, recent trauma events, or occupation-related stressors (Christensen et al., 2020; Hovens et al., 2015; Petereit-Haack et al., 2020). Another study by Negele et al. (2015) found that 75.6% of chronically depressed patients had reported clinically significant histories of childhood trauma, with repeated traumatic experiences being significantly associated with more severe depressive symptoms. There also exists a noticeable comorbidity between major depressive disorder (MDD) and posttraumatic stress disorder (PTSD), another disorder commonly found among immigrants, as research suggests that approximately half of those diagnosed with PTSD also meet the criteria for MDD (Bustamante et al., 2017; Flory & Yehuda, 2015).

Given prior research on depression, it is not surprising that migrants are at increased risk for depression, with an estimated 15.6% of immigrants reporting prevalent depressive symptoms (Foo et al., 2018). Foo and colleagues found that education level, employment status, and length of residency in the host country significantly influenced the severity of depressive symptoms. Newly arrived, unemployed migrants with low educational attainment were particularly at higher risk of depression. The association between low educational attainment and depression also applies to migrants' experiences in navigating the complex U.S. healthcare system. A study using the 2007 California Health Interview Survey (CHIS), which surveyed 51,000 adults, found that immigrants generally have lower health literacy, particularly among Latino and Asian American and Pacific Islander (AAPI) groups (Zhou et al., 2019).

Specifically, inadequate health literacy is associated with difficulty in understanding health information and lower medication adherence, thereby increasing the risk of ineffective healthcare treatment, increased costs and health disparities, higher rates of mortality, and poorer overall health (Liu et al., 2020). Health literacy has also been found to be negatively correlated with depressive symptoms among Asian immigrants in the United States (Lee et al., 2015). In other words, the less one is familiar with the services and policies of a foreign country's health care system, the more likely they are to experience symptoms of depression. Coffman and Norton (2010) found depressive symptoms to be a significant problem among recent Latino immigrants. Similar to the study by Lee et al. (2015), Coffman and Norton reported that lower health literacy and greater immigration demands predicted higher depression scores. Using the Center for Epidemiologic Studies Depression Scale (CES-D), they found that depressive symptoms commonly associated with poor health literacy included the lack of hopeful feelings for the future and thinking that life had been a failure (Coffman & Norton, 2010). They suggest that this may be due to feelings of isolation and separation from family and loved ones, the lack of acclimation and feelings of acceptance in the host country, problems in finding adequate resources and support, and the overwhelming general demands of resettlement.

Conversely, Ikonte et al. (2020), found that the prevalence of depression was lower among U.S. immigrants compared to US-born individuals; this may be due to the general underreporting of immigrant mental illnesses from U.S. mental health professionals, as well as the reluctance of immigrants to seek help from mental health services (Ikonte et al., 2020; Mohammadifirouzeh et al., 2023). The authors attribute the underrepresentation of immigrants in mental health services to cultural barriers such as the lack of English proficiency, stigmatization of mental health treatment, adherence to one's own cultural beliefs, and the lack of trust in health care providers. Additionally, studies have found that Asian American immigrants tend to underreport feelings of sadness or depressed mood, as they avoid seeking professional help until the depressive symptoms become severe and chronic (Lee et al., 2020).

Other Mental Health Disorders

Several other mental health disorders are prevalent among immigrants. For instance, a meta-analysis by Selten et al. (2020) found that migrants from both first and second generations are at a heightened risk of developing a non-affective psychotic disorder. The risk factors for developing non-affective psychotic disorder among immigrants include going through the process of migration during early childhood and living in areas with low levels of diversity. It is essential to evaluate the prevalence and risks of immigrants developing psychotic disorders, as individuals with psychosis and a comorbid PTSD diagnosis, tend to exhibit more severe symptoms of psychosis, psychological distress, and an overall reduced quality of physical and mental well-being (Fan et al., 2008; Steel et al., 2011).

Conduct disorder is another mental disorder that has several risk factors among immigrants. Conduct disorder is characterized by persistent patterns of aggression or violations of age-appropriate norms during childhood and adolescence (American Psychiatric Association, 2022). Children diagnosed with conduct disorders tend to be at high risk of developing substance use disorders, dropping out of school, unemployment, incarceration, and early mortality (Breslau et al., 2009; Laub & Vaillant, 2000). A cross-national study by Breslau (2011) examining the risk of conduct disorders among several generations of Mexican immigrants in the U.S. found that its prevalence steadily increased across the generations following migration to the host country. In other words, children who were born and raised in the United States had a greater risk of developing conduct disorder than their first-generation immigrant parents, who were also at a greater risk of conduct disorders compared to the general population of Mexico.

POLICY AND PRACTICE RECOMMENDATIONS

In addition to the stressors they face regularly, immigrants lack access to the mental health care needed for accurate treatment, thus perpetuating the risk factors for mental illnesses, mistrust in healthcare providers, and traumatic experiences across multiple generations (Derr, 2016). A meta-analysis by Derr (2016) indicated that 3% to 6% of immigrants in the United States utilized mental health services, which is notably lower than their US-born counterparts, 13% of whom utilized these services. Immigrants who utilized mental health services highlighted the importance of "informal channels", such as family, friends, and religious communities, when recognizing their own need for mental health treatment. This underscores the need for culturally sensitive and responsive training among healthcare providers, as well as trauma-informed care, in order to make accurate assessments of the mental status of immigrants in a way that promotes respect and mindfulness toward their respective cultures (Cipta et al., 2024).

The lack of culturally responsive training among healthcare professionals significantly contributes to poorer physical and mental health outcomes, as well as underrepresentation among immigrants and minorities in U.S. healthcare (Brach & Fraser, 2016). Culturally responsive training entails that healthcare providers guide their clinical decisions based on the patients' and their families' cultural and lingual preferences, values, traditions, religious beliefs, and socioeconomic conditions (Stubbe, 2020). By achieving this level of cultural competence, wherein the patient's perspective on health and treatment preferences are given the same amount of respect and consideration as the clinician's recommendations, healthcare professionals may provide services to diverse populations effectively and compassionately, potentially addressing the issue of mistrust and stigmatization of healthcare among immigrants (Hays et al., 2006; Pearson et al., 2007). With the rapidly expanding Hispanic population in the United States, the need for culturally responsive training and education steadily increases, with Hispanic patients expressing a preference for healthcare services that are more family-oriented, personal, and spiritual in their practices (Fang et al., 2016).

Another recommended practice for promoting sufficient psychological support among migrants with traumatic experiences would be the integration of a trauma-informed care curriculum when training mental healthcare providers (Vukčević et al., 2016). The lack of training in trauma-informed care, combined with the lack of cultural sensitivity and responsiveness, may result in clinicians misinterpreting migrant patients' behaviors and misdiagnosing them based on stereotypes (Murray et al., 2010; Stone & Moskowitz, 2011; Sundvall et al., 2015). A study by Yeomans and Forman (2009) found that clinicians tend to diagnose PTSD as a broad characterization of the traumatic experiences of people from different cultures when other, more prevalent symptoms, such as depression, anxiety, and somatization, may be more appropriate (Yeomans & Forman, 2009; Eshun & Gurung, 2009). These findings further indicate the urgent need for clinicians to undergo transcultural training to avoid broad, stereotype-informed evaluations.

With the ever-increasing rate of immigrants and refugees in the United States, many of whom are victims or have been exposed to the traumas of war, persecution, and the challenges of migration, there is an urgent need for transcultural mental health assessments and trauma-informed care (Wylie et al., 2018). Psychological evaluations are not just essential for immigrant proceedings; they are a necessity as the assessment of an incoming migrant's social and psychological functioning, and well-being may be used to ensure that the individual is physically and mentally capable of withstanding the arduous tasks of resettlement and acculturation in the host country (Mercado et al., 2022). Immigration support agencies, such as the U.S. Citizenship and Immigration Services (USCIS), also rely on psychological evaluations to ensure adequate care for migrants seeking legal relief. Several studies have also acknowledged the growing need for psychiatric evaluations for immigrants and asylum seekers, as there is an increasing recognition of the psychiatric needs of immigrants and how their mental health statuses affect their abilities to adjust (Meffert et al., 2010). Studies have also demonstrated how transcultural approaches to trauma-informed care can be used to improve assessment and screening processes, thus leading to more effective mental health treatment for immigrants and their families (Adeponle et al., 2015).

A comprehensive baseline evaluation of mental health services for immigrants and refugees in the UK by Wylie et al. (2018) found several recurring, complex issues faced by mental health care providers when assessing mental health disorders among immigrant and refugee families who have experienced trauma. They outline the general lack of training in cultural competence and transcultural care among practitioners, which are vital when taking narrative histories among patients, as they ensure that patients are comfortable and at ease while engaging in difficult conversations while also reducing the possibility of re-triggering trauma (Betancourt et al., 2017; Murray et al., 2010). Unfortunately, the integration of such training, as well as the use of transcultural trauma assessments, is reportedly time-consuming, with hospital staff often overlooking its importance, leading to insufficient time given to properly evaluate clients and provide treatment recommendations in a way that is culturally informed (Ferrari et al., 2016). However, if properly educated on the importance of cultural humility and trauma-informed care, healthcare providers can ensure their physical and mental well-being and reduce the likelihood of intergenerational trauma among immigrants.

SUMMARY

This chapter examined the psychological effects of migration into a new country, specifically immigrant stress and trauma as they adjust to a new country. It discussed common mental health conditions experienced by immigrant populations, including anxiety, depression, and PTSD. The traumatic experiences of immigrants are not limited to the adverse conditions that motivated them to move out of their home countries, as the process of migration and their experiences afterward introduce a host of other stressors. The feelings of loss and separation from one's country of origin, combined with the daily hardships of integration and acculturation, increase the risk of mental disorders that may persist across multiple generations. In addition to the stressors they face regularly, many immigrants lack access to adequate mental health care. This results in untreated trauma and the amplifying of the negative impact of daily stressors. This highlights the need for culturally sensitive and responsive training among healthcare providers, as well as trauma-informed care, to make accurate assessments of the mental needs of immigrants in a way that promotes respect and mindfulness toward their respective cultures.

REFERENCES

Adeponle, A. B., Groleau, D., & Kirmayer, L. J. (2015). Clinician reasoning in the use of cultural formulation to resolve uncertainty in the diagnosis of psychosis. *Culture, Medicine and Psychiatry*, *39*(1), 16–42. DOI: 10.1007/s11013-014-9408-5 PMID: 25310907

Alegría, M., Álvarez, K., & DiMarzio, K. (2017). Immigration and Mental Health. *Current Epidemiology Reports*, *4*(2), 145–155. DOI: 10.1007/s40471-017-0111-2 PMID: 29805955

American Psychiatric Association. (2022). Diagnostic and Statistical Manual of Mental Disorders. American Psychiatric Association Publishing., , DSM-5-TR.DOI: 10.1176/appi.books.9780890425787

Arbona, C., Olvera, N., Rodriguez, N., Hagan, J., Linares, A., & Wiesner, M. (2010). Acculturative Stress Among Documented and Undocumented Latino Immigrants in the United States. *Hispanic Journal of Behavioral Sciences*, *32*(3), 362–384. DOI: 10.1177/0739986310373210 PMID: 25484488

Atwoli, L., Stein, D. J., Koenen, K. C., & McLaughlin, K. A. (2015). Epidemiology of posttraumatic stress disorder: Prevalence, correlates and consequences. *Current Opinion in Psychiatry*, *28*(4), 307–311. DOI: 10.1097/YCO.0000000000000167 PMID: 26001922

Atwoli, L., Stein, D. J., Williams, D. R., Mclaughlin, K. A., Petukhova, M., Kessler, R. C., & Koenen, K. C. (2013). Trauma and posttraumatic stress disorder in South Africa: Analysis from the South African Stress and Health Study. *BMC Psychiatry*, *13*(1), 182. DOI: 10.1186/1471-244X-13-182 PMID: 23819543

Atxotegui, J. (2000). *Los duelos de la migración: Una aproximación psico-patológica y psicosocial*. https://www.semanticscholar.org/paper/Los-duelos-de-la-migraci%C3%B3n%3A-una-aproximaci%C3%B3n-y-Atxotegui/635c7af7084be5d623a5a6d32c2c107d9ad3e7d5

Bailey, C. A., & Widener, K. (2022). The nexus between immigration status, policy, and proceedings, and mental health. *Current Opinion in Psychology*, *47*, 101411. DOI: 10.1016/j.copsyc.2022.101411 PMID: 35914487

Barber-Rioja, V., Akinsulure-Smith, A. M., & Vendzules, S. (2022). *Mental health evaluations in immigration court: A guide for mental health and legal professionals*. NYU Press. https://books.google.com/books?hl=en&lr=&id=Gr5HEAAAQBAJ&oi=fnd&pg=PA1&dq=mental+health+evaluations+in+immigration+court&ots=Kio2lcqG8e&sig=ClVyjPeNZkO0o08WkJHdHO4KlUM

Barber Rioja, V., & Rosenfeld, B. (2018). Addressing Linguistic and Cultural Differences in the Forensic Interview. *International Journal of Forensic Mental Health, 17*(4), 377–386. DOI: 10.1080/14999013.2018.1495280

Bas-Sarmiento, P., Saucedo-Moreno, M. J., Fernández-Gutiérrez, M., & Poza-Méndez, M. (2017). Mental Health in Immigrants Versus Native Population: A Systematic Review of the Literature. *Archives of Psychiatric Nursing, 31*(1), 111–121. DOI: 10.1016/j.apnu.2016.07.014 PMID: 28104048

Bennik, E. C., Ormel, J., & Oldehinkel, A. J. (2013). Life changes and depressive symptoms: The effects of valence and amount of change. *BMC Psychology, 1*(1), 14. DOI: 10.1186/2050-7283-1-14 PMID: 25566366

Benuto, L. T., Gonzalez, F. R., & Singer, J. (Eds.). (2020). *Handbook of Cultural Factors in Behavioral Health: A Guide for the Helping Professional*. Springer International Publishing., DOI: 10.1007/978-3-030-32229-8

Berry, J. W. (1997). Lead Article—Immigration, Acculturation, and Adaptation. *Applied Psychology, 46*(1), 5–34. DOI: 10.1080/026999497378467

Betancourt, T. S., Newnham, E. A., Birman, D., Lee, R., Ellis, B. H., & Layne, C. M. (2017). Comparing Trauma Exposure, Mental Health Needs, and Service Utilization Across Clinical Samples of Refugee, Immigrant, and U.S.-Origin Children. *Journal of Traumatic Stress, 30*(3), 209–218. DOI: 10.1002/jts.22186 PMID: 28585740

Bhugra, D., & Becker, M. A. (2005). Migration, cultural bereavement and cultural identity. *World Psychiatry; Official Journal of the World Psychiatric Association (WPA), 4*(1), 18–24. PMID: 16633496

Bisson, J. I., Cosgrove, S., Lewis, C., & Roberts, N. P. (2015). Post-traumatic stress disorder. *BMJ (Clinical Research Ed.), h6161*, h6161. DOI: 10.1136/bmj.h6161 PMID: 26611143

Bisson, J. I., & Sakhuja, D. (2006). Adjustment disorders. *Psychiatry (Abingdon), 5*(7), 240–242. DOI: 10.1053/j.mppsy.2006.04.004

Bond, M., & Lai, T.-M. (2001). Embarrassment and code-switching into a second language. *The Journal of Social Psychology, 126*(2), 179–186. DOI: 10.1080/19401183.1986.12461512

Brach, C., & Fraser, I. (2002). Reducing disparities through culturally competent health care: An analysis of the business case. *Quality Management in Health Care, 10*(4), 15–28. DOI: 10.1097/00019514-200210040-00005 PMID: 12938253

Breslau, J. (2011). Migration From Mexico to the United States and Conduct Disorder: A Cross-national Study. *Archives of General Psychiatry*, *68*(12), 1284. DOI: 10.1001/archgenpsychiatry.2011.140 PMID: 22147845

Breslau, J., Borges, G., Hagar, Y., Tancredi, D., & Gilman, S. (2009). Immigration to the USA and risk for mood and anxiety disorders: Variation by origin and age at immigration. *Psychological Medicine*, *39*(07), 1117. DOI: 10.1017/S0033291708004698 PMID: 19000338

Bustamante, L. H. U., Cerqueira, R. O., Leclerc, E., & Brietzke, E. (2017). Stress, trauma, and posttraumatic stress disorder in migrants: A comprehensive review. *Revista Brasileira de Psiquiatria : Orgão Oficial da Associação Brasileira de Psiquiatria, Asociación Psiqui´trica de la América Latina*, *40*(2), 220–225. DOI: 10.1590/1516-4446-2017-2290 PMID: 29069252

Carlson, E. B., Palmieri, P. A., Field, N. P., Dalenberg, C. J., Macia, K. S., & Spain, D. A. (2016). Contributions of risk and protective factors to prediction of psychological symptoms after traumatic experiences. *Comprehensive Psychiatry*, *69*, 106–115. DOI: 10.1016/j.comppsych.2016.04.022 PMID: 27423351

Chong, A., & Chong, M. Z. (2023). Feeling the heat? Fear of failure and performance. *Kyklos*, *76*(1), 3–17. DOI: 10.1111/kykl.12316

Christensen, M. C., Florea, I., Loft, H., & McIntyre, R. S. (2020). Efficacy of vortioxetine in patients with major depressive disorder reporting childhood or recent trauma. *Journal of Affective Disorders*, *263*, 258–266. DOI: 10.1016/j.jad.2019.11.074 PMID: 31818787

Chu, T., Keller, A. S., & Rasmussen, A. (2013). Effects of Post-migration Factors on PTSD Outcomes Among Immigrant Survivors of Political Violence. *Journal of Immigrant and Minority Health*, *15*(5), 890–897. DOI: 10.1007/s10903-012-9696-1 PMID: 22976794

Cipta, D. A., Andoko, D., Theja, A., Utama, A. V. E., Hendrik, H., William, D. G., Reina, N., Handoko, M. T., & Lumbuun, N. (2024). Culturally sensitive patient-centered healthcare: A focus on health behavior modification in low and middle-income nations-insights from Indonesia. *Frontiers in Medicine*, *11*, 1353037. DOI: 10.3389/fmed.2024.1353037 PMID: 38681051

Coffman, M. J., & Norton, C. K. (2010). Demands of Immigration, Health Literacy, and Depression in Recent Latino Immigrants. *Home Health Care Management & Practice*, *22*(2), 116–122. DOI: 10.1177/1084822309347343

Cohodes, E. M., Kribakaran, S., Odriozola, P., Bakirci, S., McCauley, S., Hodges, H. R., Sisk, L. M., Zacharek, S. J., & Gee, D. G. (2021). Migration-related trauma and mental health among migrant children emigrating from Mexico and Central America to the United States: Effects on developmental neurobiology and implications for policy. *Developmental Psychobiology*, *63*(6), e22158. DOI: 10.1002/dev.22158 PMID: 34292596

Costa, J. R. A. D., Lima, J. V. D., & Almeida, P. C. D. (2003). Stress no trabalho do enfermeiro. *Revista da Escola de Enfermagem da USP*, *37*(3), 63–71. DOI: 10.1590/S0080-62342003000300008 PMID: 14686049

Crouch, J. L., Hanson, R. F., Saunders, B. E., Kilpatrick, D. G., & Resnick, H. S. (2000). Income, race/ethnicity, and exposure to violence in youth: Results from the national survey of adolescents. *Journal of Community Psychology*, *28*(6), 625–641. DOI: 10.1002/1520-6629(200011)28:6<625::AID-JCOP6>3.0.CO;2-R

De Arellano, M. A., Andrews, A. R., Reid-Quiñones, K., Vasquez, D., Doherty, L. S., Danielson, C. K., & Rheingold, A. (2018). Immigration trauma among Hispanic youth: Missed by trauma assessments and predictive of depression and PTSD symptoms. *Journal of Latina/o Psychology*, *6*(3), 159–174. DOI: 10.1037/lat0000090 PMID: 31840010

Derr, A. S. (2016). Mental Health Service Use Among Immigrants in the United States: A Systematic Review. *Psychiatric Services (Washington, D.C.)*, *67*(3), 265–274. DOI: 10.1176/appi.ps.201500004 PMID: 26695493

Elmore, A. L., & Crouch, E. (2020). The Association of Adverse Childhood Experiences With Anxiety and Depression for Children and Youth, 8 to 17 Years of Age. *Academic Pediatrics*, *20*(5), 600–608. DOI: 10.1016/j.acap.2020.02.012 PMID: 32092442

Eshun, S., & Gurung, R. A. (Eds.). (2009). *Culture and mental health: Sociocultural influences, theory, and practice*. John Wiley & Sons. DOI: 10.1002/9781444305807

Essayagh, F., Essayagh, M., Essayagh, S., Marc, I., Bukassa, G., El Otmani, I., Kouyate, M. F., & Essayagh, T. (2023). The prevalence and risk factors for anxiety and depression symptoms among migrants in Morocco. *Scientific Reports*, *13*(1), 3740. DOI: 10.1038/s41598-023-30715-8 PMID: 36878989

Evans, B., & Hass, G. (2018). *Forensic Psychological Assessment in Immigration Court: A Guidebook for Evidence-Based and Ethical Practice*. Routledge., DOI: 10.4324/9781315621197

Fan, X., Henderson, D. C., Nguyen, D. D., Cather, C., Freudenreich, O., Evins, A. E., Borba, C. P., & Goff, D. C. (2008). Posttraumatic stress disorder, cognitive function and quality of life in patients with schizophrenia. *Psychiatry Research, 159*(1–2), 140–146. DOI: 10.1016/j.psychres.2007.10.012 PMID: 18423611

Fang, M. L., Sixsmith, J., Sinclair, S., & Horst, G. (2016). A knowledge synthesis of culturally- and spiritually-sensitive end-of-life care: Findings from a scoping review. *BMC Geriatrics, 16*(1), 107. DOI: 10.1186/s12877-016-0282-6 PMID: 27193395

Ferrari, M., Ahmad, F., Shakya, Y., Ledwos, C., & McKenzie, K. (2016). Computer-assisted client assessment survey for mental health: Patient and health provider perspectives. *BMC Health Services Research, 16*(1), 516. DOI: 10.1186/s12913-016-1756-0 PMID: 27663508

Flory, J. D., & Yehuda, R. (2015). Comorbidity between post-traumatic stress disorder and major depressive disorder: Alternative explanations and treatment considerations. *Dialogues in Clinical Neuroscience, 17*(2), 141–150. DOI: 10.31887/DCNS.2015.17.2/jflory PMID: 26246789

Foo, S. Q., Tam, W. W., Ho, C. S., Tran, B. X., Nguyen, L. H., McIntyre, R. S., & Ho, R. C. (2018). Prevalence of Depression among Migrants: A Systematic Review and Meta-Analysis. *International Journal of Environmental Research and Public Health, 15*(9), 1986. DOI: 10.3390/ijerph15091986 PMID: 30213071

Gamez, A. M. (2024). *Overcoming Adversity*. Self-Publishing.

García-Sierra, R., Fernández-Cano, M. I., Manresa-Domínguez, J. M., Feijoo-Cid, M., Moreno Gabriel, E., Arreciado Marañón, A., Ramos-Roure, F., Segura-Bernal, J., & Torán-Monserrat, P. (2020). Psychological Distress and Somatization in Immigrants in Primary Health Care Practices. *Health Care, 8*(4), 557. DOI: 10.3390/healthcare8040557 PMID: 33322209

Garcini, L. M., Domenech Rodríguez, M. M., Mercado, A., Silva, M., Cadenas, G., Galvan, T., & Paris, M. (2023). Anti-immigration policy and mental health: Risk of distress and trauma among deferred action for childhood arrivals recipients in the United States. *Psychological Trauma: Theory, Research, Practice, and Policy, 15*(7), 1067–1075. DOI: 10.1037/tra0001228 PMID: 35482682

Gonsalves, C. J. (1992). Psychological stages of the refugee process: A model for therapeutic interventions. *Professional Psychology, Research and Practice, 23*(5), 382–389. DOI: 10.1037/0735-7028.23.5.382

Grove, C. L., & Torbiörn, I. (1985). A new conceptualization of intercultural adjustment and the goals of training. *International Journal of Intercultural Relations*, *9*(2), 205–233. DOI: 10.1016/0147-1767(85)90008-2

Guardia, D., Salleron, J., Roelandt, J.-L., & Vaiva, G. (2017). Prévalence des troubles psychiatriques et addictologiques auprès de trois générations successives de migrants: Résultats d'une étude menée en population générale. *L'Encéphale*, *43*(5), 435–443. DOI: 10.1016/j.encep.2016.06.008 PMID: 27644920

Hays, R.D., Ngo-Metzger, Q., Sorkin, D.H., Telfair, J., Weidmer, B.A., Weech-Maldonado, R., & Hurtado, M.P. (2006). Cultural Competency and Quality of Care: Obtaining the Patient's Perspective.

Hovens, J. G. F. M., Giltay, E. J., Spinhoven, P., Van Hemert, A. M., & Penninx, B. W. J. H. (2015). Impact of Childhood Life Events and Childhood Trauma on the Onset and Recurrence of Depressive and Anxiety Disorders. *The Journal of Clinical Psychiatry*, *76*(07), 931–938. DOI: 10.4088/JCP.14m09135 PMID: 25699690

Hyland, P., Shevlin, M., Fyvie, C., & Karatzias, T. (2018). Posttraumatic Stress Disorder and Complex Posttraumatic Stress Disorder in *DSM-5* and *ICD-11*: Clinical and Behavioral Correlates. *Journal of Traumatic Stress*, *31*(2), 174–180. DOI: 10.1002/jts.22272 PMID: 29577450

Ikonte, C. O., Prigmore, H. L., Dawson, A. Z., & Egede, L. E. (2020). Trends in prevalence of depression and serious psychological distress in United States immigrant and non-immigrant populations, 2010—2016. *Journal of Affective Disorders*, *274*, 719–725. DOI: 10.1016/j.jad.2020.05.010 PMID: 32664007

Kaminer, D., Grimsrud, A., Myer, L., Stein, D. J., & Williams, D. R. (2008). Risk for post-traumatic stress disorder associated with different forms of interpersonal violence in South Africa. *Social Science & Medicine*, *67*(10), 1589–1595. DOI: 10.1016/j.socscimed.2008.07.023 PMID: 18774211

Kouyoumdjian, H., Zamboanga, B. L., & Hansen, D. J. (2003). Barriers to community mental health services for Latinos: Treatment considerations. *Clinical Psychology : a Publication of the Division of Clinical Psychology of the American Psychological Association*, *10*(4), 394–422. DOI: 10.1093/clipsy.bpg041

Kroening, A. L. H., & Dawson-Hahn, E. (2019). Health Considerations for Immigrant and Refugee Children. *Advances in Pediatrics*, *66*, 87–110. DOI: 10.1016/j.yapd.2019.04.003 PMID: 31230701

Laub, J. H., & Vaillant, G. E. (2000). Delinquency and Mortality: A 50-Year Follow-Up Study of 1,000 Delinquent and Nondelinquent Boys. *The American Journal of Psychiatry, 157*(1), 96–102. DOI: 10.1176/ajp.157.1.96 PMID: 10618019

Lechner, E. (2007). Imigração e saúde mental. *Migrações*, 79–101. https://estudogeral.uc.pt/handle/10316/33297

Lee, H. Y., Rhee, T. G., Kim, N. K., & Ahluwalia, J. S. (2015). Health Literacy as a Social Determinant of Health in Asian American Immigrants: Findings from a Population-Based Survey in California. *Journal of General Internal Medicine, 30*(8), 1118–1124. DOI: 10.1007/s11606-015-3217-6 PMID: 25715993

Lee, M., Bhimla, A., & Ma, G. X. (2020). Depressive Symptom Severity and Immigration-Related Characteristics in Asian American Immigrants. *Journal of Immigrant and Minority Health, 22*(5), 935–945. DOI: 10.1007/s10903-020-01004-7 PMID: 32221768

LeMaster, J. W., Broadbridge, C. L., Lumley, M. A., Arnetz, J. E., Arfken, C., Fetters, M. D., Jamil, H., Pole, N., & Arnetz, B. B. (2018). Acculturation and post-migration psychological symptoms among Iraqi refugees: A path analysis. *The American Journal of Orthopsychiatry, 88*(1), 38–47. DOI: 10.1037/ort0000240 PMID: 28253013

Lewis, S. J., Koenen, K. C., Ambler, A., Arseneault, L., Caspi, A., Fisher, H. L., Moffitt, T. E., & Danese, A. (2021). Unravelling the contribution of complex trauma to psychopathology and cognitive deficits: A cohort study. *The British Journal of Psychiatry, 219*(2), 448–455. DOI: 10.1192/bjp.2021.57 PMID: 34538875

Lindert, J., Ehrenstein, O. S. V., Priebe, S., Mielck, A., & Brähler, E. (2009). Depression and anxiety in labor migrants and refugees – A systematic review and meta-analysis. *Social Science & Medicine, 69*(2), 246–257. DOI: 10.1016/j.socscimed.2009.04.032 PMID: 19539414

Liu, C., Wang, D., Liu, C., Jiang, J., Wang, X., Chen, H., Ju, X., & Zhang, X. (2020). What is the meaning of health literacy? A systematic review and qualitative synthesis. *Family Medicine and Community Health, 8*(2), e000351. DOI: 10.1136/fmch-2020-000351 PMID: 32414834

Maguire, J., Sizer, H., Mifsud, N., & O'Donoghue, B. (2020). Outcomes for migrants with a first episode of psychosis: A systematic review. *Schizophrenia Research, 222*, 42–48. DOI: 10.1016/j.schres.2020.05.048 PMID: 32561236

McAuliffe, M., & Triandafyllidou, A. (2021). *World Migration Report 2022*. International Organization for Migration. https://publications.iom.int/system/files/pdf/WMR-2022-EN_1.pdf

McLaughlin, K. A., Koenen, K. C., Hill, E. D., Petukhova, M., Sampson, N. A., Zaslavsky, A. M., & Kessler, R. C. (2013). Trauma Exposure and Posttraumatic Stress Disorder in a National Sample of Adolescents. *Journal of the American Academy of Child and Adolescent Psychiatry*, *52*(8), 815–830.e14. DOI: 10.1016/j.jaac.2013.05.011 PMID: 23880492

Meffert, S. M., Musalo, K., McNiel, D. E., & Binder, R. L. (2010). The role of mental health professionals in political asylum processing. *The Journal of the American Academy of Psychiatry and the Law*, *38*(4), 479–489. PMID: 21156906

Mehta, C., Theodore, N., Mora, I., & Wade, J. (2002). *Chicago's undocumented immigrants: An analysis of wages, working conditions, and economic contributions*. https://www.semanticscholar.org/paper/Chicago%27s-undocumented-immigrants%3A-An-analysis-of-Mehta-Theodore/6457030c1296887962916ce526723bfb408e73a8

Melander, C., & Shmulyar Gréen, O. (2023). Language brokering as acts of care: Experiences of young migrants born in Poland and Romania living in Sweden. *Nordic Social Work Research*, *13*(4), 577–588. DOI: 10.1080/2156857X.2023.2199417

Mercado, A., Antuña, C. S., Bailey, C., Garcini, L., Hass, G. A., Henderson, C., Koslofsky, S., Morales, F., & Venta, A. (2022). Professional guidelines for psychological evaluations in immigration proceedings. *Journal of Latina/o Psychology*, *10*(4), 253–276. DOI: 10.1037/lat0000209

Miao, X.-R., Chen, Q.-B., Wei, K., Tao, K.-M., & Lu, Z.-J. (2018). Posttraumatic stress disorder: From diagnosis to prevention. *Military Medical Research*, *5*(1), 32. DOI: 10.1186/s40779-018-0179-0 PMID: 30261912

Miller, K. K., Brown, C. R., Shramko, M., & Svetaz, M. V. (2019). Applying Trauma-Informed Practices to the Care of Refugee and Immigrant Youth: 10 Clinical Pearls. *Children (Basel, Switzerland)*, *6*(8), 94. DOI: 10.3390/children6080094 PMID: 31434278

Mohammadifirouzeh, M., Oh, K. M., Basnyat, I., & Gimm, G. (2023). Factors Associated with Professional Mental Help-Seeking Among U.S. Immigrants: A Systematic Review. *Journal of Immigrant and Minority Health*, *25*(5), 1118–1136. DOI: 10.1007/s10903-023-01475-4 PMID: 37000385

Mölsä, M., Kuittinen, S., Tiilikainen, M., Honkasalo, M.-L., & Punamäki, R.-L. (2017). Mental health among older refugees: The role of trauma, discrimination, and religiousness. *Aging & Mental Health*, *21*(8), 829–837. DOI: 10.1080/13607863.2016.1165183 PMID: 27080403

Munir, S., & Takov, V. (2024). Generalized Anxiety Disorder. In *StatPearls*. StatPearls Publishing., https://www.ncbi.nlm.nih.gov/books/NBK441870/

Murray, K. E., Davidson, G. R., & Schweitzer, R. D. (2010). Review of refugee mental health interventions following resettlement: Best practices and recommendations. *The American Journal of Orthopsychiatry*, *80*(4), 576–585. DOI: 10.1111/j.1939-0025.2010.01062.x PMID: 20950298

Negele, A., Kaufhold, J., Kallenbach, L., & Leuzinger-Bohleber, M. (2015). Childhood Trauma and Its Relation to Chronic Depression in Adulthood. *Depression Research and Treatment*, *2015*, 1–11. DOI: 10.1155/2015/650804 PMID: 26693349

Osooli, M., Ohlsson, H., Sundquist, J., & Sundquist, K. (2023). Major depressive disorders in young immigrants: A cohort study from primary healthcare settings in Sweden. *Scandinavian Journal of Public Health*, *51*(3), 315–322. DOI: 10.1177/14034948211019796 PMID: 34120516

Pearson, A., Srivastava, R., Craig, D., Tucker, D., Grinspun, D., Bajnok, I., Griffin, P., Long, L., Porritt, K., Han, T., & Gi, A. A. (2007). Systematic review on embracing cultural diversity for developing and sustaining a healthy work environment in healthcare. *International Journal of Evidence-Based Healthcare*, *5*(1), 54–91. DOI: 10.1111/j.1479-6988.2007.00058.x PMID: 21631782

Penninx, B. W., Pine, D. S., Holmes, E. A., & Reif, A. (2021). Anxiety disorders. *Lancet*, *397*(10277), 914–927. DOI: 10.1016/S0140-6736(21)00359-7 PMID: 33581801

Perreira, K. M., & Ornelas, I. (2013). Painful Passages: Traumatic Experiences and Post-Traumatic Stress among U.S. Immigrant Latino Adolescents and their Primary Caregivers. *The International Migration Review*, *47*(4), 976–1005. DOI: 10.1111/imre.12050 PMID: 24385676

Petereit-Haack, G., Bolm-Audorff, U., Romero Starke, K., & Seidler, A. (2020). Occupational Risk for Post-Traumatic Stress Disorder and Trauma-Related Depression: A Systematic Review with Meta-Analysis. *International Journal of Environmental Research and Public Health*, *17*(24), 9369. DOI: 10.3390/ijerph17249369 PMID: 33327657

Pignon, B., Amad, A., Pelissolo, A., Fovet, T., Thomas, P., Vaiva, G., Roelandt, J.-L., Benradia, I., Rolland, B., & Geoffroy, P. A. (2018). Increased prevalence of anxiety disorders in third-generation migrants in comparison to natives and to first-generation migrants. *Journal of Psychiatric Research*, *102*, 38–43. DOI: 10.1016/j.jpsychires.2018.03.007 PMID: 29597072

Portes, A. (2001). Introduction: The debates and significance of immigrant transnationalism. *Global Networks*, *1*(3), 181–194. DOI: 10.1111/1471-0374.00012

Qureshi, A., & Eiroa-Orosa, F. (2013). *Training for overcoming health disparities in mental health care: Interpretive-relational cultural competence*. Hogrefe Publishing. https://repository.uel.ac.uk/download/ffe867cdf7cf37eb40320e3a4b7f3a159f97b4f100cfc503a8c1b5d4dd739f5c/280351/Qureshi%2C%20Eiroa-Orosa%20-%202012%20-%20Cultural%20Variations%20in%20Psychopathology.%20From%20Research%20to%20Practice.pdf

Rasmussen, A., Crager, M., Baser, R. E., Chu, T., & Gany, F. (2012). Onset of Posttraumatic Stress Disorder and Major Depression Among Refugees and Voluntary Migrants to the United States. *Journal of Traumatic Stress*, *25*(6), 705–712. DOI: 10.1002/jts.21763 PMID: 23184423

Richter-Levin, G., & Xu, L. (2018). How could stress lead to major depressive disorder? *IBRO Reports*, *4*, 38–43. DOI: 10.1016/j.ibror.2018.04.001 PMID: 30155523

Rintell, L. S., Buchholz, K. R., & Gladstone, T. R. G. (2021). Depression. In W. O'Donohue & M. Zimmermann (Eds.), *Handbook of Evidence-Based Prevention of Behavioral Disorders in Integrated Care* (pp. 101–137). Springer International Publishing. DOI: 10.1007/978-3-030-83469-2_6

Salas-Wright, C. P., Kagotho, N., & Vaughn, M. G. (2014). Mood, anxiety, and personality disorders among first and second-generation immigrants to the United States. *Psychiatry Research*, *220*(3), 1028–1036. DOI: 10.1016/j.psychres.2014.08.045 PMID: 25223256

Sangalang, C. C., Becerra, D., Mitchell, F. M., Lechuga-Peña, S., Lopez, K., & Kim, I. (2019). Trauma, Post-Migration Stress, and Mental Health: A Comparative Analysis of Refugees and Immigrants in the United States. *Journal of Immigrant and Minority Health*, *21*(5), 909–919. DOI: 10.1007/s10903-018-0826-2 PMID: 30244330

Schouler-Ocak, M. (Ed.). (2015). *Trauma and Migration: Cultural Factors in the Diagnosis and Treatment of Traumatised Immigrants*. Springer International Publishing., DOI: 10.1007/978-3-319-17335-1

Selten, J.-P., Van Der Ven, E., & Termorshuizen, F. (2020). Migration and psychosis: A meta-analysis of incidence studies. *Psychological Medicine*, *50*(2), 303–313. DOI: 10.1017/S0033291719000035 PMID: 30722795

Shibley, M. G., & Holt, M. (2022). *Conducting immigration evaluations: A practical guide for mental health professionals*. Routledge. https://api.taylorfrancis.com/content/books/mono/download?identifierName=doi&identifierValue=10.4324/9781003139973&type=googlepdf

Simich, L. (2006). Hidden Meanings of Health Security: Migration Experiences and Systemic Barriers to Mental Well-Being among Non-status Migrants in Canada. *International Journal of Migration, Health and Social Care*, *2*(3/4), 16–27. DOI: 10.1108/17479894200600024

Steel, C., Haddock, G., Tarrier, N., Picken, A., & Barrowclough, C. (2011). Auditory Hallucinations and Posttraumatic Stress Disorder Within Schizophrenia and Substance Abuse. *The Journal of Nervous and Mental Disease*, *199*(9), 709–711. DOI: 10.1097/NMD.0b013e318229d6e8 PMID: 21878787

Sternberg, R. M., Nápoles, A. M., Gregorich, S., Paul, S., Lee, K. A., & Stewart, A. L. (2016). Development of the Stress of Immigration Survey: A Field Test Among Mexican Immigrant Women. *Family & Community Health*, *39*(1), 40–52. DOI: 10.1097/FCH.0000000000000088 PMID: 26605954

Stone, J., & Moskowitz, G. B. (2011). Non-conscious bias in medical decision making: What can be done to reduce it? *Medical Education*, *45*(8), 768–776. DOI: 10.1111/j.1365-2923.2011.04026.x PMID: 21752073

Stubbe, D. E. (2020). Practicing Cultural Competence and Cultural Humility in the Care of Diverse Patients. *Focus - American Psychiatric Publishing*, *18*(1), 49–51. DOI: 10.1176/appi.focus.20190041 PMID: 32047398

Subu, M. A., Holmes, D., Arumugam, A., Al-Yateem, N., Maria Dias, J., Rahman, S. A., Waluyo, I., Ahmed, F. R., & Abraham, M. S. (2022). Traditional, religious, and cultural perspectives on mental illness: A qualitative study on causal beliefs and treatment use. *International Journal of Qualitative Studies on Health and Well-being*, *17*(1), 2123090. DOI: 10.1080/17482631.2022.2123090 PMID: 36097886

Subudhi, C. (2014). Culture and mental illness. *Social Work Practice in Mental Health: Cross-Cultural Perspectives, 141*, 132–140. https://www.researchgate.net/profile/Chittaranjan-Subudhi-2/publication/270762975_Culture_and_Mental_Illness/links/54b4adac0cf28ebe92e4818f/Culture-and-Mental-Illness.pdf

Sundvall, M., Tidemalm, D. H., Titelman, D. E., Runeson, B., & Bäärnhielm, S. (2015). Assessment and treatment of asylum seekers after a suicide attempt: A comparative study of people registered at mental health services in a Swedish location. *BMC Psychiatry*, *15*(1), 235. DOI: 10.1186/s12888-015-0613-8 PMID: 26446409

Szaflarski, M., Cubbins, L. A., & Meganathan, K. (2017). Anxiety Disorders among US Immigrants: The Role of Immigrant Background and Social-Psychological Factors. *Issues in Mental Health Nursing*, *38*(4), 317–326. DOI: 10.1080/01612840.2017.1287790 PMID: 28379742

Trabsa, A., Redolar-Ripoll, D., Vargas, L., Llimona, A., Hogg, B., Valiente-Gómez, A., Pérez, V., Moreno-Alcázar, A., & Amann, B. L. (2023). A comparison of PTSD and traumatic event rates in a clinical sample of non-refugee immigrants and native-born individuals with a psychotic disorder: A case-control study. *European Journal of Psychotraumatology*, *14*(2), 2263151. DOI: 10.1080/20008066.2023.2263151 PMID: 37846737

Vargas-Willis, G., & Cervantes, R. C. (1987). Consideration of Psychosocial Stress in the Treatment of the Latina Immigrant. *Hispanic Journal of Behavioral Sciences*, *9*(3), 315–329. DOI: 10.1177/07399863870093007

Vélez-Coto, M., Rute-Pérez, S., Pérez-García, M., & Caracuel, A. (2021). Unemployment and general cognitive ability: A review and meta-analysis. *Journal of Economic Psychology*, *87*, 102430. DOI: 10.1016/j.joep.2021.102430

Vukcevic, M., Momirovic, J., & Puric, D. (2016). Adaptation of Harvard Trauma Questionnaire for working with refugees and asylum seekers in Serbia. *Psihologija (Beograd)*, *49*(3), 277–299. DOI: 10.2298/PSI1603277V

Wang, S.-K., Feng, M., Fang, Y., Lv, L., Sun, G.-L., Yang, S.-L., Guo, P., Cheng, S.-F., Qian, M.-C., & Chen, H.-X. (2023). Psychological trauma, posttraumatic stress disorder and trauma-related depression: A mini-review. *World Journal of Psychiatry*, *13*(6), 331–339. DOI: 10.5498/wjp.v13.i6.331 PMID: 37383283

Wilson, F. E., Hennessy, E., Dooley, B., Kelly, B. D., & Ryan, D. A. (2013). Trauma and PTSD rates in an irish psychiatric population: A comparison of native and immigrant samples. *Disaster Health*, *1*(2), 74–83. DOI: 10.4161/dish.27366 PMID: 28228990

Wylie, L., Van Meyel, R., Harder, H., Sukhera, J., Luc, C., Ganjavi, H., Elfakhani, M., & Wardrop, N. (2018). Assessing trauma in a transcultural context: Challenges in mental health care with immigrants and refugees. *Public Health Reviews*, *39*(1), 22. DOI: 10.1186/s40985-018-0102-y PMID: 30151315

Yeomans, P. D., & Forman, E. M. (2009). Cultural factors in traumatic stress. In Eshun, S., & Gurung, R. A. R. (Eds.), *Culture and mental health: Sociocultural influences, theory, and practice* (pp. 221–244). Wiley Blackwell., DOI: 10.1002/9781444305807.ch11

Zangeneh, M., & Al-Krenawi, A. (Eds.). (2019). *Culture, Diversity and Mental Health—Enhancing Clinical Practice*. Springer International Publishing., DOI: 10.1007/978-3-030-26437-6

Zhou, A. Q., Lee, H. Y., & Lee, R. M. (2019). Who has low health literacy and does it matter for depression? Findings from aggregated and disaggregated racial/ ethnic groups. *Cultural Diversity & Ethnic Minority Psychology*, *25*(1), 73–81. DOI: 10.1037/cdp0000210 PMID: 30714769

Chapter 3
Language Barriers in the Mexican Immigrant Population

John Park
https://orcid.org/0009-0000-3289-4158
California Baptist University, USA

Jasmine Morando
https://orcid.org/0009-0007-3420-1467
California Baptist University, USA

Junior Joseph Anguiano
https://orcid.org/0009-0009-5980-0698
California Baptist University, USA

Ashley L. Alvarado
California Baptist University, USA

ABSTRACT

The Latino immigrant population in the US plays a major role in society. The US Census Bureau (2022) reports that a substantial number of Spanish speaking individuals report having limited English proficiency (LEP). Furthermore, LEP patients report language barriers as the greatest challenge to receiving healthcare service which may negatively impact their treatment and may lead to negative health outcomes. This chapter provides a brief overview of the Latino immigrant population, the challenges they experience, both societally and personally, as they navigate the immigration process in the US. Specifically, this chapter addresses the concerns and issues related to administering psychological evaluations for the LEP individuals. We expound upon the various challenges that may arise in the interaction between

DOI: 10.4018/979-8-3693-7944-8.ch003

the LEP client and the provider. Clinical implications and recommendations are suggested for the assessor for mitigating communication and cultural disparities for this population.

VIGNETTE

Paloma is trying to sleep but struggles to do so during the late hours of the night on the couch of her cousin's living room in California. It is the first week of December, and she feels pretty uneasy and uncomfortable, tossing and turning, searching for some relief. She finally calms herself down as much as possible and attempts to settle the constant anxiety that floods her mind. Worries and fears consume her as she wrestles with these questions. *"Will he find me here?" "Should I leave right now?" "I don't feel safe at all." "How long will I have enough money and food for my baby and me?" "Will they take the baby if I am found by the police?"* These thoughts are uncontrollable and endless. She hardly manages to sleep before her cousin wakes her up at 4:00 AM to get ready for work cleaning motel rooms.

Paloma is 7 months pregnant with her second child and has been in the United States for 6 months. After being physically and sexually assaulted by her boyfriend and his gang in Michoacán, Mexico, Paloma's mother arranged for her to cross the border into the United States. It was during her time in the Sonoran Desert that she believed she was pregnant. While hiding under piles of rocks to evade border patrol helicopter search efforts, she felt the excruciating pain of her abdominal wall ripping and blood coming out between her legs. She kept her pain a secret from the "coyotes" her parents paid to take her to Arizona.

Although she gets paid under the table by the motel manager and her cousin promised that she could live in the one-bedroom apartment with her once the baby is born, for the past 2 months, Paloma has felt hopeless and in utter despair nearly every day. She can hardly keep any weight on for herself, let alone for the baby's health. On the rare occasion that there isn't overtime available at the motel, she can't even concentrate for long enough to progress in learning English or thinking about how to survive in the United States. She has started to wonder more often whether the second story of the motel is high enough to jump from to end the torment for her and her child. Paloma's greatest fear is that if she gives birth to the baby, the doctors will deport her and separate her from her child. She fears that her child will be left screaming for help and being faced with the real possibility of never being able to see her child again.

INTRODUCTION

In the fictional story depicted above, Paloma is an example of one of many individuals who may experience real-life challenges and difficulties with immigration. Immigration has been pivotal in the U.S.'s history and development (Bolter, 2022; Gutiérrez, 2019). With people immigrating from all countries, the United States has been and is still known as the "melting pot" of the world. Nearly 14% of the United States population was born in another country, numbering more than 44 million people in 2017, according to a Pew Research Center analysis of the U.S. Census Bureau's American Community Survey (Connor & Budiman, 2019). That percentage was slightly higher than in the previous five years (Passel & Krogstad, 2024).

It is well known that the U.S. has long had more immigrants than any other country. In fact, the U.S. is home to one-fifth of the world's international migrants (Gutiérrez, 2019; Mosilmani & Passel, 2024; United Nations, 2020). These immigrants come from almost every country worldwide (Mosilmani & Passel, 2024; United Nations, 2020). It is by far the largest destination country for international migrants, with 51 million migrants in 2020, equal to 18% of the world's total migration population (United Nations, 2020). In 2022, Mexico was the top country of birth for immigrants who arrived last year, with about 150,000 people (Batalova, 2024; Mosilmani & Passel, 2024). Mexico is also the largest country of origin for U.S. immigrants (Batalova, 2025; Batalova, 2024; Mosilmani & Passel, 2024). Mexico is also the top country of birth for U.S. immigrants; in 2022, roughly 10.6 million immigrants living in the U.S. were born there, making up 23% of all U.S. immigrants (Mosilmani & Passel, 2024). The following largest origin groups were those from India (6%), China (5%), the Philippines (4%), and El Salvador (3%) (Mosilmani & Passel, 2024). However, immigration from Mexico has slowed since 2007, and the Mexican-born population in the U.S. has dropped from 29% in 2010 to 23% in 2022 (Gonzalez-Barrera, 2021; Mosilmani & Passel, 2024). The Hispanic population in the U.S. reached 62.1 million in 2020, accounting for 19% of all Americans (Funk & Lopez, 2022) and making it the nation's second-largest racial or ethnic group, behind white Americans and ahead of Black Americans, according to the U.S. Census Bureau (2024).

In terms of geographic location, over half of Mexican immigrants in the United States resided in California (36 percent) or Texas (22 percent) during 2018-2022 (Batalova, 2024; Israel & Batalova, 2020). In other regions of the U.S., Mexican immigrants resided in Illinois (slightly less than 6%) or Arizona (slightly less than 5%). Six states, Florida, Washington, Georgia, Nevada, North Carolina, and New York, comprised 13%. The top counties of residence for Mexican immigrants were Los Angeles County, California, Harris County, Texas, and Cook County, Illinois (Batalova, 2024; Krogstad et al., 2023). This data shows how a substantial Mexican immigrant population appears to reside in cities or states that may be considered more urban than rural (Batalova, 2024; Krogstad et al., 2023). Data also shows that about 78% of Hispanic immigrants have lived in the U.S. for over 10 years, an increase from 64% in 2010. Panamanian (87%) and Mexican (86%) immigrants are the most likely to have lived in the U.S. for more than 10 years (Batalova, 2024; Krogstad et al., 2023; Moslimani et al., 2023).

Vignette

Eduardo, a 19 year old Mexican male, is working with his parents on their farm. He has lived in Mexico for his whole life, and loves his country and family. He is one of five children, and his parents have owned a small farm since he was born. However, recently in his town, there have been serious problems where there have been many instances of gang violence and crime. People in the community have gone missing or they have been murdered. Even though crime has been rampant, the police or law enforcement have not done much to address these issues. Eduardo, as well as his whole family, are concerned and have been walking on egg shells. Moreover, his parents are older, and he often thinks about what their future may look like as they are barely able to keep food on the table. Eduardo is also concerned and is thinking about his own future as well. Recently, a friend has been telling him about a "life changing" opportunity to join a local gang. All he would have to do is collect "fees" from different people, and make sure things are orderly in his designated area. He has heard about these gangs, and his parents are fearful since the gang is suspected of killing their uncle in the recent past. His parents, fearing the safety of his son, urges him to go to America where he can work and send money back home to his family. Eduardo does not want to leave his parents behind due to his fears for his parents' safety as well as his siblings. Either way, whether he decides to join the gang or leave to the US, it feels like a no win situation. He feels that he is not safe here at home or in America where immigrants are vilified and hated. Much less, the journey and the cost to go to America would require so much money, an amount that his family does not have. Eduardo drinks himself to sleep as he grapples with these choices.

Reasons for Immigration

The story above is a fictional depiction of an example of various life circumstances that some individuals may experience in their native country. It is commonly understood that there are significant factors and motivations for an individual to migrate to another country (Gutiérrez, 2019; National Immigration Forum, 2019). These reasons may include but are not limited to improved environmental conditions, improved financial needs, getting out of poverty, enhancing family or social relationships, and increased professional, academic, or life opportunities (Batalova, 2024; Gutiérrez, 2019; Schumacher et al., 2024). Nonetheless, a study by Schumacher and colleagues (2024) found that despite being employed, two-thirds of Hispanic immigrants (67%) have annual household incomes under $40,000, leading to significant challenges in meeting basic needs.

More specifically, immigrating to the US may be due to a more immediate and imminent threat or concern. A study by Batalova (2024) reported that Mexican immigration experienced a recent uptick due to the impacts of COVID-19, including economic difficulties in Mexico. According to Illimen (2023), migrant laborers are immigrating into the U.S. due to "economic deprivation, governmental failure in supervising decent living standards (i.e., healthcare, education, housing, wages, and investments) and smuggling (i.e., human and drug trafficking)". Additionally, Illimen asserts a historical association between the United States and entrepreneurship, prosperity, materialism, and consumerism, which drives Mexican immigration (2023, p. 260). Thus, studies document that Mexicans may resort to immigrating to the US, not for the choice of a better or improved lifestyle, but more likely for survival and/or to escape out of poverty.

Challenges Experienced in the United States

A common perception or misperception is that the U.S. provides abundant resources and opportunities to individuals who migrate from another country. With the view of such unlimited resources and opportunities, it may be assumed that success is bound to occur for the immigrant. While there may be some truth to this notion, immigrants do encounter difficulties and challenges, like all people, that may pose a serious concern to their well-being and safety. Such challenges may include, financial instability, housing insecurity, exposure to higher crime and violence rates, victimization, lack of social support, and medical or health issues (Schumacher et al., 2024).For the purposes of this chapter, we narrow our focus to the specific challenges that Mexican immigrants experience in the U.S. healthcare system due to language barriers. Moreover, we also look into the specific challenges that may occur in the legal setting when psychological evaluations are conducted with LEP individuals for various legal or immigration purposes.

LANGUAGE BARRIERS IN IMMIGRANT COMMUNITIES

Language is an essential modality of verbal communication for all individuals; living a fulfilling life, interacting, and socializing with others is necessary. Without language, verbal communication would be lacking, negatively impacting all aspects of life (Rao et a., 2024). In various groups and communities, people communicate with one another in their native language (Rao et al., 2024). This serves the purpose of building and maintaining connections within the social and cultural group, finding unity and commonality among the social circle that the individual is a part of, and providing an outlet for cultural expression and bond (Rao et al., 2024). What happens when a group of people cannot communicate in the common language of the country they reside in? We explore this question in this section.

Of course, not everyone in the U.S. can speak English fluently. In the U.S., about 26 million people have limited English proficiency (LEP), meaning their English speaking skills are limited and may pose a challenge when communicating with English-speaking individuals (Gonzalez-Barrera et al., 2024). The Department of Health and Human Services (DHSS) identifies individuals with LEP as those who do not speak English as their primary language and who have a limited ability to read, write, speak, or understand English (Haldar et al., 2023; Funk & Lopez, 2022). This may suggest that different individuals may have varying capacities to speak or understand the English language. However, the varying limitations may point to a gap in communication, which can lead to miscommunication or misunderstanding (Haldar et al., 2023; Funk & Lopez, 2022). This, as well as its consequences, will be further expounded in subsequent sections. To further elaborate, it has been reported that most LEP adults in the US fluently speak Spanish (62%), followed by Chinese (7%), Vietnamese (3%), Arabic (2%), and Tagalog (2%), with the remainder speaking a variety of different languages from regions across the world (Gonzalez-Barrera, 2024).

From these statistics, it can be safely asserted that Mexican immigrants are less likely to be proficient in English than the overall U.S. foreign-born population (Gonzalez-Barrera, 2024; Haldar et al., 2023; Funk & Lopez, 2022). In 2023, about 65 percent of Mexican immigrants ages five and over reported speaking English less than "very well," compared to 47 percent of all immigrants. Approximately 6 percent of Mexicans spoke only English at home, compared to 17 percent of the foreign-born population (Batalova, 2024). There are a variety of factors, whether cultural, psychosocial, or environmental, that contribute to this language and communication discordance. Schumacher and colleagues (2024) found that two-thirds of Hispanic immigrants who have LEP reported experiencing language-related challenges. Specifically, about eight in ten (nine in ten undocumented Hispanic immigrants) report confusion and uncertainty regarding healthcare programs that aid in financial support.

It is commonly believed that immigrants maintain a sense of their cultural identity and a sense of community by preserving or maintaining their native language (Bhugra & Becker, 2005). This may lead some people to continue to speak in their native tongue without actively learning the language of the country they reside in (Rao et al., 2024). For the Mexican population, it has been reported that Spanish use at home or in their families remains high (Funk & Lopez, 2022; Krogstad et al., 2023). About 94% of Hispanic immigrants spoke Spanish at home or their residence in 2019 (Funk & Lopez, 2022). Although it may not be the main factor, this may contribute to the decrease in the English language acquisition or limited English language skills of Mexican immigrants in the U.S. With a strong Latino representation in the U.S. and the prominent role they play in U.S. society, the language barrier that exists, to a certain degree, can also be viewed as a societal dilemma for the U.S. population as a whole due to the challenges and consequences it poses for the U.S. society as a whole.

Consequences of Language Barriers

Language barriers are not only a communication issue or problem but also contribute to severe physical and mental health concerns. It is well-accepted that the Mexican immigrant community continues to grow each year in the U.S., which places a spotlight on this topic (Batalova, 2024). Currently, Spanish is the second most spoken language in the U.S., which speaks to the significant role that the Latino population plays in U.S. society (Dietrich & Hernandez, 2022; Gonzalez-Barrera & Lopez, 2013; Shin & Kominski, 2010). Across the various aspects of life, it has been shown that language barriers or limited English proficiency may pose a challenge to the individual across various settings, leading to lower quality of life, negative consequences due to miscommunication, and poor health outcomes when compared to those who do not have language barriers (Schumacher et al., 2024). According to the Pew Research Center, 44% of the participants in a 2021 survey said that language barriers are a primary contributor to Hispanic Americans having worse health outcomes than other adults in the U.S. (Funk & Lopez, 2022). This is due to the fact that language barriers contribute to miscommunication of medical information, misdiagnosis, poorer treatment adherence, and ultimately mistreatment (Schumacher et al., 2024; United States Census Bureau, 2020).

Due to these various challenges, the Latino community may experience higher levels of health disparities and problems, which can impact their overall quality of life. Moreover, specifically for the Latino community, it has been stated that "stigma, low health literacy, lack of knowledge, and misconceptions about depression are considered pervasive barriers contributing to the disparities Latino adults with limited English proficiency (LEP) face in accessing and receiving high-quality depression care" (Cabassa et al., 2010, p. 747).

It is essential to note that the language barrier that exists in the Latino population is broad and pervasive in Latino communities in the U.S. About half of adults with LEP say they encountered at least one language barrier in a healthcare setting in the last three years that contributed to miscommunication or the inaccurate communication of health information (Al Shamsi et al., 2020). This includes about a third of LEP adults who say there was a time in the past three years when difficulty speaking or reading English posed a significant challenge as it made it hard for them to fill out necessary medical forms for a health care provider (34%) or communicate with medical office staff (33%), three in ten who reported difficulty understanding a health care provider's instruction (30%), and about 25% who reported experiencing challenges with communication which made it difficult to fill a prescription or understand how to schedule a medical appointment (25%)(Rao et al., 2024). These statistics represent the overarching difficulties and challenges that exist for the Mexican immigrant population regarding navigating the U.S. healthcare system.

Not only do Mexican immigrants have to deal with the realities of adjusting to a new country, but they are at higher risk of experiencing negative consequences to their health. According to Valdes (2020), children of immigrant families are challenged by perceived English language limitations, directly limiting future educational opportunities. According to Ortega et al. (2015), undocumented and recent immigrants have challenges accessing and utilizing health care due to U.S. policy. Moreover, it is also important to note that the U.S. healthcare system experiences significant issues, as this population accounts for a substantial financial responsibility on the healthcare system due to various problems related to the lack of insurance or other financial issues (Lopes et al., 2024).

Access to Medical Care

A common and very concerning challenge is access to medical care for the Mexican immigrant community (Martinez-Donate et al., 2017). This becomes even more of an obstacle due to the language barriers that may exist with these individuals. It is also documented that the Latino LEP patients themselves report language barriers as the greatest challenge to receiving medical or mental health services, which compromises the quality of healthcare treatment and leads to the contribution to poorer health outcomes (Carrasquillo et al., 1999; Twersky et al., 2024).

Over the past decade, many studies have examined the healthcare interactions between LEP Hispanic patients and the non-LEP medical physicians who treat them (Gonzalez-Barrera, et al., 2024; Escobedo et al., 2023; Oh et al., 2020; Twersky et al., 2024). These studies reveal patterns and outcomes that allude to healthcare disparities. Moreover, Funk and Lopez (2022) document that LEP patients report their views that doctors do not provide the best treatment, appropriate medications, or valuable resources due to doctors' negative assumptions or lack of cultural competency about the Mexican community. This has been shown to lead to mistreatment, misdiagnoses, and, ultimately, poorer health outcomes for this community. Thus, researchers emphasize how LEP patients are at higher risk of receiving compromised care, especially in the medical and mental health settings, which may be another reason for the reluctance of these individuals to reach out for medical or professional help (Twersky et al., 2024).

The U.S. government has provisions for various institutions, including the healthcare setting, to provide translation and interpretation services to LEP individuals. While this has been a vital milestone in the U.S., it has fallen short in terms of its primary goal of increasing or improving communication between LEP patients and their healthcare providers. Despite available resources, such as interpreter aids and other translation services, research points to continual difficulties in the healthcare system to address the language discordance among the LEP patients and the Healthcare Provider (HP), which contributes to miscommunication of the diagnosis and treatment, lack of treatment adherence, patient attrition, and ultimately adverse health outcomes (Batalova, 2024; Funk & Lopez, 2022; Krogstad et al., 2023). This also illustrates that LEP individuals do not feel comfortable with a third party providing communication and prefer to have a family or friend provide such communication (Pandey et al., 2021).

Regarding mental health access, the Substance Abuse and Mental Health Services Administration (2018) reports that 56.8% of young Latino adults in the age range of 18 to 25 years did not receive treatment despite serious mental health issues, such as excessive anxiety, depression, and bipolar disorder. Many factors contribute to the lack of mental health (MH) treatment received, including the following: language barriers, poverty, negative stigma, lack of cultural competence, and legal status. These are a few of the documented factors related to why Latinos may not seek MH treatment (National Alliance on Mental Illness, 2018). However, studies have consistently shown that the language barrier serves as the main factor for LEP individuals not accessing mental health care (Al Shamsi et al., 2020; Pandey et a;., 2021; Twersky et al., 2024).

It cannot be ignored that unstable residency or immigration status also may contribute to the lack of healthcare access for LEP individuals. It has been reported that the "fear of deportation likely contributed to conflict between the LEP patient and physician (Schumacher et al., 2024). Deportation is a constant reality for undocumented immigrants as it "often precludes access to health care and may lead to negative perceptions of the health care environment" (Smith et al., 2009, p. 1049). The amount of personal information required when applying for services also becomes a barrier due to an individual lacking a social security number or legal immigration status. Thus, there is uncertainty about what type of personal information is needed and if it will expose a person's immigration status while attempting to apply for health insurance or healthcare services (Schumacher et al., 2024; Stutz et al., 2020).

The fear of deportation due to their undocumented status discourages some Latinos from applying for any type of services and resources available, such as medical care (Halder et al., 2023; Pillai & Artiga, 2023; Schumacher et al., 2024; Doshi, 2020). Furthermore, there is a lack of awareness of the resources available to these individuals, regardless of their legal status, which only compounds such challenges (Halder et al., 2023; Schumacher et al., 2024). For example, most immigrants, whether undocumented or documented, in the United States may be eligible for the Affordable Care Act, which provides health coverage without a waiting period and without a social security number, and other government benefits (Halder et al., 2023; KFF, 2025Ortega et al., 2015). People may be unaware of certain benefits or be overburdened with fear, which contributes to the barriers to healthcare services (Haldar et al., 2023; Pillai & Artiga, 2023; KFF, 2025).

Sociocultural Factors Contributing to Barriers

Culture plays a major role in perpetuating a belief that these barriers are a necessity for survival in the U.S., especially for LEP individuals (Pillai & Artiga, 2023). On top of that, there is also a cultural aspect playing a role for Latino individuals and their hesitancy with receiving mental health (MH) care, as any mental health concern or problem may be associated with weakness in a person (Caballero et al., 2017; Forcén et al., 2023; Grieb et al., 2023). Negative stigma shared by family and peers discourages people from seeking MH services (Eno Louden et al., 2023). Latinos face social criticism from family and peers due to MH challenges, as family members and loved ones may view people who receive mental health services as those who do not receive family or social support (Eno Louden et al., 2023). The implication may be that these individuals need more family connection or support, rather than mental health services (Caballero et al., 2017; Eno Louden et al., 2023; Forcén et al., 2023; Grieb et al., 2023)..

Depending on a person's culture, MH services are frowned upon for a variety of reasons (Caballero et al., 2017; DeFeitas et al., 2018; Eno Louden et al., 2023; Luque et al., 2018). People who seek mental health services do not want to be seen as “weak” or “insane,” which may often be the case in a more traditional Latino cultural orientation. DeFreitas et al. (2018) describe common stigma beliefs as being blamed for one's mental illness, being seen as never recovering from it, and being seen as dangerous to self and others. The stigma behind MH services affects both how people are seen and how they feel (Caballero et al., 2017; DeFeitas et al., 2018;

Eno Louden et al., 2023; Luque et al., 2018). For example, society may see that people who attend therapy and see a psychiatrist are "mentally unfit" (Eno Louden et al., 2023). The fear of criticism by family and peers can create alienation between people and shame (Caballero et al., 2017; DeFeitas et al., 2018; Eno Louden et al., 2023; Luque et al., 2018).

Generally speaking, Latino individuals adhere to a collectivistic and hierarchical value system that influences how individuals may interact and communicate with others (Krys et al., 2022). For example, children may feel family or parental obligations to support the needs of their families (Caballero et a;., 2017). There is a common saying, 'Mi casa es sucasa,' which speaks to the collective and interdependent nature of the Latino family (Krys et al., 2022). Moreover, it is commonly accepted that the Latino individuals adhere to attitudinal familism, which highlights the commitment of an individual to their family and family relationships (Cohen, 2013; Valdivieso-Mora et al., 2016). This approach emphasizes the important role of family cohesion, bonds, obligations, and responsibility (Cohen, 2013; Valdivieso-Mora et al., 2016).

We also find that Latino individuals reflect their cultural dynamics in communication with people outside of their family system (Cohen, 2013; Valdivieso-Mora et al., 2016; Santisteban et al., 2012). Some other examples of cultural dynamics in communication may be the following: being submissive to authority figures, demonstrating agreeableness despite contrary views and opinions, and restraining from expressing one's perspective (Elder et al., 2009; Forcen et al., 2023; Magana, 2020). This has been shown to carry over and impact how the Latino individual may interact and communicate with various professionals in the U.S., as it may lead to increased submissive behaviors, communicating agreeableness despite contrary perspectives, and experiencing less autonomy in decision making (Castro et al., 2023; Davis et al., 2011; Elder et al., 2009; Forcen et al., 2023; Magaña, 2020). Supporting this, studies document a strong level of acquiescence and social desirability in response characteristics of patients from a Latino background (Davis et al., 2018). For example, an LEP client may agree to a medical procedure without fully understanding the risks and benefits of treatment due to the fears, pressures, and stressors associated with communicating with English speaking professionals (Castro et al., 2023; Davis et al., 2011; Davis et al., 2018; Elder et al., 2009; Forcen et al., 2023; Magaña, 2020)..

It has been documented that LEP individuals experience higher levels of migration trauma (Twersky et al., 2024), acculturative stress (Baeza-Rivera et al., 2022), and discrimination (Rao et al., 2024), which contribute to increased mental health problems, such as depressionanxiety, panic attacks, attention deficit/hyperactivity disorder, conduct disorder, and posttraumatic stress disorder (PTSD) in adults and children (Caballero et al., 2017; Cabassa et al., 2012; Rogers, 2025; Sentell et al.,

2007; Twersky et al., 2025). In addition, the current political climate in the U.S. increases the stigma and negative perceptions of the Latino immigrant communities as they may be viewed as 'undeserving' of health care and government services and some think they should be deported (Caballero et al., 2017; DeFeitas et al., 2018; Eno Louden et al., 2023; Luque et al., 2018). It has also been noted that negative stereotypes exist about Latino individuals that may impact the quality of healthcare that they receive (Funk & Lopez, 2022; Lightfoot et al., 2019; Rivera, 2023). Such examples may include the sexual promiscuous behaviors of Latino men, the assumption of the hypersexuality of Latino females, and other xenophobic prejudices related to race or language, housing or employment discrimination, and/or anti-immigrant policies at state and federal levels (Funk & Lopez, 2022; Lightfoot et al., 2019; Rivera, 2023).

The negative impact of these sociocultural dynamics and inaccuracies in communication has persisted in various institutions in the U.S. that continue to contribute to negative health outcomes in the U.S. healthcare system (Al Shamsi et al., 2020; Batalova, 2024; Funk & Lopez, 2022; Krogstad et al., 2023). It has also been documented that LEP or language discordant patients reported levels of mistrust and perceived discrimination, which also contribute to lower quality of care (Magana, 2020) With these various challenges and problems at many levels, including the family, culture, society, and the government, we can see how and why LEP individuals may experience challenges with the U.S. healthcare system and other resources that may be beneficial to them. It can be assumed that this continues to pose a major obstacle to the LEP population in the U.S.

Language Barriers in Psychological Evaluations for Immigration Cases

Psychological evaluations play an important role in many aspects of the healthcare setting, the legal system, and other institutions: to ensure proper treatment and diagnosis, to promote safety and well-being of the individual and the members of society, and for other important decisions pertaining to legal, criminal, and other facets of life (Miller, 2013; Neal et al., 2020; Wahass, 2005). Specifically, for immigration cases, such evaluations are conducted to assess for competency, for safety and risk to self, others, and society, and for other measures to ensure the individual is "fit" to reside in the U.S (Mercado et al., 2022; NeMoyer et al. 2019).

When a psychological evaluation is conducted, a licensed forensic or clinical psychologist with the appropriate training and experience is required (Aldalur et al., 2022; Mercado et al., 2022; NeMoyer et al. 2019). These evaluations consist of a thorough and comprehensive assessment and evaluation process where historical data and present information are gathered on the individual, his or her family, and personal background (Aldalur et al., 2022; Mercado et al., 2022; NeMoyer et al. 2019). Information may consist of, and is not limited to, the following: medical history, family background, psychiatric history, social and interpersonal functioning, education and employment background, developmental history, clinical psychodiagnostic assessment, and past and current psychological functioning (Aldalur et al., 2022; Mercado et al., 2022; NeMoyer et al. 2019). Standardized assessment tools may be utilized to assess for specific pathological concerns, characterological issues, and to clarify if there is a psychiatric disturbance (Aldalur et al., 2022; Mercado et al., 2022; NeMoyer et al. 2019). Such evaluations may evaluate various facets of one's mental health, including anxiety and mood disorders, personality disorders, severe mental illness, substance use disorders, and other psychiatric conditions (Aldalur et al., 2022; Mercado et al., 2022; NeMoyer et al. 2019).

These evaluations also assess to see if such conditions, if they do exist or relate to the individual, pose a serious concern for the individual's welfare and functioning in society (Aldalur et al., 2022; Mercado et al., 2022; NeMoyer et al. 2019). Questions that may need clarification might be the following. Can this individual function in society without being a harm to others in society? Does the individual have the capacity and the insight to engage in behaviors and activities that are acceptable and do not pose a legal or criminal concern? Will members of society be at risk due to this individual being present in society? Are there any limitations or concerns that would warrant specific support or professional help for this individual to function in society? Thus, it is not so much the mental health condition that may disqualify an individual from functioning in society; the question for the evaluator is to see if such condition may pose a significant impairment and concern for his or her functioning, which poses a major concern or danger to society and its members.

The American Psychological Association (2015) estimates that there are approximately 106,000 licensed psychologists in the U.S. Out of these licensed psychologists, only 5.5% are able to provide psychological services in Spanish (Delgado et al., 2018; Smith, 2018). Moreover, out of the 5.5% licensed psychologists, there are even fewer who may be trained to provide psychological evaluations for the Mexican LEP immigrant community (Delgado et al., 2018; Smith, 2018). Thus, language barriers become even more critical and detrimental when they pertain to a specialized service like a psychological evaluation (Al Shamsi et al., 2020). Due to the important nature of such evaluations, making sure that communication between the LEP individual and the evaluator is clear is critical in such settings. If this is compromised in any sense, it may significantly impact the evaluation and assessment of the LEP individual (Al Shamsi et al., 2020; Delgado et al., 2018; Smith, 2018).

During this evaluation process, especially for the LEP patient population, it is essential for the evaluator and the client to effectively communicate to ensure mutual reciprocal understanding due to the nature of the interaction (Gadon et al.,

2007; Pillai & Artiga, 2023). From the patient perspective, we acknowledge the emotional and stressful experience of being seen in the medical or clinical setting due to the potentially life-altering clinical interaction that will be communicated by the healthcare providers. Any individual who is in the clinical setting could experience strong emotions and feelings, but for LEP individuals, these feelings, emotions, and fears may be heightened due to the challenges of communication and being in a setting that they are not comfortable in. (Al Shamsi et al., 2020; Twersky et al., 2024). Thus, strong negative and anxious emotions may be felt during these encounters, such as fear, anxiety, claustrophobia, and dehumanization, leading to a difficult personal experience. It has been shown that effective communication can help to mitigate and provide support for the patient's difficult experience by improving their understanding of the health or clinical information that is communicated (Wynia et al., 2010).

Additionally, miscommunication of information may lead to inaccurate transmission of personal data (Haldar et al., 2023; Funk & Lopez, 2022; Schumacher et al., 2024). For example, a relatively common pattern may occur, where Latinos do not understand the questions that they are asked, but may signal to the evaluator that they do understand for the purpose of appearing cooperative and not defying the authority figure (Magaña, 2020; Ramirez et al., 2017; Smith et al, 2009; Walters et al., 2021). Misinformation or the lack of proper communication has the possibility of leading to an inaccurate assessment or evaluation, which can spurn negative consequences for the individual being evaluated (Magaña, 2020; Ramirez et al., 2017; Smith et al, 2009; Walters et al., 2021). These consequences may entail an inaccurate diagnosis of the individual, a pathological understanding of the client, which may warrant legal action, or clinical recommendations that would suggest a false narrative of the individual, which can lead to life-altering circumstances for the individual and their families.

The experience of immigration, assimilation, and acculturation is pervasive in the journey of Latino immigrant families (Abraído-Lanza, 2016; Davis et al., 2011). Professionals must consider and recognize the importance of providing an environment where language concordance, cultural sensitivity, and respect are highlighted to reduce stigma and prejudice related to any concerns (Ahad et al., 2023; Caballero et al., 2017). Furthermore, it is encouraged that during these clinical interactions, the clinician or evaluator recognize that the LEP Latino individual may be at greater risk of experiencing trauma and may present with PTSD symptomology or other mental health concerns due to a variety of life situations and circumstances Caballero et al., 2017; Cabassa et al., 2012; Rogers, 2025; Sentell et al., 2007; Twersky et al., 2025). It is emphasized that evaluators raise their awareness and increase their cultural competency to address such difficulties (Rivera, 2023). Bridging the language barrier gaps can significantly improve the communication process between the provider and the LEP individual (Squires, 2018). By improving or mitigating the language discordance, the consequences of miscommunication or the lack of communication can be addressed in a positive manner (Squires, 2018). In this section, we discuss the different approaches and considerations that may serve to bridge this gap.

Provision of Resources

First, we recommend that the provider uses resources and assessment tools that can help facilitate effective communication with the LEP individual. This may consist of standardized assessment tools, questionnaires, or inventories that are in Spanish and English. We recommend that the provider make accessible various patient resources that may help facilitate understanding of the various medical conditions, terminology, and treatments that are relevant. Such resources may come in the form of institutional or educational websites with accurate translation, pamphlets, brochures, and possibly using various online modalities (i.e., online and multi-media modules, or websites) that may be conducive and user-friendly to the LEP patients (Koff et al., 1999; Hansbury et al., 2022).

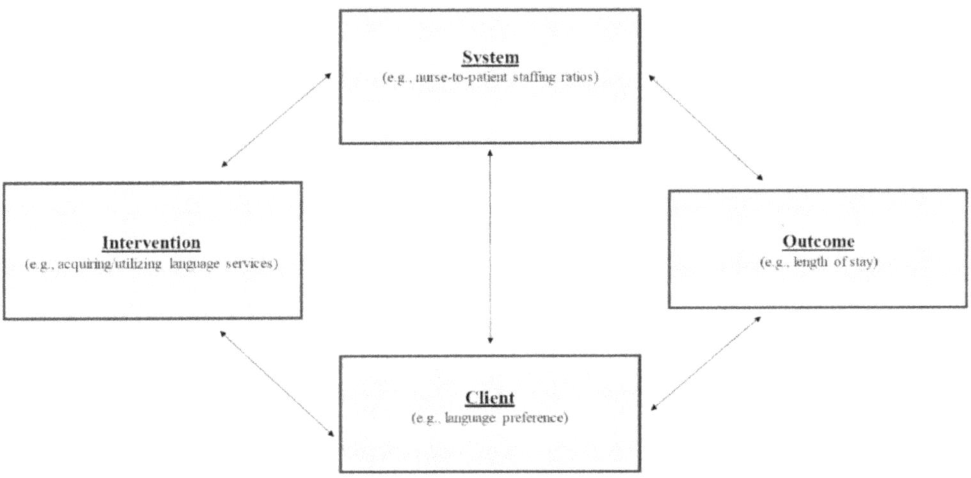

It is recommended that these resources specifically address the various levels of health literacy as they are pertinent to the evaluation process and the unique cultural needs of Spanish speaking patients (Christy et al., 2021; Soto Mas et al., 2018; Stonbraker et al., 2015). We believe that this approach has the potential to inform and educate patients, promoting greater independence and autonomy of the LEP patients which will ultimately lead to a more accurate evaluation of the LEP individual (Twersky et al., 2024). The effort invested in the development and provision of such resources has been shown to lead to improved patient communication, improved relationships, and overall increased satisfaction of the LEP patients (Sliwinski et al., 2024). Moreover, we also note that the LEP population may have challenges and barriers with locating basic health information from their country of origin, navigating the U.S. healthcare system, and understanding basic communication from other professionals (Cabassa et al., 2010).

Sliwinski and colleagues (2024) note the importance of a Quality Health Outcomes Model (QHOM) that demonstrate the relationship between four elements: system, intervention, outcomes, and client (as shown in Figure 1). The authors suggest that though research has explored the relationship between intervention (e.g., interpreter services and LEP materials) and outcomes (e.g., disparities between LEP and English proficient patients), there is limited research on the impact of systems (e.g., nurse to patient ratio) has on interventions and outcomes. The study found that factors such as using professional interpreters, bilingual staff, and system-level factors such as work environments, and staffing may be critical to facilitating effective care to LEP patients. Though healthcare systems can make efforts to accommodate LEP patients, system-level factors are an area of great importance when considering provision of resources. We encourage the provision of resources that may address some of these concerns.

A Comprehensive Language Training Course

It has been documented that language concordant services are most effectively addressed when the provider speaks the same language as the patient (Dunlap et al., 2015; Lopez-Vera et al., 2023). We encourage, when possible, that these psychological evaluations be conducted by a fluent Spanish speaking professional rather than a non-fluent Spanish speaking professional (Aldalur et al., 2022 Weber et al., 2022). Fluency in the language can be important in allowing for more nuanced and aligned communication between the LEP individual and the evaluator (Aldalur et al., 2022). A bilingual provider and/or a ‘‘culturally concordant’’ provider might be more advantageous for the native Spanish speakers in asking more thorough questions or having a more in-depth conversation about treatment options (Wallace et al., 2009). When questioning and assessing, there may be subtle cultural or linguistic discrepancies, and a non-fluent translator or interpreter may not be able to communicate as concisely as a fluent Spanish-speaking professional (Bauer & Alegria, 2010, Wand et al., 2020). In the current healthcare system, the disparities in the number of fluent Spanish-speaking professionals constitute a significant challenge that has not been sufficiently addressed and will persist (Escobedo et al., 2023; Quiroz et al., 2024). Due to this, it may not always be possible to have language fluency alignment between LEP individuals and their evaluators (Escobedo et al., 2023; Quiroz et al., 2024; Wilson et al., 2005). We encourage the various institutions and organizations involved to accommodate such situations.

We also encourage the provision and the incentivization of the medical staff and team to engage in a comprehensive language training course that provides specific feedback and training in effective communication in the Spanish language. A pilot study (Han et al., 2009) in emergency departments has documented the positive impact of a 6-month language training program for healthcare providers. The study revealed a significant decrease in major medical errors, misunderstanding of symptoms, and vocabulary use, and an improvement in the "quality of bidirectional, interactive communication" between clinicians and LEP patients (Han et al., 2009). Moreover, Nguyen and colleagues (2024) incorporated interpreter and limited-English proficiency (LEP) patient training into the medical and physician assistant student curriculum to improve equitable care provisions and healthcare disparities. They found that both the medical students and interpreter, felt that they benefited from pre-interview recommendations and post-session feedback when working with LEP patients (Nguyen et al., 2024). The medical students reported feeling more confident working with medical interpreters and LEP patients after the clinical sessions (Nguyen et al., 2024). Integrating interpreter and language training courses as noted in the studies above, can aid providers in strengthening communication skills and confidence when treating linguistically diverse populations.

There may be restrictions on and limitations of resources and time in various healthcare and clinical settings, which may impact such recommendations. However, we emphasize the importance and relevance of incorporating such programs and training to build a culturally competent team that can address the needs of a diverse patient population. It has been shown that language-concordant care is more efficient and contributes to reduced healthcare expenditures and adverse outcomes (Eamranond et al., 2011; Freimuth & Quinn, 2004; Lopez-Vera et al., 2023) Taking such measures can effectively improve the evaluation process of the LEP individual and evaluator, which not only benefits the LEP individuals but also has a long-reaching positive impact on the U.S. society (Twersky et al., 2024).

Use of Bilingual Interpreters

During the evaluation process, we encourage using professional, fluent, bilingual interpreters to assist with communication between the LEP individual and the evaluator if necessary. Research shows that using professional interpreters, as opposed to ad hoc interpreters, improves communication and clinical outcomes (Heath et al., 2023; Karliner et al., 2007; Lee et al., 2017). During such clinical or professional interactions, the incongruency of verbal communication between the client and the evaluator has been shown to lead to inaccurate information communication, as mentioned earlier (Heath et al., 2023; Karliner et al., 2007; Lee et al., 2017). This concern can be a significant problem as such evaluations require precise and accurate reporting of data, which serves as the basis for the assessment of the client. Health and colleagues (2023) conducted a literature search exploring the utilization of interpreters to facilitate communication between health care providers and non-native speaking patients. They found that in-person professional interpreter resulting in highest satisfaction and communication of non-native speaking patients (Heath et al., 2023). This, in turn, reaffirms that any interpreter is better than none and relational interpreters can be a valuable interpreter resource for patients (Heath et al., 2023).

In many instances, LEP patients are accompanied by family members or utilize a translation service that aids in communicating LEP individuals with medical physicians, lawyers, or other professionals (Wilson, 2005). As an alternative to a professional interpreter, children or relatives often act as so-called 'language brokers' in healthcare. Nielsen et al. (2020) note that patients feel comfortable using relatives as interpreters because patients feel they know and can trust family members as opposed to professional interpreters. Family members or friends may be a trusted source (Nielsen et al., 2020), however, they may also make their subjective interpretation of information, which can affect the communication between the LEP individual and the evaluator (Nielsen et al., 2020). Studies have confirmed that "ad hoc" interpreters, such as family members or friends, may alter the communicated information in accordance with their own subjective beliefs, which may lead to a modification in the LEP individual's response (Smith et al., 2009). This has been shown to have severe limitations and concerns due to the complexity of the clinical or psychological terminology and various procedures involved in the evaluation process.

Studies have also shown that healthcare providers who learn Spanish at a basic conversational level and attempt to practice medical Spanish terminology negatively impact their LEP patients due to the linguistic differences and the inability to encourage a bidirectional communicative relationship, which contributes to adverse health outcomes, lack of treatment adherence, and overall dissatisfaction with their medical care (Al Shamsi et al., 2020; Fatahi et al., 2010; Nguyen et al., 2024). Many of these studies are conducted in clinical or medical settings; however, we believe such interactions are parallel or consistent with LEP individuals' experiences in the varied professional settings they may encounter. We see the importance of language fluency in such interactions when communicating vital information, asking and answering important personal questions about personal or family history, or evaluating for specific psychological problems pertinent to the LEP individual. A rudimentary or basic level of language comprehension may not be sufficient or appropriate for interactions that warrant a more in-depth and complex line of questioning about an individual's life experiences.

It is safe to assume that effective communication in the individual's dominant language increases patient satisfaction (AL Shamsi et al., 2024; Magana, 2020). Due to the importance of precise and accurate interpretation in a specialized setting, we encourage using professional bilingual translation services during medical interactions. Moreover, Title VI of the 1964 Civil Rights Act states the basis for a legal right to an interpreter, a principle reinforced by the courts and President Clinton's Executive Order #13166. Unfortunately, many patients with limited English proficiency are unaware of their legal right to a trained medical interpreter (Grubbs et al., 2006). Therefore, Latino patients should be informed about their legal right to an interpreter at no cost and be offered one if desired. Healthcare professionals do not need to obtain informed consent before disclosing protected health information to interpreters (Smith et al., 2009).

Psychological evaluations play an important role in a variety of purposes and settings. They are a unique service intended to provide psychological insights, perspectives, and recommendations, which can be used in legal, clinical, and educational settings with significant ramifications (Magaña, 2020; Ramirez et al., 2017; Smith et al, 2009; Walters et al., 2021). Due to the critical nature of such evaluations, we strongly recommend that LEP individuals, the evaluators, and all people involved thoughtfully consider the most appropriate and beneficial approach to conducting and implementing such evaluations, enabling them to provide the most accurate information possible for all parties involved.

CONCLUSION

Immigrant communities in the U.S. have long been stigmatized and marginalized for a variety of reasons. However, it is recognized that immigrants have played a significant role in the U.S. (Batalova, 2024; Krogstad et al., 2023; Rao et al., 2024) Specific to Mexican immigrant communities, there exists a long history of how they have shaped many facets of U.S. society (Aldalur et al., 2022; Mercado et al., 2022; NeMoyer et al. 2019; Twersky et al., 2024). The main concern raised in this chapter is the language barriers that Mexican immigrants face in the U.S. These barriers are a major psychosocial and cultural issue that significantly impacts Mexican immigrants (Caballero et al., 2017; Forcén et al., 2023; Grieb et al., 2023; Rao et al., 2024).

In specialized settings, such as the administration of psychological evaluations, we can see how various difficulties may affect the LEP individual and the evaluator. These evaluations are a comprehensive and detailed process that requires extensive information gathering, psychological assessment, and other clinical considerations where a language barrier between the LEP individual and the evaluator may negatively impact the accuracy and legitimacy of the evaluation. In this chapter, we provide information and recommendations that may help guide professionals to conduct such evaluations with this population group.

REFERENCES

Abraído-Lanza, A. F., Echeverría, S. E., & Flórez, K. R. (2016). Latino Immigrants, Acculturation, and Health: Promising New Directions in Research. *Annual Review of Public Health*, *37*(1), 219–236. DOI: 10.1146/annurev-publhealth-032315-021545 PMID: 26735431

Ahad, A. A., Sanchez-Gonzalez, M., & Junquera, P. (2023). Understanding and Addressing Mental Health Stigma Across Cultures for Improving Psychiatric Care: A Narrative Review. *Cureus*, *15*(5), e39549. DOI: 10.7759/cureus.39549 PMID: 37250612

Al Shamsi, H., Almutairi, A. G., Al Mashrafi, S., & Al Kalbani, T. (2020). Implications of Language Barriers for Healthcare: A Systematic Review. *Oman Medical Journal*, *35*(2), e122. DOI: 10.5001/omj.2020.40 PMID: 32411417

Aldalur, A., Bridgett, T., & Pick, L. H. (2022). Psychological Assessment Reports for Linguistically Minoritized Clients: Considerations for Ethical and Professional Practice. *Professional Psychology, Research and Practice*, *53*(6), 606–614. DOI: 10.1037/pro0000462 PMID: 37744892

Archuleta, A. J., & Lakhwani, M. (2016). Posttraumatic Stress Disorder Symptoms among first-generation Latino youths in an English as a second language school. *Children & Schools*, *38*(2), 119–127. DOI: 10.1093/cs/cdw005

Baeza-Rivera, M. J., Salazar-Fernández, C., Manríquez-Robles, D., Salinas-Oñate, N., & Smith-Castro, V. (2022). Acculturative Stress, Perceived Social Support, and Mental Health: The Mediating Effect of Negative Emotions Associated with Discrimination. *International Journal of Environmental Research and Public Health*, *19*(24), 16522. DOI: 10.3390/ijerph192416522 PMID: 36554406

Batalova, J. (2024). Mexican immigrants in the United States. *Migration Policy.* https://wawww.migrationpolicy.org/article/mexican-immigrants-united-states#:~:text=Mexicans%20are%20the%20largest%20group%20of%20immigrants%20in,million%20in%202022%20but%20has%20started%20growing%20again

Batalova, J. (2025). Frequently Requested Statistics on Immigrants and Immigration in the United States. *Migration Policy*. https://www.migrationpolicy.org/article/frequently-requested-statistics-immigrants-and-immigration-united-states

Bauer, A. M., & Alegría, M. (2010). Impact of patient language proficiency and interpreter service use on the quality of psychiatric care: A systematic review. *Psychiatric Services (Washington, D.C.)*, *61*(8), 765–773. DOI: 10.1176/ps.2010.61.8.765 PMID: 20675834

Bhugra, D., & Becker, M. A. (2005). Migration, cultural bereavement and cultural identity. *World Psychiatry; Official Journal of the World Psychiatric Association (WPA)*, *4*(1), 18–24. PMID: 16633496

Bolter, J. (2022). *Immigration Has Been a Defining, Often Contentious, Element Throughout U.S. History*. Migration Policy. https://www.migrationpolicy.org/article/immigration-shaped-united-states-history

Caballero, T. M., Ross DeCamp, L., Platt, R. E., Shah, H., Johnson, S. B., Sibinga, E. M. S., & Polk, S. (2017). Addressing the mental health needs of Latino children in immigrant families. *Clinical Pediatrics*, *56*(7), 648–658. https://doi-org.libproxy.calbaptist.edu/10.1177/0009922816679509. DOI: 10.1177/0009922816679509 PMID: 27879297

Cabassa, L. J., Molina, G. B., & Baron, M. (2012). Depression Fotonovela: Development of a depression literacy tool for Latinos with limited English proficiency. *Health Promotion Practice*, *13*(6), 747–754. DOI: 10.1177/1524839910367578 PMID: 21051325

Castro, F. G., Berkel, C., & Epstein, D. R. (2023). Cultural adaptations and cultural factors in EBI implementation with Latinx communities. *Frontiers in Public Health*, *11*, 1007328. DOI: 10.3389/fpubh.2023.1007328 PMID: 37026135

Christy, S. M., Cousin, L. A., Sutton, S. K., Chavarria, E. A., Abdulla, R., Gutierrez, L., Sanchez, J., Lopez, D., Gwede, C. K., & Meade, C. D. (2021). Characterizing Health Literacy Among Spanish Language-Preferring Latinos Ages 50-75. *Nursing Research*, *70*(5), 344–353. DOI: 10.1097/NNR.0000000000000519 PMID: 33990120

Cohen, S. R. (2013). Advocacy for the "Abandonados": Harnessing cultural beliefs for Latino families and their children with intellectual disabilities. *Journal of Policy and Practice in Intellectual Disabilities*, *10*(1), 71–78. DOI: 10.1111/jppi.12021

Connor, P., & Budiman, A. (2019). *Immigrants share in the U.S. nears record high but remains below that of many other countries*. Pew Research Center. https://www.pewresearch.org/short-reads/2019/01/30/immigrant-share-in-u-s-nears-record-high-but-remains-below-that-of-many-other-countries/

Davis, R. E., Johnson, T. P., Lee, S., & Werner, C. (2018). Why Do Latino Survey Respondents Acquiesce? Respondent and Interviewer Characteristics as Determinants of Cultural Patterns of Acquiescence Among Latino Survey Respondents. *Cross-Cultural Research*, *53*(1), 87-115. (Original work published 2019)DOI: 10.1177/1069397118774504

Davis, R. E., Resnicow, K., & Couper, M. P. (2011). Survey Response Styles, Acculturation, and Culture Among a Sample of Mexican American Adults. *Journal of Cross-Cultural Psychology*, *42*(7), 1219–1236. DOI: 10.1177/0022022110383317 PMID: 21927503

Delgado-Romero, E. A., De Los Santos, J., Raman, V. S., Merrifield, J. N., Vazquez, M. S., Monroig, M. M., Bautista, E. C., & Durán, M. Y. (2018). Caught in the Middle: Spanish-Speaking Bilingual Mental Health Counselors as Language Brokers. *Journal of Mental Health Counseling*, *40*(4), 341–352. DOI: 10.17744/mehc.40.4.06

Delgado-Romero, E. A., De Los Santos, J., Raman, V. S., Merrifield, J. N., Vazquez, M. S., Monroig, M. M., & Durán, M. Y. (2018). Caught in the middle: Spanish-speaking bilingual mental health counselors as language brokers. *Journal of Mental Health Counseling*, *40*(4), 341–352.

Dietrich, S., & Hernandez, E. (2022). *Nearly 68 Million People Spoke a Language Other Than English at Home in 2019*. U.S. Census Bureau. https://www.census.gov/library/stories/2022/12/languages-we-speak-in-united-states.html

Dunlap, J. L., Jaramillo, J. D., Koppolu, R., Wright, R., Mendoza, F., & Bruzoni, M. (2015). The effects of language concordant care on patient satisfaction and clinical understanding for Spanish pediatric surgery patients. *Journal of Pediatric Surgery*, *50*(9), 1586–1589. DOI: 10.1016/j.jpedsurg.2014.12.020 PMID: 25783324

Eamranond, P. P., Davis, R., Phillips, R. S., & Wee, C. C. (2011). Patient-physician Language Concordance and Primary Care Screening Among Spanish-speaking Patients. *Medical Care*, *49*(7), 668–672. DOI: 10.1097/MLR.0b013e318215d803 PMID: 21478772

Eno Louden, J., Avila, A., del Villar, O. A. E., Jung, H., Kosyluk, K. A., & Flores, E. (2023). Self-stigma of mental illness among Latino people on the U.S.-México border. *Stigma and Health*, *8*(1), 21–30. DOI: 10.1037/sah0000365

Escobedo, L. E., Cervantes, L., & Havranek, E. (2023). Barriers in Healthcare for Latinx Patients with Limited English Proficiency: A Narrative Review. *Journal of General Internal Medicine*, *38*(5), 1264–1271. DOI: 10.1007/s11606-022-07995-3 PMID: 36720766

Forcén, F. E., Vélez Flórez, M. C., Bido Medina, R., Zambrano, J., Pérez, J. H., Rodríguez, A. M., & Santos, L. H. (2023). Deconstructing Cultural Aspects of Mental Health Care in Hispanic/Latinx People. *Psychiatric Annals*, *53*(3), 127–132. DOI: 10.3928/00485713-20230215-02 PMID: 37781171

Freimuth, V. S., & Quinn, S. C. (2004). The contributions of health communication to eliminating health disparities. *American Journal of Public Health, 94*(12), 2053–2055. DOI: 10.2105/AJPH.94.12.2053 PMID: 15569949

Funk, C., & Lopez, M. H. (2022). *A brief statistical portrait of U.S. Hispanics.* Pew Research Center. https://www.pewresearch.org/science/2022/06/14/a-brief-statistical-portrait-of-u-s-hispanics/

Gadon, M., Balch, G. I., & Jacobs, E. A. (2007). Caring for patients with limited English proficiency: The perspectives of small group practitioners. *Journal of General Internal Medicine, 22*(S2, Suppl 2), 341–346. DOI: 10.1007/s11606-007-0311-4 PMID: 17957422

Gonzalez-Barrera, A. (2021). *Before COVID-19, more Mexicans came to the U.S. than left for Mexico for the first time in years.* Pew Research Center. https://www.pewresearch.org/short-reads/2021/07/09/before-covid-19-more-mexicans-came-to-the-u-s-than-left-for-mexico-for-the-first-time-in-years/

Gonzalez-Barrera, A., Hamel, L., Artiga, S., & Presiado, M. (2024). *Language barriers in health care: findings from the KFF survey on racism, discrimination, and health.* KFF. https://www.kff.org/racial-equity-and-health-policy/poll-finding/language-barriers-in-health-care-findings-from-the-kff-survey-on-racism-discrimination-and-health/

Gonzalez-Barrera, A., & Lopez, M. H. (2013). *Spanish is the most spoken non-English language in U.S. homes, even among non-Hispanics.* Pew Research Center. https://www.pewresearch.org/short-reads/2013/08/13/spanish-is-the-most-spoken-non-english-language-in-u-s-homes-even-among-non-hispanics/

Gray, T. (2023). Teaching and learning amid demographic change: A thematic review of school responses to newcomer students in the new Latinx diaspora. *Journal of Latinos and Education, 22*(2), 745–766. DOI: 10.1080/15348431.2020.1819284

Grieb, S. M., Platt, R., Vazquez, M. G., Alvarez, K., & Polk, S. (2023). Mental Health Stigma Among Spanish-Speaking Latinos in Baltimore, Maryland. *Journal of Immigrant and Minority Health, 25*(5), 999–1007. DOI: 10.1007/s10903-023-01488-z PMID: 37213041

Grubbs, V., Chen, A. H., Bindman, A. B., Vittinghoff, E., & Fernandez, A. (2006). Effect of awareness of language law on language access in the health care setting. *Journal of General Internal Medicine, 21*(7), 683–688. DOI: 10.1111/j.1525-1497.2006.00492.x PMID: 16808766

Gutiérrez, R. (2019). *Mexican Immigration to the United States.* Oxford Research Encyclopedia of American History. https://oxfordre.com/americanhistory/view/10.1093/acrefore/9780199329175.001.0001/acrefore-9780199329175-e-146

Haldar, S., Pillai, D., & Artiga, S. (2023). *Overview of health coverage and care for individuals with limited English proficiency (LEP).* KFF. https://www.kff.org/racial-equity-and-health-policy/issue-brief/overview-of-health-coverage-and-care-for-individuals-with-limited-english-proficiency/

Han, A., Laranjo, H., & Friedman, S. M. (2009). The design and pilot of a translation aid to help ED clinicians enhance communication with Portuguese-speaking patients. *International Journal of Emergency Medicine, 2*(1), 41–46. DOI: 10.1007/s12245-008-0081-8 PMID: 19390916

Heath, M., Hvass, A. M. F., & Wejse, C. M. (2023). Interpreter services and effect on healthcare - a systematic review of the impact of different types of interpreters on patient outcome. *Journal of Migration and Health, 7*, 100162. DOI: 10.1016/j.jmh.2023.100162 PMID: 36816444

İlimen, E. (2023). The Devil's Highway: The U.S. - Mexico border crossing, global influences and politics*. *Folklor / Edebiyat, 29*(113), 253–270. https://doi-org.libproxy.calbaptist.edu/10.22559/folklor.2277

Israel, E., & Batalova, J. (2020). Mexican Immigrants in the United States. *Migration Policy.*https://www.migrationpolicy.org/article/mexican-immigrants-united-states-2019

Karliner, L. S., Jacobs, E. A., Chen, A. H., & Mutha, S. (2007). Do professional interpreters improve clinical care for patients with limited English proficiency? A systematic review of the literature. *Health Services Research, 42*(2), 727–754. DOI: 10.1111/j.1475-6773.2006.00629.x PMID: 17362215

KFF. (2025). *Key Facts on Health Coverage of Immigrants.*https://www.kff.org/racial-equity-and-health-policy/fact-sheet/key-facts-on-health-coverage-of-immigrants/

Koff, M. D., & McGowan, J. J. (1999). MedSpanish: A language tool for the emergency department. In *Proceedings of the American Medical Informatics Association Symposium,* 565–569. https://pubmed.ncbi.nlm.nih.gov/10566422

Krogstad, J. M., Passel, J. S., Moslimani, M., & Noe-Bustamante, L. (2023). *Key facts about U.S. Latinos for National Hispanic Heritage Month.* Pew Research Center. https://www.pewresearch.org/short-reads/2023/09/22/key-facts-about-us-latinos-for-national-hispanic-heritage-month/

Krys, K., Vignoles, V. L., de Almeida, I., & Uchida, Y. (2022). Outside the "Cultural Binary": Understanding Why Latin American Collectivist Societies Foster Independent Selves. *Perspectives on Psychological Science, 17*(4), 1166-1187. (Original work published 2022)DOI: 10.1177/17456916211029632

Lanesskog, D., Muñoz, J., & Castillo, K. (2020). Language is not enough: Institutional supports for Spanish speaking client-worker engagement in child welfare. *Journal of Public Child Welfare, 14*(4), 435–457. https://doi-org.libproxy.calbaptist.edu/10.1080/15548732.2019.1621235. DOI: 10.1080/15548732.2019.1621235

Lee, J. S., Pérez-Stable, E. J., Gregorich, S. E., Crawford, M. H., Green, A., Livaudais-Toman, J., & Karliner, L. S. (2017). Increased Access to Professional Interpreters in the Hospital Improves Informed Consent for Patients with Limited English Proficiency. *Journal of General Internal Medicine, 32*(8), 863–870. DOI: 10.1007/s11606-017-3983-4 PMID: 28185201

Lightfoot, A. F., Thatcher, K., Eng, E., Merino, Y., Thomas, T., Simán, F. M., Coyne-Beasley, T., & Chapman, M. V. (2019). "What I wish my doctor knew about my life": Using photovoice with immigrant Latino adolescents to explore barriers to healthcare. *Qualitative Social Work: Research and Practice, 18*(1), 60–80. https://doi-org.libproxy.calbaptist.edu/10.1177/1473325017704034. DOI: 10.1177/1473325017704034 PMID: 32973399

Lopes, L., Montero, A., Presiado, M., & Hamel, L. (2024). *Americans' Challenges with Health Care Costs.* KFF. https://www.kff.org/health-costs/issue-brief/americans-challenges-with-health-care-costs/

Lopez Vera, A., Thomas, K., Trinh, C., & Nausheen, F. (2023). A Case Study of the Impact of Language Concordance on Patient Care, Satisfaction, and Comfort with Sharing Sensitive Information During Medical Care. *Journal of Immigrant and Minority Health, 25*(6), 1261–1269. DOI: 10.1007/s10903-023-01463-8 PMID: 36840903

Magaña, D. (2020). Local Voices on Health Care Communication Issues and Insights on Latino Cultural Constructs. *Hispanic Journal of Behavioral Sciences, 42*(3), 300–323. DOI: 10.1177/0739986320927387

Martinez-Donate, A. P., Ejebe, I., Zhang, X., Guendelman, S., Lê-Scherban, F., Rangel, G., Gonzalez-Fagoaga, E., Hovell, M. F., & Amuedo-Dorantes, C. (2017). Access to Health Care among Mexican Migrants and Immigrants: A Comparison across Migration Phases. *Journal of Health Care for the Poor and Underserved, 28*(4), 1314–1326. DOI: 10.1353/hpu.2017.0116 PMID: 29176097

Mercado, A., Antuña, C. S., Bailey, C., Garcini, L., Hass, G. A., Henderson, C., Koslofsky, S., Morales, F., & Venta, A. (2022). Professional guidelines for psychological evaluations in immigration proceedings. *Journal of Latina/o Psychology*, *10*(4), 253–276. DOI: 10.1037/lat0000209

Miller, L. (2013). Psychological evaluations in the criminal justice system: Basic principles and best practices. *Aggression and Violent Behavior, 18*(1), Issue 1, p. 83-91. .DOI: 10.1016/j.avb.2012.10.005

Moslimani, M., Lopez, M. H., & Noe-Bustamante, L. (2023). *11 facts about Hispanic origin groups in the U.S.* Pew Research Center. https://www.pewresearch.org/short-reads/2023/08/16/11-facts-about-hispanic-origin-groups-in-the-us/

Moslimani, M., & Passel, J. S. (2024). *What the data says about immigrants in the U.S.* Pew Research Center. https://www.pewresearch.org/short-reads/2024/09/27/key-findings-about-us-immigrants/

National Immigration Forum. (2019). Push or Pull Factors: What Drives Central American Migrants to the U.S.? https://immigrationforum.org/article/push-or-pull-factors-what-drives-central-american-migrants-to-the-u-s/

Neal, T. M. S., Slobogin, C., Saks, M. J., Faigman, D. L., & Geisinger, K. F. (2020). Psychological Assessments in Legal Contexts: Are Courts Keeping "Junk Science" Out of the Courtroom? *Psychological Science in the Public Interest, 20*(3), 135-164. (Original work published 2019)DOI: 10.1177/1529100619888860

NeMoyer, A., Rodriguez, T., & Alvarez, K. (2019). Psychological Practice with Unaccompanied Immigrant Minors: Clinical and Legal Considerations. *Translational Issues in Psychological Science*, *5*(1), 4–16. DOI: 10.1037/tps0000175 PMID: 30882017

Nielsen, D. S., Abdulkadir, L. S., Lynnerup, C., & Sodemann, M. (2020). 'I had to stifle my feelings' – Bilingual health professionals translating for family members in a healthcare setting. A qualitative study. *Scandinavian Journal of Caring Sciences*, *34*(4), 929–937. DOI: 10.1111/scs.12800 PMID: 31830311

Oh, H., Trinh, M. P., Vang, C., & Becerra, D. (2020). Addressing Barriers to Primary Care Access for Latinos in the U.S.: An Agent-Based Model. *Journal of the Society for Social Work and Research*, *11*(2), 165–184. https://www.journals.uchicago.edu/doi/full/10.1086/708616. DOI: 10.1086/708616

Ortega, A. N., Rodriguez, H. P., & Bustamante, A. V. (2015). Policy dilemmas in Latino health care and implementation of the Affordable Care Act. *Annual Review of Public Health, 36*(1), 525–544. https://doi-org.libproxy.calbaptist.edu/10.1146/annurev-publhealth-031914-122421. DOI: 10.1146/annurev-publhealth-031914-122421 PMID: 25581154

Pandey, M., Maina, R. G., Amoyaw, J., Li, Y., Kamrul, R., Michaels, C. R., & Maroof, R. (2021). Impacts of English language proficiency on healthcare access, use, and outcomes among immigrants: A qualitative study. *BMC Health Services Research, 21*(1), 741. DOI: 10.1186/s12913-021-06750-4 PMID: 34311712

Passel, J. S., & Krogstad, J. M. (2024). *What we know about unauthorized immigrants living in the U.S.* Pew Research Center. https://www.pewresearch.org/short-reads/2024/07/22/what-we-know-about-unauthorized-immigrants-living-in-the-us/

Pillai, D., & Artiga, S. (2023). *Overview of Health Coverage and Care for Individuals with Limited English Proficiency (LEP).* KFF. https://www.kff.org/racial-equity-and-health-policy/issue-brief/overview-of-health-coverage-and-care-for-individuals-with-limited-english-proficiency/

Quiroz, A. D., Boothe, R., Cruz, H., Palnati, S. R., & Bhakta, S. (2024). Primary Care Perceptions Among Spanish-Speaking Populations: A Comprehensive Review. *Cureus, 16*(9), e68736. DOI: 10.7759/cureus.68736 PMID: 39371846

Ramirez, A. S., Willis, G., & Rutten, L. F. (2017). Understanding Spanish-Language response in a national health communication survey: *Implications for health communication research.Journal of Health Communication, 22*(5), 442–450. DOI: 10.1080/10810730.2017.1304470 PMID: 28414618

Rao, A., Pillai, D., Artiga, S., Hamel, L., Schumacher, S., Kearney, A., & Presiado, M. (2024). *Five key facts about immigrants with limited English proficiency.* KFF. https://www.kff.org/racial-equity-and-health-policy/issue-brief/five-key-facts-about-immigrants-with-limited-english-proficiency/

Rivera, T. (2023). A social-ecological approach to Latino immigrant trauma and intervention: An integrative review. *Journal of Immigrant and Minority Health, 25*(4), 916–924. https://doi-org.libproxy.calbaptist.edu/10.1007/s10903-023-01474-5. DOI: 10.1007/s10903-023-01474-5 PMID: 37004677

Rodriguez, C. (2019). Latino/a citizen children of undocumented parents negotiating illegality. *Journal of Marriage and Family, 81*(3), 713–728. https://doi-org.libproxy.calbaptist.edu/10.1111/jomf.12551. DOI: 10.1111/jomf.12551

Rogers, R. G. (2025). *The Dire Mental Health Effects of Restrictive Immigration Policies.* U.S. Committee for Refugees and Immigrants. https://refugees.org/the-dire-mental-health-effects-of-restrictive-immigration-policies/

Santisteban, D. A., Mena, M. P., & Abalo, C. (2012). Bridging Diversity and Family Systems: Culturally Informed and Flexible Family Based Treatment for Hispanic Adolescents. *Couple & Family Psychology, 2*(4), 246–263. DOI: 10.1037/cfp0000013 PMID: 24772378

Schumacher, S., Hamel, L., Artiga, S., Pillai, D., Kearney, A., & Presaido, M. (2024). Most Hispanic Immigrants Say Their Lives Are Better In The US But Face Financial And Health Care Challenges: The 2023 KFF/LA Times Survey of Immigrants. KFF January 2024.

Sentell, T., Shumway, M., & Snowden, L. (2007). Access to mental health treatment by English language proficiency and race/ethnicity. *Journal of General Internal Medicine, 22*(S2, Suppl 2), 289–293. DOI: 10.1007/s11606-007-0345-7 PMID: 17957413

Sliwinski, K., Kutney-Lee, A., McHugh, M. D., & Lasater, K. B. (2024). A Review of Disparities in Outcomes of Hospitalized Patients with Limited English Proficiency: The Importance of Nursing Resources. *Journal of Health Care for the Poor and Underserved, 35*(1), 359–374. https://pmc.ncbi.nlm.nih.gov/articles/PMC11047028/ . DOI: 10.1353/hpu.2024.a919823 PMID: 38661875

Smith, A. K., Sudore, R. L., Pérez-Stable, E. J., Smith, A. K., Sudore, R. L., & Pérez-Stable, E. J. (2009). Palliative care for Latino patients and their families: Whenever we prayed, she wept. *Journal of the American Medical Association, 301*(10), 1047–E1. https://doi-org.libproxy.calbaptist.edu/10.1001/jama.2009.308. DOI: 10.1001/jama.2009.308 PMID: 19278947

Smith, B. L. (2018). Spanish-speaking psychologists in demand. *Monitor on Psychology, 49*(6). https://www.apa.org/monitor/2018/06/spanish-speaking

Soto Mas, F., & Jacobson, H. E. (2018). Advancing Health Literacy Among Hispanic Immigrants: The Intersection Between Education and Health. *Health Promotion Practice, 20*(2), 251–257. https://www.doi.org/10.1177/1524839918761865. DOI: 10.1177/1524839918761865 PMID: 29564920

Squires, A. (2018). Strategies for overcoming language barriers in healthcare. *Nursing Management, 49*(4), 20–27. DOI: 10.1097/01.NUMA.0000531166.24481.15 PMID: 29528894

Stonbraker, S., Schnall, R., & Larson, E. (2015). Tools to measure health literacy among Spanish speakers: An integrative review of the literature. *Patient Education and Counseling, S0738-3991(*15)30020-3 . Advance online publication. https://doi .org/DOI: 10.1016/j.pec.2015.07.012

Torres, S. A., Santiago, C. D., Walts, K. K., & Richards, M. H. (2018). Immigration policy, practices, and procedures: The impact on the mental health of Mexican and Central American youth and families. *The American Psychologist*, *73*(7), 843–854. https://doi-org.libproxy.calbaptist.edu/10.1037/amp0000184. DOI: 10.1037/ amp0000184 PMID: 29504782

Twersky, S. E., Jefferson, R., Garcia-Ortiz, L., Williams, E., & Pina, C. (2024). The Impact of Limited English Proficiency on Healthcare Access and Outcomes in the U.S.: A Scoping Review. *Healthcare (Basel)*, *12*(3), 364. DOI: 10.3390/ healthcare12030364 PMID: 38338249

United Nations. (2020). International migrant stock. https://www.un.org/development/ desa/pd/content/international-migrant-stock

United States Census Bureau. (2020). *People that speak English less than very well in the United States*. Public Tableau. https://public.tableau.com/app/profile/us.census .bureau/viz/shared/TSN7T2CMX

United States Census Bureau. (2024). *How do Hispanic or Latino Groups in the United States Compare?* Census.Gov. https://www.census.gov/library/visualizations/ interactive/population-pyramid-hispanic-origin.html

Valdés, G. (2020). (Mis)educating the children of Mexican-origin people in the United States: The challenge of internal language borders. *Intercultural Education*, *31*(5), 548–561. DOI: 10.1080/14675986.2020.1794122

Valdivieso-Mora, E., Peet, C. L., Garnier-Villarreal, M., Salazar-Villanea, M., & Johnson, D. K. (2016). A Systematic Review of the Relationship between Familism and Mental Health Outcomes in Latino Population. *Frontiers in Psychology*, *7*, 1632. DOI: 10.3389/fpsyg.2016.01632 PMID: 27826269

Wahass, S. H. (2005). The role of psychologists in health care delivery. *Journal of Family & Community Medicine*, *12*(2), 63–70. PMID: 23012077

Wallace, L. S., DeVoe, J. E., Heintzman, J. D., & Fryer, G. E. (2009). Language Preference and Perceptions of Healthcare Providers' Communication and Autonomy Making Behaviors among Hispanics. *Journal of Immigrant and Minority Health*, *11*(6), 453–459. DOI: 10.1007/s10903-008-9192-9 PMID: 18814028

Wand, A. P. F., Pourmand, D., & Draper, B. (2020). Working with interpreters in the psychiatric assessment of older adults from culturally and linguistically diverse backgrounds. *International Psychogeriatrics, 32(*1), p.11-16. DOI: 10.1017/S1041610219000280

Waters, A. R., Zamora, E. R., Fluchel, M., Warner, E. L., Rosen, S., Gwilliam, V., Tavor, G. E., Morales, J. P., & Kirchhoff, A. C. (2021). A qualitative inquiry of communication based barriers to the diagnosis of pediatric cancer: Perceptions of primarily Spanish-speaking caregiver. *Patient Education and Counseling*, *504*(6), 1503–1509. DOI: 10.1016/j.pec.2021.09.028 PMID: 34598802

Weber, O., Klemp, J., Chmetz, F., Daliani, A., Diserens, E. A., & Faucherre, F. (2023). Interpreter-mediated psychiatric assessments: Metacommunication as key. *Transcultural Psychiatry*, *60*(4), 626–636. DOI: 10.1177/13634615221119383 PMID: 36083232

Wells, A., Lagomasino, I., Palinkas, L., Green, J., & Gonzalez, D. (2013). Barriers to depression treatment among low-income, Latino emergency department patients. *Community Mental Health Journal*, *49*(4), 412–418. https://doi-org.libproxy.calbaptist.edu/10.1007/s10597-012-9547-5. DOI: 10.1007/s10597-012-9547-5 PMID: 23054150

Wilson, E., Chen, A. H., Grumbach, K., Wang, F., & Fernandez, A. (2005). Effects of limited English proficiency and physician language on health care comprehension. *Journal of General Internal Medicine*, *20*(9), 800–806. DOI: 10.1111/j.1525-1497.2005.0174.x PMID: 16117746

Wynia, M. K., & Osborn, C. Y. (2010). Health literacy and communication quality in health care organizations. *Journal of Health Communication*, *15*(2), 102–115. DOI: 10.1080/10810730.2010.499981 PMID: 20845197

Chapter 4
The Land of Dreams or Muffled Screams:
An Examination on the Intersectionality of Immigration and Violent Crime Within the United States

Mikaylin J. Turner
https://orcid.org/0009-0007-2408-9838
Independent Researcher, USA

Abbie R. Nelson
Southeast Missouri State University, USA

Joshua Todd Shadwick
https://orcid.org/0000-0003-1934-4594
Southeast Missouri State University, USA

ABSTRACT

The United States is often noted as the land of immigrants. Despite this national and international nomenclature, crimes against immigrants have received less empirical examination in comparison to crimes against U.S. citizens. This disparity is an issue since this gap in the literature can potentially obscure and minimize policy and practice. It can be surmised that diminished responses to crime victims, especially violent crimes, is an issue and the inability to consider potential barriers and other contextual factors associated with language and cultural barriers impedes the effectiveness of the justice system and other social institutions. Therefore, the purpose of this chapter is to explore the importance between immigrants and violent crime.

DOI: 10.4018/979-8-3693-7944-8.ch004

INTRODUCTION

In *The Epic of America* (1931), James Truslow Adams coined the phrase American Dream. Since its creation, some have argued that the phrase has changed meaning (Churchwell, 2021). Originally, Adams intended for the phrase to mean "a dream of a social order in which each man and each woman shall be able to attain to the fullest stature of which they are innately capable, and be recognized by others for what they are, regardless of the fortuitous circumstances of birth or position." Conversely, however, the American Dream is the success story of a self-made person and their upward climb in social status (Churchwell, 2021). Thus, scholarship has argued that the American Dream went from being a concept for all individuals, regardless of nationality, to one being only for U.S. citizens (Bod, 2022). Regardless of the empirical arguments framed around the American Dream (Adams, 1931; Bod, 2022; Churchwell, 2021; Popal, 2021), individuals have continued to immigrate to the United States.

Subsequently, the United States is often noted as the land of immigrants (Foner, 2005; Ragsdale, 2013). This sentiment is exemplified on the plaque located at the Statue of Liberty, "give me your tired, your poor, your huddled masses yearning to breathe free" (NPS, n.d.) Despite this national and international nomenclature, crimes against immigrants have received less empirical examination in comparison to crimes against U.S. citizens (Xie & Baumer, 2021). This disparity is an issue since this gap in the literature can potentially obscure and minimize policy and practice for all individuals located within the United States. It can be surmised that diminished responses to crime victims, especially violent crimes, is an issue and the inability to consider potential barriers and other contextual factors (e.g., culture, language) impedes the effectiveness of the justice system and other social institutions.

For example, in 2022 it was reported that 13.8 percent, or 45 million, of the United States population were immigrants (American Immigration Council, 2022; The Immigrant Learning Center, 2021). Of those 45 million immigrants, roughly 78 percent of them are documented, leaving only 22 percent undocumented. Regardless of the documentation status, immigrants face many challenges, such as language barriers, cultural differences, and discrimination (Vesti, 2023). Work by Martinez and Rumbaut (2015), indicates that immigrants are less likely to commit serious crimes, and immigration has been shown to lead to less violent and property crimes. There is still more to know, however, regarding victimization among immigrants (Shen, 2017; Mainstreaming Hate, 2018; Anonymous, 2022; Fletcher, 2024).

Therefore, the purpose of this chapter is to explore the intersectionality between immigration and violent crime—specifically, hate crimes, domestic violence, and human trafficking. For this chapter, nomenclature will be clearly defined so that motivated individuals and institutions clearly understand how we conceptualize and apply prominent terms. For example, our definition of immigrant is "a person who comes to a country to take up permanent residence" (Merriam-Webster, n.d.). A hate crime will be defined as "a criminal offense against a person or property motivated in whole or in part by an offender's bias against a race, religion, disability, sexual orientation, ethnicity, gender, or gender identity" (FBI, 2016). Moreover, our domestic violence definition will comport with the FBI's (2017) as "The use, attempted use, or threatened use of physical force, or a weapon; or the use of coercion or intimidation; or committing a crime against property by a current or former spouse, parent, or guardian of the victim; a person with whom the victim shares a child in common; a person who is or has been in a social relationship of a romantic or intimate nature with the victim; a person who is cohabiting with or has cohabited with the victim as a spouse, parent, or guardian; or by a person who is or has been similarly situated to a spouse, parent, or guardian of the victim." Human trafficking will be defined as "a crime involving the exploitation of a person for labor, services, or commercial sex." (U.S. DOJ, 2022). Lastly, we define immigrant as any individual who is lawfully within the United States, who is not a US citizen or national (DHS, n.d.). We draw a distinction between immigrants who are here legally versus individuals who are residing here illegally, so interested parties understand we are referring to individuals who are pursuing legal platforms for residency within the United States. With obscurity removed from our working definitions we now turn toward contextual factors associated with immigration status.

More specifically, social factors such as community context (e.g., urban, rural) and social economic status are elements that researchers and motivated parties should consider when considering violent crimes among immigrants. Thus, intersectionality consisting of immigrant status and social factors should be considered as one attempts to understand victimization among this population. It should be noted that immigrants reside in all areas of the U.S. and occupy every level of the economic status continuum (Duleep & Dowhan, 2008; Moslimani & Passel, 2024). Therefore, context, like social problems, is multifaceted. The following section unpacks three violent crime areas as it relates to immigration status and other social factors. The ability to disaggregate and disentangle these crimes as it relates to immigrants is vital to understanding limitations associated with the criminal justice system and other social institutions.

VIOLENT VICTIMIZATION AMONG IMMIGRANTS

Hate Crimes

A hate crime can be challenging to define. For this discussion, the FBI's definition of hate crimes will be used. A hate crime is defined as "a criminal offense against a person or property motivated in whole or in part by an offender's bias against a race, religion, disability, sexual orientation, ethnicity, gender, or gender identity (Federal Bureau of Investigation, 2016). Although hate per se is not a crime, what a person does with that hatred is what makes it a crime. For example, charged language centered around anti-immigration has been a noted pipeline for hate crimes within the United States (Astrada & Astrada, 2019).

Hate Crime Scholarship & Statistics

Prior to 1991, no data was collected about hate crimes. In 1990, the Hate Crime Statistics Act was enacted and called for the collection of hate crime information from 1990 to 1994, specifically regarding the victim's race, religion, sexual orientation, and/or ethnicity (H.R. 1048 Hate Crime Statistics Act, 1990). This act also paved the way for all future data collection resources regarding hate crimes.

Research has shown that after some influential events, such as 9/11 or a massive influx of Hispanic immigrants, lead to an increase in hate crimes against the "offending" group (Ewing, Martinez, & Rumbaut, 2015; Finley & Esposito, 2019). For instance, in the early 2000s, large numbers of Latin American immigrants came to the United States (Immigration Policy Center, 2008). With this increase in immigrants came an increase in hate crimes. More recently, in 2022, there was an almost three percent increase in hate crimes against Hispanics within the major cities in the United States (Linares, 2023). However, looking at the past three years, from September 2021 to September 2024, there was an increase in hate crimes and then a decrease (Crime Data Explorer, 2022a; Crime Data Explorer, 2023a; Crime Data Explorer, 2024a). From 2021 to 2022, there was a total of 13,043 reported hate crimes of those hate crimes, 7,563 of which regarded the victim's race and/or ethnicity (Crime Data Explorer, 2022a). In the 2022 through 2023 data, there were 12,642 reported hate crimes, and 6,889 of them were committed because of the offender's bias against the victim's race or ethnicity (Crime Data Explorer, 2023a). From 2023 to 2024, there were 4,617 reported hate crimes, and 2,182 were based on race or ethnicity (Crime Data Explorer, 2024a).

Between September 2021 and September 2022, there was a three percent decrease in overall hate crimes and a nine percent decrease in racial hate crimes (Crime Data Explorer, 2022a; Crime Data Explorer, 2023a). Between September 2022 and

September 2023, there was a 63 percent decrease in hate crimes overall and a 68 percent decrease in racial hate crimes (Crime Data Explorer, 2023a; Crime Data Explorer, 2024a). This is not to say that hate crimes actually decreased. There is the possibility that there were just more hate crimes that went unreported or hate crimes that were categorized as something other than a hate crime by law enforcement and the variation in reporting practices across state lines (Turner, 2023). According to Wiggins (2024), reported hate crimes only account for approximately only one percent of hate crimes that actually occur. As a result, even the most obvious of hate crimes go unreported by law enforcement (Wiggins,2024). This gap in hate crime reporting is a concern for communities and institutions (IACP, 2019). For instance, in 2020, the National Crime Victimization Survey (NCVS) reported that violent crime went down from 3.4 to 2.8 victimizations for every 1,000 persons. In contrast, the FBI reported an increase in violent crime, from 3.8 per 1,000 persons to 4.0 per 1,000 persons (Bureau of Justice Statistics, 2021). Therefore, directed attention toward standardizing reporting practices is needed so that a more refined understanding of hate crimes, within the United States, can emerge.

Human Trafficking

Immigration and Customs Enforcement (ICE) states that human trafficking is a global issue that can affect anyone, regardless of their age, gender, or background (Immigration and Customs Enforcement, n.d.). According to the Department of Justice (2022), human trafficking is defined as "a crime involving the exploitation of a person for labor, services, or commercial sex" (U.S. Department of Justice, 2022). The term "smuggling" is also often used interchangeably with "human trafficking" (Pedron & de Arimateia da Cruz, 2021). The United Nations defines smuggling as "the facilitation, for financial or other material gain, of irregular entry into a country where the migrants is not a national or resident" (United Nations, n.d.). There are two specific types of human trafficking: sex trafficking and forced labor. The Department of Justice states that

Sex trafficking is the recruitment, harboring, transportation, provision, obtaining, patronizing, or soliciting of a person for the purpose of a commercial sex act in which a commercial sex act is induced by force, fraud, or coercion, or in which the person induced to perform such act has not attained 18 years of age (U.S. Department of Justice, 2022).

The Department of Justice defines forced labor as The recruitment, harboring, transportation, provision, or obtaining of a person for labor or services through the use of force, fraud, or coercion for the purpose of subjection to involuntary servitude, peonage, debt bondage, or slavery. (U.S. Department of Justice, 2022).

The main difference between human trafficking and smuggling is that human trafficking does not focus solely on one's immigration status but on their likelihood of exploitation, whereas smuggling does focus on immigration status, specifically those who enter the country "illegally" (Pedron & de Arimateia da Cruz, 2021). For continuity, the term human trafficking will be used moving forward.

HUMAN TRAFFICKING SCHOLARSHIP & STATISTICS

Human traffickers focus on individuals who are desperate and looking for a better life (Immigration and Customs Enforcement, n.d.; Hartmann, 2019). Most immigrants will do what they can to make a new life, which makes them vulnerable to being victims. Human Traffickers, also known as coyotes, promise immigrants a better life, telling them they can help them obtain a high-paying job, reconnect with their family who have already come to the United States, or other opportunities for success (Hartmann, 2019).

Human Trafficking data was not collected until 2013 (Federal Bureau of Investigation, 2019). An act created in 2008 requires the FBI to collect human trafficking data and to make differences between human trafficking and offenses regarding prostitution. It should be noted that anyone can be a victim of human trafficking, so the information available from the FBI is not entirely accurate regarding immigrants and human trafficking as they do not note the victim's immigration status. To illustrate this point, between September 2021 and September 2022, there were a total of 1,091 cases of commercial human trafficking reported in the United States (Crime Data Explorer, 2022b). Of those cases, 415 (38 percent) of the victims were of Hispanic descent. In that same period, there were 2,722 sex trafficking cases. Of those, 457 (17 percent) of the victims were Hispanic. Between September 2022 and 2023, there was a total of 841 commercial human trafficking cases (Crime Data Explorer, 2023b). Hispanic individuals were the victim in 379 (45 percent) of the cases. From September 2022 to 2023, there were 2,656 cases of sex trafficking; of those cases, 1,546 (58 percent) had a Hispanic individual as the victim. Within the past year, there were 190 commercial trafficking cases (Crime Data Explorer, 2024b), where 92 (48 percent) involved a Hispanic victim. In that same time frame, there were 760 instances of sex trafficking. Of those 760 cases, the victim in 128 (17 percent) was someone of Hispanic descent.

Moreover, between September 2021 and September 2022, there was a 23 percent decrease in commercial human trafficking cases. In that same year, there was a 2 percent decrease in sex trafficking cases. Between September 2022 and 2023, there was a 77 percent decrease in commercial human trafficking cases. In that same time frame, the rate of sex trafficking also decreased by 71 percent. It should be noted that this does not necessarily mean that human trafficking has decreased. There is the possibility that cases will go unnoticed or unreported. One could also speculate that these cases are being recorded as a different crime. Similar to hate crimes, human trafficking is complex and the ability for law enforcement and other social institutions to correctly identify these cases is needed for improved practices moving forward.

Domestic violence (IPV)

Domestic Violence is an umbrella term that encompasses many different types of abuse. As outlined in the FBI (2017) definition above, the physical, emotional, and/or sexual abuse under the term domestic violence can be committed by a current or former spouse, or parent, or guardian of the victim. This section will outline two distinct types of domestic violence that immigrants experience intimate partner violence (IPV), and child abuse. The following section outlines information pertinent to these crimes such as protective elements and risk factors.

Domestic Violence Scholarship & Statistics

Intimate partner violence (IPV) is a major public health issue, that The Centers for Disease Control and Prevention (CDC) defines as including "physical violence, sexual violence, stalking and psychological aggression (including coercive tactics) by a current or former intimate partner (e.g., spouse, boyfriend/girlfriend, dating partner, or ongoing sexual partner)" (Breiding, 2015). Estimates reveal one in four women and 1 in 10 men in the United States (U.S.) experience intimate partner violence victimization (IPV-V) in their lifetime (CDC, 2024; Smith et al., 2018). The National Organization for Women reports that the rates of IPV for immigrant women is almost 3 times the national average (NOW, 2024). Only one systematic review has been conducted to look at the rates of IPV-V and intimate partner violence perpetration (IPV-P) among all immigrants in the US (Morrison et al., 2024). Morrison et al. (2024) found IPV-V rates ranging from 3.8% to 46.9% in the past year and ranges from 13.9%-93% for a lifetime. IPV-P rates ranged from 3-24.8%. Within the 24 articles that were analyzed, the rates varied depending on factors such as how IPV was measured, if a random or convenience sample was used, and the different immigrant populations included. For example, one study used a sample of 55 Iraqi women in Detroit and found a 93% prevalence for controlling behavior abuse (Barkho et al., 2011). Latino women (n=1,038) reported a lifetime IPV rate of 43.5% using a random sample (Ingram, 2007). Overall rates of IPV appear to be higher for immigrants than non-immigrant populations in the US, at least for some populations. There are a variety of factors that may contribute to this prevalence which will be discussed after explaining the consequences of IPV.

IPV is concerning due to its high prevalence, and dire consequences not only to the survivor but also to society. The costs to society of intimate partner rape, physical assault, and stalking are estimated at $3.6 trillion over the lifetime of a survivor (Peterson et al., 2018). This includes costs associated with medical and mental health care services, lost productivity, and criminal justice responses (Peterson et al., 2018). IPV has a devastating effect on survivors mental and physical health. The effect of IPV on mental health is well documented by a systematic review and meta-analysis that confirm the association between IPV, depression, posttraumatic stress disorder, anxiety, and bidirectional relationships between IPV and hard drug and marijuana use (Bacchus et al., 2018; Lagdon et al., 2014). In addition, mental health consequences such as eating disorders, sleep disturbances, suicidal behavior, sexual problems, problems with concentration, somatization, personality, and bipolar disorders as well as social, educational, and occupational difficulties have been associated with IPV (Gallegos et al., 2021; Mazza et al., 2021; Trevillion et al., 2012). A large cross-sectional public-health survey across 16 US states and two territories identified many physical health issues related to IPV (Breiding et al., 2008). These include a greater likelihood of high cholesterol, heart disease, stroke, joint disease, current asthma, HIV risk factors, and activity limitations when compared to those who did not experience IPV (Breiding et al., 2008). Immigrants in the US are experiencing IPV at high rates and are experiencing consequences to their bodies and minds as a result. It is important to note that immigrant men are survivors of abuse but the pronoun she will be used more below due to women being the primary samples of the studies included.

Factors that Impact Immigrants Experience of IPV

The vulnerable experience of being an immigrant in a new country and working to start a new life, places the immigrant in a unique position with factors that have the potential to impact domestic violence. Using the ecological systems framework can help to organize the risk and protective factors on the micro individual level, the interpersonal or communal level, and the macro or societal level (Crawford, 2020).

For the survivor population overall risk factors for IPV and perpetration include low income, low education, high stress, alcohol use, and lack of social support (Spencer et al., 2022). Immigrant survivors share these factors but also have specific factors related to their immigration status such as being undocumented, not having family in the US, language barriers, and acculturation status (Erez et al., 2009; Kim, 2019; Njie-Carr et al., 2020; Sabri et al., 2018). The perpetrator of IPV is often trying to gain power and control over the victim in any way possible.

Coming to a new country and not having legal status already puts immigrants in a position of powerlessness. The abuser can further exploit this status by threatening to report them to authorities (Erez et al., 2009). The immigrant power and control wheel created by the National Center on Domestic and Sexual Violence (2024) gives further examples of how immigrant abusers may use emotional and physical abuse directly related to immigration issues such as isolating her from others who speak her language, failing to file papers to legalize her status, threatening to report her if she works, hiding or destroying important papers such as ID cards or property from her country of origin, and threatening to report children to the Immigration and Naturalization Service (INS). Being in a position where she does not have financial freedom or even speak the language of the country she is in, can put her at a greater risk to be stuck in an abusive situation and not have the ability to access the resources she needs in order to escape (Njie-Carr et al., 2020). In addition, the process of acculturation can also be a risk factor for abuse (Kim, 2019). As the survivor starts to learn about the new culture in the US, make connections with others, and becomes aware of the different freedoms' women are experiencing, they may start to gain empowerment and independence that can become a threat to the abuser and thus exacerbate abuse (Erez et al., 2009; Sabri et al., 2018). On the other hand, this newfound independence can also be a protective factor for women. Having financial resources, education, and access to resources such as a phone, money, and a car they can drive have been shown to be protective factors against immigrant abuse (Njie-Carr et al., 2020; Sabri et al., 2018).

Just like on the individual level, the relationships or lack thereof and connections in the community impact the risk and protective factors of survivors. Support from friends, co-workers, neighbors, and children can have a great impact on a woman's ability to survive and eventually be able to leave an abusive relationship (Njie-Carr et al., 2020; Sabri et al., 2018). In addition to informal supports that served as a protective factor, those that had access to formal support such as therapists and healthcare providers, found that it supported them in connecting with resources to leave the relationship as well as cope and heal with the emotional trauma from the abuse (Sabri et al., 2018). Conversely if survivors experienced a lack of support from their communities, this became a risk factor. In the interviews done by Sabri et al. (2018), with immigrant and refugee survivors that identified as Asian, Latina, and African, they outlined how family members would often get involved and try to convince women to stay with their abusers, especially if they came from cultures that had strong ideas about the position of men being superior to that of women. Without support from family and friends, it was hard for women to have the internal or external resources to cope within a relationship or leave if that was an option. Another risk factor related to the community was women's fear of the police. If women were afraid of the police and wanted to avoid contact with the criminal justice system, this was a risk factor, as they would be less likely to report or reach out for help when needed (Akinsulure-Smith, 2013; Sabri et al., 2018).

The individual, communal, and relationship factors are all influenced by the macro systems of the overall culture and structure of society (Crawford, 2020). Immigrants find themselves in a position of navigating not only the culture from the country they immigrated from, but also the influence of the US culture once immigrated. Known risk factors at this level include patriarchal norms and religion (Akinsulure-Smith, 2013; Njie-Carr et al., 2020; Sabri et al., 2018). If an immigrant comes from a culture in which patriarchal norms are strong and women are expected to have traditional roles in the home such as serving the man, this can be a risk factor for abuse (Njie-Carr et al., 2020). For example, if the couple comes from a culture in which women are not supposed to express opinions and then the woman in the relationship expresses her disagreement with her husband, there is a greater chance that will turn to abuse as the man will see that as more disrespectful than if he was surrounded by a culture that accepted opinions of women as valid (Akinsulure-Smith, 2013). Religion and faith can play a role as a risk or protective factor. In cultures that use religion to justify why women should stay in an abusive relationship, women can feel pressured to stay for fear they would be upsetting "God" if they were to leave (Sabri et al., 2018). On the other hand, survivors have reported faith as a strong coping skill that helped them address the pain of the abuse and survive (Njie-Carr et al., 2020; Sabri et al., 2018). Laws and religion in the US that are more pro-women and provide stronger protections against abuse provide a protective mechanism for immigrants (Erez et al., 2009; Sabri et al., 2018). Particularly women who immigrate from cultures that have not had the same history or waves of feminism that have fought for the rights that are in the US, seeing that displayed around them may be the first time they are exposed to the possibility of women being in relationships without abuse or deserving of protection. The risk and protective factors at the individual, relational, and macro levels, have an impact of immigrant IPV perpetration, escaping, and healing. Couched within the domestic violence, IPV nexus is the documented connection between IPV and child abuse (Goddard & Bedi, 2010). Subsequently, we now turn toward a discussion on child abuse and immigration.

Child Abuse Scholarship & Statistics

Child abuse is a type of abuse that falls under the umbrella of domestic violence. It can include overt acts such as physical, sexual, or psychological abuse, or covert acts such as neglect or failure to provide appropriate supervision (Leeb, 2008). It is estimated that per year about one in seven children experience child abuse or neglect in the United States (Finkelhor et al., 2015). Broken down by gender, one in four girls and one in 13 boys are estimated to experience child abuse (National Children's Alliance, 2024). Just like IPV, the numbers reported are likely much lower than the actual numbers due to the taboo nature of child abuse and that children do not always have the power or voice to report abuse. The Migration Policy Institute (MPI) reports that in 2023 there were 17,890,000 children under the age of 18 living in the US with at least one immigrant parent. Of that number 86% were born in the US (MPI, 2024). Almost 90% of these children are US citizens and more than half are bilingual (Urban Institute, 2019). Over half (57%) of the immigrant children in 2017 had a parent from Mexico, Central or South America with the rest from a variety of different countries and regions such as East and Southeast Asia, Middle East, Africa, Canada, Australia, and New Zealand (Urban Institute, 2019). Statistics on child abuse of immigrants can be difficult to find as official rates of child abuse in the US do not specify information on immigrant status (LeBrun et al., 2015). Individual studies have looked at rates for certain populations and their involvement with the child welfare system. Data from the National Survey of Child and Adolescent Well-Being (NSCAW) that used a nationally representative sample of children who were subjects of reports to Child Protective Services found that 8.6% of the reports were children living with a foreign-born parent (Dettlaff & Earner, 2012). Of those 67.2% were Hispanic, 14.8% White, 10% Black, and 7.5% Asian (Dettlaff & Earner, 2012). The NSCAW also showed that immigrant children are more likely to experience emotional abuse but nearly eight times less likely to experience physical neglect (Dettlaff & Earner, 2012). A systematic review over 17 studies to determine rates of abuse for migrant and immigrant children found lifetime prevalences for physical maltreatment ranged from 9-65% and child sexual abuse from 5-20% (Jud et al., 2020). Those rates included only 3 studies with US samples. There is not strong evidence for exact numbers and types of abuse, but we can see from the above information that immigrant children are experiencing child abuse.

Although most immigrant children do live with a parent, there has been a growing number of unaccompanied minors crossing the southern border of the US. More than 600,000 have immigrated since 2012 from Central American countries primarily Guatemala, El Salvador, and Honduras, with almost 130,000 arriving in 2022 (Young et al., 2024). Exact numbers of abuse for this population are hard to find since it is an ever-growing concern and is highly politicized in the US. However, the Department of Health and Human Services between 2014-2018 received more than 4,500 complaints of sexual abuse against unaccompanied minors (Trimble 2019). Most of these were alleged from other minors but 178 accusations were against adult staff at government housing facilities who would be considered the caregivers of the youth at that time. It is also known that unaccompanied minors face abuse before coming to the US, but once again the exact numbers are unknown due to lack of reporting and access to data in other countries whose process on child abuse reporting vary (UNHCR, 2024).

Consequences

Child abuse has a devasting effect on society and the individual lives and well-being of victims and their families. First, for the societal impact, child maltreatment places a huge economic burden on the US. Across their lifetime it is estimated that the "substantiated" cases to Child and Protective Services of child abuse and neglect will incur 592 billion dollars of economic burden associated with the consequences of child abuse including death (Klika et al., 2020). Child abuse can impact the children in the immediate causing consequences such as physical and emotional injuries as well as have an impact on their future health and well-being as adults. In regard to physical health, child abuse has been associated with higher risk for long term and future health problems such as diabetes, lung disease, malnutrition, vision problems, heart attack, arthritis, high blood pressure, headaches, cancer, stroke, bowel disease, and chronic fatigue syndrome (Widom et al., 2012; Monnat & Chandler, 2015; Afifi et al., 2016). A meta- analysis and systematic review by Norman et al. (2012) found statistically significant associations between child abuse and neglect and depressive disorders, drug use, suicide attempts, sexually transmitted infections and risky sexual behavior. Other psychological consequences include risk of cognitive problems (Bick & Nelson, 2016). The extreme stress of child maltreatment can change the brain's response to trauma as well as result in posttraumatic stress disorder (PTSD), which can lead to further mental health and behavioral consequences (Sege et al., 2017). There is also a correlation between child abuse and future criminal activities and involvement with the juvenile justice system (Herrenkohl et al., 2017). Immigrant child abuse survivors not only experience the above consequences of child abuse, but also may already experience mental and physical risks from the status of being a refugee or migrant. Studies on refugee and migrant youth have shown an elevated risk in developing mental health problems such as PTSD and depression (Blackmore et al., 2020, Curtis et al., 2018; Reavell & Fazil, 2017). The consequences of child abuse have a great impact on immigrant survivors physical and mental well-being in addition to impacts on the society in which they live.

FACTORS THAT IMPACT IMMIGRANTS EXPERIENCE OF CHILD ABUSE

Research has shown a variety of risk and protective factors associated with child abuse. Protective factors that show moderate or strong association with improved well-being for child abuse survivors have been identified at the individual, relational, and community levels (Child Welfare Information Gateway, 2015; 2019). These include individually having a sense of purpose, self-regulation, relational, and problem-solving skills. Relationally having connection with positive peers and parents that have parental competencies and well-being themselves is protective. On the community level protective factors include having a positive school environment, living in a stable situation, and being in a community that has a positive environment (Child Welfare Information Gateway, 2015). Risk factors include parental stress, substance use, and poverty (Child Welfare Information Gateway, 2019). Studies about immigrant families show overlaps in some of the risk and protective factors as well as unique factors to immigration. On the individual level, among immigrant and non-immigrant families high stress is the risk factor reported most frequently (LeBrun et al., 2015). The reasons for this stress would be different for immigrant families as they are coping with not only the daily family stressors but the unique stressors that come from acculturation and relocation (Segal & Mayadas,2005). Other individual level risk factors include living in a step or single parent home (Alink et al., 2013; Euser et al., 2011), in a family with low levels of education (Alink et al., 2013; Euser et al., 2011), being a part of a large family, and living in a home with domestic violence against a caregiver (Dettlaff & Earner, 2012).

Although not all immigrants are refugees, being a refugee is a type of immigrant. Timshel et al. (2017), conducted a systematic review of risk and protective factors associated with family related violence in refugee families that settle in Western countries. They and other research found individual parental factors such as the history of child abuse for the parent and the cultural discipline practices could present as risk factors (LeBrun et al., 2015). Protective factors specifically related to immigration were the longer a family was in the US, less severe abuse was associated, having a foreign-born mother, higher educational levels, and a two-parent household (LeBrun et al., 2015).

Acculturation stress hypothesis predicts that immigrants may be at a higher risk in the first years of immigration due to the stress of acculturation and the process of learning the new norms and culture of the new place of settlement. Timshel et al. (2017) identified a combination of parental trauma and acculturation stress as community level risk factors. In addition, on the community and relational level, lack of social support is a risk factor for immigrants especially when they are leaving their family and friends from the country of origin and have not have time to build new ones yet upon resettling (Dettlaf et al., 2009). On the flip side, maintaining a connection with the immigrant family's culture of their family of origin can work as a protective factor (Dettlaff & Earner, 2012). Social connection seems to be key and may impact why living in a neighborhood with higher immigrant and ethnic diversity serves as a protective factor (LeBrun et al., 2015), as being surrounded by other immigrants could provide more opportunities for families to connect with other families more readily and find social support. One of the greatest macro level risk factors is lack of access to medical, social, and community resources due to public policies and laws that exclude immigrants (LeBrun et al., 2015). They may be excluded due to direct policies or cultural barriers such as not knowing where to find services or the unavailability of culturally competent services.

Many unaccompanied immigrant children are fleeing from abuse in their own countries to seek protection in the United States. A study that conducted interviews with 404 unaccompanied minors to explore what was pushing them to migrate found that 48% of the children came to escape violence from organized crime in their region and 21% had survived domestic violence (UNHCR, 2024). Another study found that girls reported experiencing more domestic abuse than boys who were unaccompanied minors (Schmidt, 2022). Therefore, they are child abuse survivors before even coming to the US. There are many risks for continued abuse as they journey alone to the US and are detained at the border. Within 72 hours of being caught on the border by Customs and Border Protection, the minors are sent to shelter funded by the Office of Refugee Resettlement (ORR) where they receive medical care, food, shelter, case management, education and therapy until they are released to a relative in the US or sent back to their country depending on the situation (Young et al., 2024). The shelters work to screen for trafficking and make sure that the children are going to end up with an appropriate caregiver, but recent reports have shown that many of these minors are at risk of ending up in abusive and exploitative situations (Dreier, 2023).

Laws Related to Domestic Violence and Immigration

There is a long history behind the development and implementation of policies and the involvement of the criminal justice system with domestic violence. Before the 1900's the US was still under the colonial system of English Common Law that stated it was not illegal for husbands to abuse wives (Barner & Carney, 2011). Laws began to be passed against domestic violence in the late 1800's to early 1900's, and the social casework model developed where short jail sentences and psychiatric treatment were offered to offenders and casework to victims (Dobash & Dobash, 2003). The criminal justice approach to IPV treatment increased in the 1980's and 90's as law enforcement became trained to deal with DV, and included increased use of protective orders, victim advocacy, batterer's intervention programs as a condition of probation, and coordinated community responses (Danis, 2003). Governmental support for domestic violence first came with the passing of the Victims of Crime Act (1984) and the Violence Against Women Act (VAWA) (1994) that invoked the power of state on women's behalf providing more resources to criminal justice and social services for domestic violence (Messing et al., 2015). Although VAWA provided added supports to this important issue, it was not until the reauthorization of 2013 that more protection and rights were given to immigrant women included the Trafficking Victims Protection Act, decrease backlog of untested rape kits, more protection for college students, tribal women, and LGBTQ survivors (National Resource Center on DV(NRCDV), 2013). More specifically for immigrants, if they are abused by a family member who is a US citizen, they can self-petition for lawful status on their own without needing the abuser as a sponsor (NNEDV, 2024). In addition, immigrant survivors can apply for a U visa if they are willing to assist law enforcement in the investigation or prosecution of the crime (Homeland Security, n.d.). The reauthorization in 2022 under the Biden administration included help for children who have been exposed to domestic violence by updating the SMART Prevention Program and the CHOOSE Youth Program to reduce dating violence (House, 2022).

Immigrant children that are US citizens would be protected under the many child abuse protection laws that exist such as The Victims of Child Abuse Act and Child Abuse Prevention and Treatment Act (Office of Justice Programs, n.d.). Children that are unaccompanied minors or immigrants that do not have legal status but have been abused, abandoned, or neglected by a parent can apply for Special Immigrant Juvenile (SIJ) status. This is an immigration classification that may allow for the immigrant children to apply for lawful permanent resident status or “a Green Card”) (USCIS, 2014). This could be very helpful to child survivors so that they can have access to education, jobs, and resources while they are healing from the abuse and moving forward with their lives.

CONCLUSION

To conclude, immigration is a cornerstone feature of the United States (Adams, 1931; Bod, 2022). This attribute has remained a constant over time regardless of political rhetoric or community conjecture (Astrada & Astrada, 2019). Subsequently, more is still needed to be understood as it relates to immigration and violent crime, such as the impact immigration status has on hate crime victimization. In addition, the ability to better unpack and address violence in the household between intimate partners and violence directed toward children regardless of immigration status, is important for individuals and institutions.

As a result, this chapter unpacked this topic so community stakeholders, researchers, and practitioners can have a better understanding surrounding this topic. The ability to highlight contextual information and gaps in recording practices illustrates potential areas of improvement. For example, research has noted the additional barriers present to immigrants when engaging with the criminal justice system and other social institutions (Dettlaff & Earner, 2012; Erez et al., 2009). This line of research highlights the need to be more receptive to the needs of all parties regardless of age, language, or cultural factors. The following section details proposed policy recommendations. Directly following policy recommendations will be avenues for future research.

Policy Recommendations

Policy recommendations are framed as individual and organizational. The reason for this approach is to highlight ways individuals can assist with addressing this issue from a "grass roots" movement perspective. Organizational-based policy recommendations are meant to improve organizational practices and potential law changes. The ability to better serve individuals, regardless of immigration status, not only impacts individuals, communities, and institutions but generations to come as well. In essence, we are advocating that the huddled masses have a voice across social platforms and are truly counted by institutions. The following expands on individual- and institutional-level policy recommendations.

For instance, FEMA (n.d.) advocates that individuals interested in addressing human trafficking should help expand awareness within communities and understand vulnerabilities within various communities. Motivated individuals should understand that asylum seekers, refugees, and marginalized individuals (i.e., immigrants) are at elevated risk for trafficking practices (Hope for Justice, 2024; Nazer & Greenbaum, 2020). Therefore, individual practices should extend beyond just wearing blue (FEMA, n.d.) to focused conversations and actions that identify those at the highest risk with human trafficking and other victimization. The crux being to create an environment that is welcoming for all individuals regardless of how they fall on the immigration spectrum.

Institutional policy recommendations should be thought about from a private and public sector perspective. More specifically, refinement to policy should not be limited to only public sector institutions such as, criminal justice organization responses. Instead, interested parties should examine ways other social institutions (e.g., hospitals, safe houses, etc.) can improve practices alongside private organizations and non-profits such as *Hope For Justice* and *United We Dream*. Partnership, coloration, and communication are key elements to achieving pro-social outcomes across a variety of social problems.

Although strides have been made to provide legal and political protection to immigrant survivors, more is needed. The National Network to End Domestic Violence (2024) identifies the need for a comprehensive immigration reform that would strengthen and develop policies to support the following: increase the number of visas available annually, include child and elder abuse as qualifying crimes, improve survivors' access to critical safety net benefits, ensure that children and dependent spouses can petition independently for legal status, ensure that organizations assisting undocumented immigrants are not criminally penalized. It is also imperative to create policies and environments among law and immigration enforcement in which immigrants are not afraid to come forward to report the abuses against them. A survey sent out in 2017 to 715 advocates and attorneys from 46 states were asked about their experiences working with immigrant survivors (Tahirih Justice Center, n.d.). The results showed 78% of advocates reported that survivors had concerns about contacting the police, 75% have concerns about going to court for matters related to their abuser, and 43% worked with immigrant survivors who dropped civil or criminal cases because of fear. Many cultures view involving the criminal justice system as a last resort (Akinsulure-Smith et al., 2013). Therefore, more collaborations and coalitions need to be made between those working in immigrant communities and the criminal justice system to build trust. Messing et al. point out that survivors need greater trust that they will receive help from police than their fear of being deported to report abuse (2015). More training is needed for law enforcement to understand the ways in which abusers will try to manipulate the system against the abuser so that they are more equipped to handle these situations (Sabri, 2018).

Policy can also be created to provide more protection for unaccompanied minors. In 2008 as a part of the zero-tolerance policy, thousands of kids were separated from their parents at the border and many still have not be reunified (Klika, 2020). This policy cannot be allowed to continue as it causes extreme trauma to families and leaves children more vulnerable to other abuses. It is also important to implement policies that provide more support and monitoring of unaccompanied minors after their release from shelters to new caregivers in the US to ensure that abuse does not continue to ensue (Young et al., 2024). With this information in mind, we now turn toward future research areas.

Future Research

A need for future research concerning violent offenses and the immigrant population is necessary to know how to best address these important issues from a micro and macro level. For example, finding the exact statistics of immigrant IPV is challenging due the large ranges that have been found in studies (Morrison et al., 2024). Therefore, it is recommended that larger, more random samples be used to get more accurate prevalence estimates. More standardization of IPV measures and a broader definition if IPV may better include IPV related to immigration. More research is needed to understand the risk and protective factors for men survivors of abuse. Only one meta-analysis was found that included the experience of male survivors (Spencer et al., 2022). The factors that protect and put men at risk for abuse may be different not only by being a male but also depending on what culture they are immigrating from. Therefore, research could expand on more country and culture specific information for men and women. Similarly to IPV rates of abuse for immigrant children can be hard to determine since national level statistics do not include immigrant status. Research therefore has used samples from places like the child welfare system but have found that immigrants are underrepresented in those agencies (Dettlaff & Earner, 2012).

Taken collectively, this chapter unpacks information associated with violent victimization among immigrants. The discussion provided should not be viewed as exhaustive. Instead, it only starts to unfold what is known in relation to unique factors associated with immigrants residing within the United States and three complex crime types that need further examination. In addition, the authors advocate that future discussions should also include other crime categories so individual-and institutional-level responses can be more refined to better serve the needs of this unique population (Kenny et al., 2020; Kuussisto & Kuusisto, 2015; Schultze-Krumbholz et al., 2022; Maynard et al., 2016). Put simply, new information removes restraints so that immigrants can be better heard and understood across social institutions and communities within the United States.

REFERENCES

Adams, J. T. (1931). *The epic of America*. Little Brown.

Afifi, T., MacMillan, H., Boyle, M., Cheung, K., Taillieu, T., Turner, S., & Sareen, J. (2016). Child abuse and physical health in adulthood. *Health Reports*, *27*, 10–18. PMID: 26983007

Akinsulure-Smith, A. M., Chu, T., Keatley, E., & Rasmussen, A. (2013). Intimate partner violence among West African immigrants. *Journal of Aggression, Maltreatment & Trauma*, *22*(1), 109–129. DOI: 10.1080/10926771.2013.719592 PMID: 23730146

Alink, L. R. A., Euser, S., IJzendoorn, M. H., & Bakermans-Kranenburg, M. J. (2013). Is elevated risk of child maltreatment in immigrant families associated with socioeconomic status? Evidence from three sources. *International Journal of Psychology*, *48*(2), 117–127. DOI: 10.1080/00207594.2012.734622 PMID: 23597011

American Immigration Council. (2022). *Take a look: How immigrants drive the economy in United States of America*. Retrieved from https://map.americanimmigrationcouncil.org/locations/national/

Anonymous. (2022). *When immigration becomes a tool in intimate partner violence*. BWJP. Retrieved from https://bwjp.org/when-immigration-becomes-a-tool-in-intimate-partner-violence/?gad_source=1&gclid=Cj0KCQjwhb60BhClARIsABGGtw9hIGTRz9tOX_lk6mP-2O_9asvXzIyRQ3KZ6zNptugl4kNqrH6jaB8aAqVEEALw_wcB

Anti-Defamation League. (2018). *Mainstreaming hate: The Anti-immigrant movement in the U.S.* https://www.adl.org/resources/report/mainstreaming-hate-anti-immigrant-movement-us

Astrada, S. B., & Astrada, M. L. (2019). Truth in Crisis: Critically Re-Examining Immigration Rhetoric and Policy under the Trump Administration. *Harv. Latinx L. Rev.*, *22*, 7.

Bacchus, L. J., Ranganathan, M., Watts, C., & Devries, K. (2018). Recent intimate partner violence against women and health: A systematic review and meta-analysis of cohort studies. *BMJ Open*, *8*(7), e019995. DOI: 10.1136/bmjopen-2017-019995 PMID: 30056376

Barkho, E., Fakhouri, M., & Arnetz, J. E. (2011). Intimate partner violence among Iraqi immigrant women in metro Detroit: A pilot study. *Journal of Immigrant and Minority Health*, *13*(4), 725–731. DOI: 10.1007/s10903-010-9399-4 PMID: 20924789

Barner, J. R., & Carney, M. M. (2011). Interventions for intimate partner violence: A historical review. *Journal of Family Violence*, *26*(3), 235–244. DOI: 10.1007/s10896-011-9359-3

Baxter, A. M., & Nowrasteh, A. (2021). *A brief history of U.S. immigration policy from the colonial period to the present day*. Cato.org. https://www.cato.org/policy-analysis/brief-history-us-immigration-policy-colonial-period-present-day

Bick, J., & Nelson, C. A. (2016). Early adverse experiences and the developing brain. Neuropsychopharmacology, 41, 177–196. Retrieved from https://www.nature.com/articles/ npp2015252. DOI: 10.1038/npp.2015.252

Blackmore, R., Gray, K. M., Boyle, J. A., Fazel, M., Ranasinha, S., Fitzgerald, G., Misso, M., & Gibson-Helm, M. (2020). Systematic Review and Meta-analysis: The Prevalence of Mental Illness in Child and Adolescent Refugees and Asylum Seekers. *Journal of the American Academy of Child and Adolescent Psychiatry*, *59*(6), 705–714. DOI: 10.1016/j.jaac.2019.11.011 PMID: 31778780

Bod, E. (2022). *The evolution of the American Dream*. The Collector. https://www.thecollector.com/american-dream-evolution/

Breiding, M. J., Basile, K. C., Smith, S. G., Black, M. C., & Mahendra, R. R. (2015). *Intimate partner violence surveillance: Uniform definitions and recommended data elements* (version 2.0). National Center for Injury Prevention and Control, Centers for Disease Control and Prevention. https://www.cdc.gov/violenceprevention/pdf/ipv/intimatepartnerviolence.pdf

Breiding, M. J., Black, M. C., & Ryan, G. W. (2008). Chronic disease and health risk behaviors associated with intimate partner violence—18 U.S. States/Territories, 2005. *Annals of Epidemiology*, *18*(7), 538–544. DOI: 10.1016/j.annepidem.2008.02.005 PMID: 18495490

Bureau of Justice Statistics. (2021). *The National Crime Victimization Survey and Uniform Crime Reporting program: A complementary picture of crime in 2020*. https://bjs.ojp.gov/sites/g/files/xyckuh236/files/media/document/cv20_ncvs_ucr_supplement.pdf

Caputo, T. (2024). Mob of teens on bikes in DTLA brutally attacks, robs man seeking asylum in U.S. ABC 7 Eyewitness News. Retrieved from https://abc7.com/post/mob-teens-bikes-downtown-los-angeles-brutally-attacks-robs-immigrant-seeking-asylum-us/15175704/

CDC. (2024, October 17). About intimate partner violence. Https://www.cdc.gov/intimate-partner-violence/about/index.html?CDC_AAref_Val=https://www.cdc.gov/violenceprevention/intimatepartnerviolence/index.html

Child Abuse | Overview | Office of Justice Programs. (n.d.). Retrieved October 26, 2024, from https://www.ojp.gov/feature/child-abuse/overview

Child Welfare Information Gateway. (2015). Promoting protective factors for victims of child abuse and neglect: A guide for practitioners. Retrieved from https://www.Childwelfare.gov/pubs/factsheets/victimscan/

Child Welfare Information Gateway. (2019). Long-term consequences of child abuse and neglect. Washington, DC: U.S. Department of Health and Human Services, Administration for Children and Families, Children's Bureau. Retrieved from https://cwig-prod-prod-drupal-s3fs-us-east-1.s3.amazonaws.com/public/documents/long_term_consequences.pdf

Children on the Run—Full Report. (n.d.). UNHCR US. Retrieved October 23, 2024, from https://www.unhcr.org/us/media/children-run-full-report

Churchwell, S. (2021). *A brief history of the American Dream*. Bush Presidential Center., Retrieved from https://www.bushcenter.org/catalyst/state-of-the-american-dream/churchwell-history-of-the-american-dream

U.S. Citizenship and Immigration Services (USCIS, 2014). Immigration relief for abused children, Special Immigrant Juvenile Status. Retrieved from Immigration_Relief_for_Abused_Children-FINAL.pdf (uscis.gov)

Crawford, M. (2020). Ecological Systems Theory: Exploring the Development of the Theoretical Framework as Conceived by Bronfenbrenner Article Details. *Journal of Public Health Issues and Practices*, *4*(2), 170. DOI: 10.33790/jphip1100170

Crime Data Explorer. (2022a). https://cde.ucr.cjis.gov/LATEST/webapp/#/pages/explorer/crime/hate-crime

Crime Data Explorer. (2022b). https://cde.ucr.cjis.gov/LATEST/webapp/#/pages/explorer/crime/crime-trend

Crime Data Explorer. (2023a). https://cde.ucr.cjis.gov/LATEST/webapp/#/pages/explorer/crime/hate-crime

Crime Data Explorer. (2023b). https://cde.ucr.cjis.gov/LATEST/webapp/#/pages/explorer/crime/crime-trend

Crime Data Explorer. (2024a). https://cde.ucr.cjis.gov/LATEST/webapp/#/pages/explorer/crime/hate-crime

Crime Data Explorer. (2024b). https://cde.ucr.cjis.gov/LATEST/webapp/#/pages/explorer/crime/crime-trend

Danis, F. S. (2003). The criminalization of domestic violence: What social workers need to know. *Social Work*, *48*(2), 237–246. DOI: 10.1093/sw/48.2.237 PMID: 12718419

Decker, S. H. (2015). Human trafficking: Contexts and connections to conventional crime. *Journal of Crime and Justice*, *38*(3), 291–296. DOI: 10.1080/0735648X.2015.1039792

Dettlaff, A. J., & Earner, I. (2012). Children of Immigrants in the Child Welfare System: Characteristics, Risk, and Maltreatment. *Families in Society*, *93*(4), 295–303. DOI: 10.1606/1044-3894.4240

DHS. (n.d.) *Office of Homeland Security Statistics: Glossary*. U.S. Department of Homeland Security. Retrieved from https://ohss.dhs.gov/glossary#:~:text=Immigrant%3A%20Any%20person%20lawfully%20in,101(a)(15)

Dobash, R. E., & Dobash, R. P. (2003). *Women, Violence and Social Change*. Routledge. https://books.google.com/books?id=NWOIAgAAQBAJ

Dreier, H., & Luce, K. (2023). Alone and exploited, migrant children work brutal jobs across the US. The New York Times, 28.

Duleep, H. O., & Dowhan, D. J. (2008). Research on Immigrant Earnings. Social Security Administration. *Social Security Bulletin*, *68*(1). https://www.ssa.gov/policy/docs/ssb/v68n1/v68n1p31.html

Erez, E., Adelman, M., & Gregory, C. (2009). Intersections of Immigration and Domestic Violence: Voices of Battered Immigrant Women. *Feminist Criminology*, *4*(1), 32–56. DOI: 10.1177/1557085108325413

Euser, E. M., van IJzendoorn, M. H., Prinzie, P., & Bakermans-Kranenburg, M. J. (2011). Elevated Child Maltreatment Rates in Immigrant Families and the Role of Socioeconomic Differences. *Child Maltreatment*, *16*(1), 63–73. DOI: 10.1177/1077559510385842 PMID: 21041234

Ewing, W., Martinez, D., & Rumbaut, R. (2015). *The criminalization of immigration in the United States*. American Immigration Council. Retrieved from https://www.americanimmigrationcouncil.org/research/criminalization-immigration-united-states

FBI. (2016). *Hate crimes*. Retrieved from https://www.fbi.gov/investigate/civil-rights/hate-crimes

FBI. (2017). *Domestic violence.* Retrieved from https://ucr.fbi.gov/leoka/2017/resource-pages/leoka_definitions_-2017#:~:text=Domestic%20violence%E2%80%93The%20use%2C%20attempted,who%20is%20or%20has%20been

FBI. (2019). *Human trafficking.* https://ucr.fbi.gov/crime-in-the-u.s/2019/crime-in-the-u.s.-2019/additional-data-collections/human-trafficking

FBI. (2022). *Hate Crime Explorer.*https://cde.ucr.cjis.gov/LATEST/webapp/#/pages/explorer/crime/hate-crime

FBI. (2023). *Hate Crime Explorer.*https://cde.ucr.cjis.gov/LATEST/webapp/#/pages/explorer/crime/hate-crime

FBI. (2024). *Hate Crime Explorer.*https://cde.ucr.cjis.gov/LATEST/webapp/#/pages/explorer/crime/hate-crime

Feliz, W. (2019). *Sorry Donald Trump, immigration is still associated with less crime and safer communities.* Immigration Impact. Retrieved from https://immigrationimpact.com/2016/04/29/donald-trump-immigration-crime-facts/?gad_source=1&gclid=Cj0KCQjwhb60BhClARIsABGGtw_Hl3LsVQYU1_osri_DKeIiLAPa7kYHfSXU2KRnQn_s631uXVMGtEQaAg0kEALw_wcB#.XlKNAmhKiM8

FEMA. (n.d.) Five ways we can work together to prevent human trafficking. Retrieved from https://www.fema.gov/blog/5-ways-we-can-work-together-prevent-human-trafficking

Finkelhor, D., Turner, H. A., Shattuck, A., & Hamby, S. L. (2015). Prevalence of Childhood Exposure to Violence, Crime, and Abuse: Results from the National Survey of Children's Exposure to Violence. *JAMA Pediatrics, 169*(8), 746–754. DOI: 10.1001/jamapediatrics.2015.0676 PMID: 26121291

Finley, L., & Esposito, L. (2020). The immigrant as bogeyman: Examining Donald Trump and the right's anti-immigrant, anti-PC rhetoric. *Humanity & Society, 44*(2), 178–197. DOI: 10.1177/0160597619832627

Finley, L., & Esposito, L. (2020). The immigrant as bogeyman: Examining Donald Trump and the right's anti-immigrant, anti-PC rhetoric. *Humanity & Society, 44*(2), 178–197. DOI: 10.1177/0160597619832627

Finno-Velasquez, M., Sepp, S. M., Lopez, A., Aquino, E., Cherie, N., & Ortiz-Upston, M. (2023). Child maltreatment prevention interventions for Latinx immigrant populations: A systematic review. Journal of Public Child Welfare, 17(4), 845-878. https://doi.org/<link linkTarget="URL" linkWindow=""DOI: 10.1080/15548732.2022.2118929

Fletcher, M. J. (2024). *Unveiling the shadows: Human trafficking amidst immigration struggles in 2024*. BWJP. Retrieved from https://bwjp.org/unveiling-the-shadows-human-trafficking-amidst-immigration-struggles-in-2024/?gad_source=1&gclid=Cj0KCQjws560BhCuARIsAHMqE0F5PX51xaP8QO1LxAZlvK339_3zmuyO31BpwEEWJFytO5jJzvg7KIUaAoJjEALw_wcB

Foner, N. (2005). *In a new land: A comparative view of immigration*. New York University Press.

Gallegos, A. M., Trabold, N., Cerulli, C., & Pigeon, W. R. (2021). Sleep and interpersonal violence: A systematic review. *Trauma, Violence & Abuse*, *22*(2), 359–369. DOI: 10.1177/1524838019852633 PMID: 31131736

Goddard, C., & Bedi, G. (2010). Intimate partner violence and child abuse: A child-centred perspective. *Child Abuse Review*, *19*(1), 5–20. DOI: 10.1002/car.1084

Hartmann, M. (2019, November). *Human trafficking and immigrants*. The Exodus Road. https://theexodusroad.com/human-trafficking-and-u-s-immigration/?utm_term=&utm_campaign=&utm_source=adwords&utm_medium=ppc&hsa_tgt=dsa-19959388920&hsa_grp=123537986530&hsa_src=g&hsa_net

Herrenkohl, T. I., Jung, H., Lee, J. O., & Kim, M.-H. (2017). Effects of child maltreatment, cumulative victimization experiences, and proximal life stress on adult crime and antisocial behavior. Retrieved from https://www.ncjrs.gov/ pdffiles1/nij/grants/250506.pdf

Homeland Security. (n.d.). *Immigration Options for Victims of Crime*. Retrieved October 18, 2024, from https://www.dhs.gov/immigration-options-victims-crime

Hope For Justice. (2024). Who is vulnerable to human trafficking. Retrieved from https://hopeforjustice.org/news/who-is-vulnerable-to-human-trafficking/#:~:text=Asylum%20seekers%2C%20displaced%20people%20and,be%20factors%20that%20create%20refugees

House, T. W. (2022, March 16). *Fact Sheet: Reauthorization of the Violence Against Women Act (VAWA)*. The White House. https://www.whitehouse.gov/briefing-room/statements-releases/2022/03/16/fact-sheet-reauthorization-of-the-violence-against-women-act-vawa/

H.R. (1990). *1048 - 101st Congress (1989-1990)*. Hate Crime Statistics Act.

Immigration and Customs Enforcement. (n.d.). *Human trafficking*. https://www.ice.gov/features/human-trafficking

Immigration Policy. (2024). NNEDV. Retrieved October 18, 2024, from https://nnedv.org/content/immigration-policy/

Ingram, E. M. (2007). A Comparison of Help Seeking Between Latino and Non-Latino Victims of Intimate Partner Violence. *Violence Against Women, 13*(2), 159–171. DOI: 10.1177/1077801206296981 PMID: 17251503

International Association of Chiefs of Police. (2019). *Enhance the response to hate crimes.*https://www.theiacp.org/sites/default/files/2019-04/IACP_Hate%20Crimes_Full%Report.pdf

Jud, A., Pfeiffer, E., & Jarczok, M. (2020). Epidemiology of violence against children in migration: A systematic literature review. *Child Abuse & Neglect, 108*, 104634. DOI: 10.1016/j.chiabu.2020.104634 PMID: 32745801

Kapadia, F. (2024). Protecting immigrant children: A public health of consequence, March 2024. *American Journal of Public Health, 114*(3), 267–269. DOI: 10.2105/AJPH.2023.307569 PMID: 38382023

Kenny, K. S., Merry, L., Brownbridge, D. A., & Urquia, M. L. (2020). Factors associated with cyber-victimization among immigrants and non-immigrants in Canada: A cross-sectional nationally-representative study. *BMC Public Health, 20*(1), 1–13. DOI: 10.1186/s12889-020-09492-w PMID: 33066741

Klika, J. B., Rosenzweig, J., & Merrick, M. (2020). Economic Burden of Known Cases of Child Maltreatment from 2018 in Each State. *Child & Adolescent Social Work Journal, 37*(3), 227–234. DOI: 10.1007/s10560-020-00665-5

Kuusisto, T., & Kuusisto, R. (2015). Cyber world as a social system. In *Cyber security: Analytics, technology and automation* (pp. 31–43). Springer International Publishing. DOI: 10.1007/978-3-319-18302-2_2

Lagdon, S., Armour, C., & Stringer, M. (2014). Adult experience of mental health outcomes as a result of intimate partner violence victimization: A systematic review. *European Journal of Psychotraumatology, 5*(1), 24794. DOI: 10.3402/ejpt.v5.24794 PMID: 25279103

League, A. D. (2018). *Mainstreaming hate: The anti-immigrant movement in the US*. Anti-Defamation League.

LeBrun, A., Hassan, G., Boivin, M., Fraser, S.-L., Dufour, S., & Lavergne, C. (2015). Review of child maltreatment in immigrant and refugee families. *Canadian Journal of Public Health = Revue Canadienne de Santé Publique, 106*(Suppl 7), eS45. https://doi.org/DOI: 10.17269/CJPH.106.4838

Lee, M., & Weber, P. (2023). *The Texas Shooter in a racist Walmart attack is going to prison. here's what to know about the case*. AP News. https://apnews.com/article/el-paso-walmart-texas-crusius-bf7d25f3567959ee8b121deabcf1d9a1

Leeb, R. T., Paulozzi, L., Melanson, C., Simon, T., & Arias, I. (2008) Child Maltreatment Surveillance: Uniform Definitions for Public Health and Recommended Data Elements, Version 1.0. Atlanta (GA): Centers for Disease Control and Prevention, National Center for Injury Prevention and Control.

Linares, A. (2023). *Rise in hate crimes includes a "significant increase" against Latinos*. College of Social Sciences and Humanities. https://cssh.northeastern.edu/rise-in-hate-crimes-includes-a-significant-increase-against-latinos/

Lou, C., Adams, G., Bernstein, H., Baird, C., Feng, A., Hagerman, L., & Lei, S. (2019). *Part of us: A data-driven look at children of immigrants*. Urban Institute.

Mason-Bish, H. (2015). Beyond the silo: Rethinking hate crime and intersectionality. In N. Hall, A. Corb, P. Giannasi, & J. G. D. Grieve (Eds.), *The Routledge International Handbook on Hate Crime* (pp. 24-33). essay, Routledge, Taylor & Francis Group.

Maynard, B. R., Vaughn, M. G., Salas-Wright, C. P., & Vaughn, S. (2016). Bullying victimization among school-aged immigrant youth in the United States. *The Journal of Adolescent Health*, *58*(3), 337–344. DOI: 10.1016/j.jadohealth.2015.11.013 PMID: 26903431

Mazza, M., Marano, G., Del Castillo, A. G., Chieffo, D., Monti, L., Janiri, D., Moccia, L., & Sani, G. (2021). Intimate partner violence: A loop of abuse, depression and victimization. *World Journal of Psychiatry*, *11*(6), 215–221. DOI: 10.5498/wjp.v11.i6.215 PMID: 34168968

Merriam-Webster. (n.d.). *Immigrant definition & meaning*. Merriam-Webster. Retrieved from https://www.merriam-webster.com/dictionary/immigrant#:~:text=im%C2%B7%E2%80%8Bmi%C2%B7%E2%80%8Bgrant,to%20take%20up%20permanent%20residence

Migration Policy Institute. (2024). *Children in U.S. Immigrant Families*. (2013, November 13). Retrieved from https://www.migrationpolicy.org/programs/data-hub/charts/children-immigrant-families

Monnat, S. M., & Chandler, R. F. (2015). Long-term physical health consequences of adverse childhood experiences. *The Sociological Quarterly*, *56*(4), 723–752. DOI: 10.1111/tsq.12107 PMID: 26500379

Moore, R. (2023). *Man who killed 23 at El Paso Walmart pleads guilty to hate crimes*. The Texas Tribune. https://www.texastribune.org/2023/02/08/el-paso-walmart-shooting-pleads-guilty/

Morrison, A. M., Campbell, J. K., Sharpless, L., & Martin, S. L. (2024). Intimate Partner Violence and Immigration in the United States: A Systematic Review. *Trauma, Violence & Abuse*, *25*(1), 846–861. DOI: 10.1177/15248380231165690 PMID: 37078533

Moslimani, M., & Passel, J. S. (2024). What the data says about immigrants in the U.S. Pew Research Center. Retrieved from https://www.pewresearch.org/short-reads/2024/09/27/key-findings-about-us-immigrants/#:~:text=Where%20do%20most%20U.S.%20immigrants,%25)%20and%20West%20(33%25).

National Center on Domestic and Sexual Violence (NCDSV). (2024, October 18). *Immigrant Power and Control Wheel*. Retrieved from https://www.familyjusticecenter.org/wp-content/uploads/2017/10/Immigrant-Power-_-Control-Wheel-Domestic-Abuse-Intervention-Project.pdf

National Children's Alliance. (2024). *National Statistics on Child Abuse*. Retrieved October 20, 2024, from https://www.nationalchildrensalliance.org/media-room/national-statistics-on-child-abuse/

National Organization for Women (NOW). (2024, October 17). Intimate partner violence undocumented and immigrant women. https://now.org/wp-content/uploads/2017/06/Learn-More-IPV-and-Immigrant-Womenpdf.pdf

National Resource Center on Domestic Violence (NRCDV). (2021). *Public Policy & Advocacy* Retrieved August 6, 2021, from https://nrcdv.org/public-policy

Nazer, D., & Greenbaum, J. (2020). Human trafficking of children. *Pediatric Annals*, *49*(5), e209–e214. DOI: 10.3928/19382359-20200417-01 PMID: 32413148

Njie-Carr, V. P., Sabri, B., Messing, J. T., Suarez, C., Ward-Lasher, A., Wachter, K., Marea, C. X., & Campbell, J. (2020). Understanding Intimate Partner Violence among Immigrant and Refugee Women: A Grounded Theory Analysis. *Journal of Aggression, Maltreatment & Trauma*, *30*(6), 792–810. DOI: 10.1080/10926771.2020.1796870 PMID: 34483645

Norman, R. E., Byambaa, M., De, R., Butchart, A., Scott, J., & Vos, T. (2012). The Long-Term Health Consequences of Child Physical Abuse, Emotional Abuse, and Neglect: A Systematic Review and Meta-Analysis. *PLoS Medicine*, *9*(11), e1001349. DOI: 10.1371/journal.pmed.1001349 PMID: 23209385

NPS. (n.d.) Statue of Liberty: The New Colossus. Retrieved from https://www.nps.gov/stli/learn/historyculture/colossus.htm#:~:text=%22Give%20me%20your%20tired%2C%20your,refuse%20of%20your%20teeming%20shore

Ojito, M. A. (2014). *Hunting season: Immigration and murder in an All-American town*. Beacon Press.

Oladipo, G. (2024). Racism is embedded in our society': how attacks on immigrants in Ohio highlight US disinformation crisis. The Guardian. Retrieved from https://www.theguardian.com/us-news/2024/sep/18/trump-republicans-springfield-aurora-political-disinformation

Park, T., Mullins, A., Zahir, N., Salami, B., Lasiuk, G., & Hegadoren, K. (2021). Domestic Violence and Immigrant Women: A Glimpse Behind a Veiled Door. *Violence Against Women*, *27*(15–16), 2910–2926. DOI: 10.1177/1077801220984174 PMID: 33506739

Pearson, L. B. (1957). *The Four Faces of Peace. The Nobel Peace Prize 1957*. The University of Oslo.

Pedron, S. M., & da Cruz, J. D. A. (2021). US Immigration and Human Traffifficking Overlap. International Social Science Review (Online), 97(4), 0_1-19.

Popal, F. (2021). *Surviving or thriving? what it takes for immigrants to succeed.* Bush Presidential Center., https://www.bushcenter.org/catalyst/state-of-the-american-dream/popal-what-it-takes-to-make-it-in-america

Ragsdale, S. (2013). Immigrants in the United States of America. *Advances in Historical Studies*, *2*(03), 167–174. DOI: 10.4236/ahs.2013.23021

Reavell, J., & Fazil, Q. (2017). The epidemiology of PTSD and depression in refugee minors who have resettled in developed countries. *Journal of Mental Health (Abingdon, England)*, *26*(1), 74–83. DOI: 10.1080/09638237.2016.1222065 PMID: 27684305

Sabri, B., Nnawulezi, N., Njie-Carr, V. P. S., Messing, J., Ward-Lasher, A., Alvarez, C., & Campbell, J. C. (2018). Multilevel risk and protective factors for intimate partner violence among African, Asian, and Latina immigrant and refugee women: Perceptions of effective safety planning interventions. *Race and Social Problems*, *10*(4), 348–365. DOI: 10.1007/s12552-018-9247-z PMID: 31289602

Schultze-Krumbholz, A., Pfetsch, J. S., & Lietz, K. (2022). Cyberbullying in a multicultural context—Forms, strain, and coping related to Ethnicity-Based Cybervictimization. *Frontiers in Communication*, *7*, 846794. DOI: 10.3389/fcomm.2022.846794

Segal, U. A., & Mayadas, N. S. (2005). Assessment of issues facing immigrant and refugee families. *Child Welfare*, *84*(5), 563–583. PMID: 16435651

Sege, R. D., Amaya-Jackson, L., Flaherty, E. G., Idzerda, S. M., Legano, L. A., Leventhal, J. M., & Sege, R. D. (2017). Clinical considerations related to the behavioral manifestations of child maltreatment. *Pediatrics*, *139*(4), e20170100.

Shelley, L. (2013). Human trafficking as a form of transnational crime. In *Human trafficking* (pp. 116–137). Willan.

Shen, A. (2017). *What we know (and don't know) about immigrants and violent crime*. The Trace. https://www.thetrace.org/2017/02/immigrants-violent-crime-facts-donald-trump/?gad_source=1&gclid=Cj0KCQjwhb60BhClARIsABGGtw8XHP94atHLfCqxKeRuIdlG2m2jLQKo5p5yVm_dz7pUdFFYrpDaaBgaAuvOEALw_wcB

Smith, S. G., Zhang, X., Basile, K. C., Merrick, M. T., Wang, J., Kresnow, M., & Chen, J. (2018). *The National Intimate Partner and Sexual Violence Survey (NISVS): 2015 Data Brief*. National Center for Injury Prevention and Control, Centers for Disease Control and Prevention.

Southern Poverty Law Center. (2009). *Climate of fear: Latino immigrants in Suffolk County, N.Y.* https://www.splcenter.org/20090831/climate-fear-latino-immigrants-suffolk-county-ny

Southern Poverty Law Center. (2019). *Terror from the right*. https://www.splcenter.org/terror-from-the-right

Spencer, C. M., Stith, S. M., & Cafferky, B. (2022). What Puts Individuals at Risk for Physical Intimate Partner Violence Perpetration? A Meta-Analysis Examining Risk Markers for Men and Women. *Trauma, Violence & Abuse*, *23*(1), 36–51. DOI: 10.1177/1524838020925776 PMID: 32431231

Timshel, I., Montgomery, E., & Dalgaard, N. T. (2017). A systematic review of risk and protective factors associated with family related violence in refugee families. *Child Abuse & Neglect*, *70*, 315–330. DOI: 10.1016/j.chiabu.2017.06.023 PMID: 28683372

Trevillion, K., Oram, S., Feder, G., & Howard, L. M. (2012). Experiences of domestic violence and mental disorders: A systematic review and meta-analysis. *PLoS One*, *7*(12), e51740. DOI: 10.1371/journal.pone.0051740 PMID: 23300562

Turner, M. (2023). *Red and blue, who's hating who: An Examination of differences in hate crimes within traditional red and blue states*. ProQuest. https://www.proquest.com/openview/9ab583d83f6d5b8b1b22c708dacbb8ee/1?pq-origsite=gscholar&cbl=18750&diss=y

United Nations. (n.d.). *Migrant smuggling*. https://www.unodc.org/unodc/en/human-trafficking/migrant-smuggling/migrant-smuggling.html

United States Department of Justice. (2022). *Human trafficking*. United States Department of Justice. https://www.justice.gov/humantrafficking

U.S. Citizenship and Immigration Services. (2024). *DHS implements keeping families together*. https://www.uscis.gov/newsroom/news-releases/dhs-implements-keeping-families-together

U.S. Department of Homeland Security. (2017). *Deferred action for parents of Americans and lawful permanent residents recession memo ("Dapa"): Homeland Security*. https://www.dhs.gov/publication/deferred-action-parents-americans-and-lawful--residents-recession-memo-dapa

U.S. Department of Justice. (2023). *Texas man sentenced to 90 consecutive life sentences for 2019 mass shooting at Walmart in El Paso, Texas, killing 23 people and injuring 22 others*. https://www.justice.gov/opa/pr/texas-man-sentenced-90-consecutive-life-sentences-2019-mass-shooting-walmart-el-paso-texas

Vesti. (2023). *Immigration and refugees: Understanding the challenges and opportunities*. LinkedIn. https://www.linkedin.com/pulse/immigration-refugees-understanding-challenges-opportunities/

Warsi, Z. (2023). Hundreds of immigrants have reported sexual abuse at Ice facilities. Most cases aren't investigated. PBS News. Retrieved from https://www.pbs.org/newshour/nation/hundreds-of-immigrants-have-reported-sexual-abuse-at-ice-facilities-most-cases-arent-investigated

Widom, C. S., Czaja, S. J., Bentley, T., & Johnson, M. S. (2012). A prospective investigation of physical health outcomes in abused and neglected children: New findings from a 30-year follow-up. *American Journal of Public Health, 102*(6), 1135–1144. DOI: 10.2105/AJPH.2011.300636 PMID: 22515854

Wiggins, K. (2024). What Congress should do about hate crime statistics. https://www.lawfaremedia.org/article/what-congress-should-do-about-hate-crime-statistics#:~:text=To%20improve%20hate%20crime%20statistics,impose%20hate%20crime%20reporting%20mandates

Xie, M., & Baumer, E. P. (2021). Immigrant status, citizenship, and victimization risk in the United States: New findings from the National Crime Victimization Survey (NCVS). *Criminology, 59*(4), 610–644. DOI: 10.1111/1745-9125.12278 PMID: 35177865

Young, J., Binford, W., Bochenek, M. G., & Greenbaum, J. (2024). Health Risks of Unaccompanied Immigrant Children in Federal Custody and in US Communities. *American Journal of Public Health*, *114*(3), 340–346. DOI: 10.2105/AJPH.2023.307570 PMID: 38330256

Chapter 5
Care and Connection via Day Labor Centers and Others Like Them:
Providing Informal Sources of Critical Support for (Im)Migrants

Julie Goodman-Bowling
https://orcid.org/0009-0002-7753-6850
California Baptist University, USA

ABSTRACT

Care and Connection via Day Labor Centers and Others Like Them: Creating Informal Sources of Critical Support for (Im)Migrants In this chapter, the role of day labor centers, and others like them, is considered as a potential source of critical support for (im)migrant workers. Through an ethnographic study of a particular day labor center alongside recent scholarship, this chapter discusses the core challenges of labor migration, the precariousness of day labor in particular, and how labor centers (and others like them) can offer tangible and emotional support for (im)migrants. Centers like these may expand to offer psychological and social services, medical care, and access to important physical provisions. In so doing, (im)migrants may improve their resiliency, knowing that they have an emotionally and physically supportive space from which to draw strength and resources, and ultimately, improve their chances for positive mental health outcomes as they contribute to their families and communities.

DOI: 10.4018/979-8-3693-7944-8.ch005

INTRODUCTION

Labor migration has come to characterize an essential part of global financial processes that has rapidly expanded in recent decades. Around the world, employers are compelled to prioritize profit, minimize costs, and increase output. The most negotiable element in the production of goods and services is in the labor; as a result, employers compete for workers – particularly those who are cheap and flexible (Constable, 2014). Migrant workers in the United States are employed in several sectors – from domestic work (maids, healthcare workers, nannies, and gardeners) to factories and fields (meat-packing plants, garment production, and seasonal farming) (Bonacich & Appelbaum, 2000; Striffler, 2005; Holmes, 2013; Horton, 2016). Increasingly, a source of necessary labor in the U.S. are migrant day laborers, workers who set out each day in hopes of finding a job to provide for themselves and potentially the families and communities whom they have left behind in pursuit of wage labor (Goodman-Bowling, 2018). The challenges that migrant workers face on a regular basis include racism, discrimination, wage-theft, maltreatment, and risking their very health as they serve in precarious and, often, dangerous occupations. Further, they face uncertainty each day as jobs may not be available or they may be rejected for any number of reasons, including appearance, lack of language or insufficient skill or experience.

Migrant day laborers, the population for which the ethnographic data for this chapter are drawn, are usually found waiting for jobs on local street corners outside of home improvement stores, nurseries, or paint shops – locations related to the type of work that day laborers are typically hired to do. They may also assemble informally on street corners, outside convenience stores, or in some public grounds in view of potential employers. As a primarily undocumented workforce, migrant day laborers are vulnerable and susceptible to labor violations and discriminatory practices. And yet, given that day labor is a unique, and inexpensive form of labor, the demand for workers has grown alongside an increasingly hostile economic environment where the demand for low-wage labor is high. Migrant workers, then, have been drawn to these positions, however precarious (Martin et al., 2007; Goodman-Bowling, 2018).

Based on ethnographic research alongside recent scholarship, this chapter centralizes the benefits of migrant labor centers and other gathering spaces like them to help mitigate the many physical and psychological challenges that migrants endure. (Martin et al., 2007; Theodore, 2023). During the two-year span upon which this ethnographic study is based, between 2016 and 2018, the researcher learned about the harrowing situations that migrants faced when crossing the U.S. – Mexico border, their motivation to flee their homelands for the hope of safety and security, and the agony of living apart from their families – including their spouses, children, and parents. Clearly, for many, these are traumatic experiences and have had numerous effects on their daily lives and their hopes for the future. Indeed, for some, engaging in the interview process alone proved therapeutic as several workers thanked the researcher for asking such in-depth and meaningful questions about their migration experience. They commented that it allowed them time to reflect on the gravity of what they had been through and what they continually experienced being far from home[1] (Goodman-Bowling, 2018).

Without a solid community of belonging, a psychological sense of security, and regular emotional support, migrant workers may fall victim to feelings of isolation, depression, and distress. Many migrant workers experience these challenges while simultaneously feeling pressure to perform financially and to fulfill their roles as men and women with dependents who are counting on them to succeed. Stress, which is a major factor for migrant workers (Organista, 2008; Organista et al., 2013), also contributes to physical health problems for which migrant workers may have little ability to address for fear of missing out on work opportunities or the cost of accessing healthcare.

The Day Labor Center (DLC), the location where the core ethnographic study discussed in this chapter took place, proved to be a space where migrant workers *could* find support in several ways. The DLC is a grass-roots collective of primarily migrant day laborers in Southern California who joined forces in 2011 to create a space for laborers to safely gather without the fear of apprehension, the constant competition for jobs like those at other, more informal gathering spaces (typically street corners and parking lots), and who desired to pull together communal support. In collaboration with the local city Police Department, the DLC organized workers, hired a formal director, and became a location of laborers, community partners, and an informal cultural community space. Over time, the DLC grew to include educational opportunities wherein migrant workers learned about labor rights and how to address violations. Several volunteer organizations visited the Day Labor Center, offering food and even spiritual encouragement on a regular basis. In coming together as a collective at the Day Labor Center, migrant workers insisted on a minimum wage for all workers, changing the expectation for employers that they could compete with potential workers for lower wages (Theodore, 2020).

Further, their collectivism resulted in various activities that would create opportunities for workers to garner a large sum of money at one time through a daily lottery. This was a strategy to support one another financially to pay a large bill (rent) or purchase a particular asset (an expensive tool) or serve an important need (funerals, coming-of-age celebrations). And as a culturally inclusive space, migrants often gathered at the Day Labor Center simply for fellowship as they found a kinship group, sharing in their mutual challenges, victories, and shared experiences as migrants in a host community[2]. These exchanges were invaluable and contributed to the prevention of psychological distress for those who regularly participated.

Finally, one of the core advantages of this Center was the director, Ricardo, who often served as a leader, coordinator, and mentor for new arrivals – recent migrants *and* workers who were new to day labor. His investment of time and energy helped each person have an opportunity to feel known, seek guidance, and ask for help. Ricardo maintained a make-shift food pantry, coordinated networking among workers to help expand the advantage of potential jobs, and spent each day engaging with workers of whom he knew all of them by name. In these acts and others like them, migrant workers felt connected and known, and even missed if they did not show up for a while. The value of this kind of relational care is immeasurable and can prove a positive game-changer for many migrant workers on the brink of isolation and distress. First, this chapter will address the many challenges that immigrants face, particularly those in the day labor sector, but also extend to the general shared experiences among im/migrants drawing on research and the qualitative data collection from migrant workers at the Day Labor Center. Then, using the Day Labor Center as a model, the importance of migrant workers centers and others like them will be addressed as they can provide critical services for the care of im/migrant workers, community members, and their families. Finally, suggestions for medical and psychological attention and support will be provided in hopes of applying the research and data to on-the-ground, tangible support to address the health and well-being of migrant workers who make up a vast of part of America's communities and labor force around the nation.

CHALLENGES MIGRANT WORKERS FACE

Migrant workers face a plethora of challenges as a result of their experiences of migration in general, the lack of available, accessible, helpful resources, and extended separation from their families and home communities. One of the most pressing stresses for migrant day laborers includes the structural vulnerabilities they frequently face (Organista & Ngo, 2019). The psychological distress of being apart from family and dealing with the everyday stress of eking out a living to support themselves and their families has many negative effects on their mental health. Further, occupational hazards are common as the types of jobs that migrant workers are typically hired to do are precarious, sometimes dangerous, and are provided without protections often afforded in other labor sectors. Maltreatment by bosses and supervisors may also contribute to the stressful nature of this work. Finally, problems arise that are connected to these core issues including low wage living, food insecurity, and an increased risk of experiencing illness and disease for which they cannot afford care. This section will elaborate on the challenges migrants face that contribute to their overall psychological and physical distress.

Structural Vulnerabilities: Discrimination and Racism

Migrant day laborers are a vulnerable population. Migrant workers may face any number of what has been anthropologically described as *structural vulnerabilities,* referring to experiences of exclusionary political policies, discrimination based on illegality, and exploitation as a result of one's legal status (Quesada et al., 2014; Golash-Boza, 2009; Negi, 2013; Organista et al., 2013; Raythod, 2016; Theodore et al., 2009; Walter et al., 2004). Several workers at the Day Labor Center discussed their encounters with racism on the job even though the DLC was situated in a very accepting community, which will be addressed later in this chapter. One worker shared about his experience with racism as a "felt experience" – one that is based on assumptions which are made about migrants. Another described how the terms "dirty," "wetback," and "illegals" all spoke to misconceptions about migrant workers, based on something as arbitrary as their skin color, language skills (and accents) and their line of work. Several workers attested to having had people shout at the workers en masse at the DLC to "go home!" or "*mojados!*" though the researcher never witnessed this type of exchange (Goodman-Bowling, 2018).

One of the most telling stories of experiencing racism on the job was told by Andy, who had been on a job for several hours, working on a landscaping project outside on a very hot day. When he asked the employer for water, they took a dirty milk jug from the recycle bin, rinsed it with hose water, and then refilled it and gave it to Andy to drink. He described this experience, noting that he felt like a dog who was expected to drink dirty water; he felt insulted and angry that he could be treated this way. On a similar occasion, Andy accepted a job which was negotiated to include lunch. After four hours of hard labor, the employer provided a cheap, fast-food hamburger, gave the receipt to Andy and said he would deduct the cost from his earnings. Andy referred to these experiences as his "two humiliations," a horrible way to remember these life-changing instances (Goodman-Bowling, 2018, p. 78).

Workers may also be discriminated against for other criteria including age, gender, and appearance. Younger males are most likely to get offered employment as they are assumed to be stronger and have more energy to complete difficult jobs. Of the two women who regularly visited the Center in search of work, it was assumed that they would only be interested in cleaning jobs, even though one of the ladies shared that she most enjoyed demolition jobs. For others, it was apparent that the lighter their skin color, the greater chances they had of getting hired. Even one's appearance of cleanliness, hygiene, and appropriateness may play a factor in hire-ability. Taking pride in one's appearance was a high value for workers at the DLC as they knew it would be a factor in whether or not they might be hired. When Stan, a young, casual worker who came to the DLC to find temporary employment, showed up dressed in pajamas, the other workers were appalled. Stan claimed he didn't have enough time to get dressed since he wanted to get to the DLC on time to be eligible to participate in the lottery. Several of the workers noted that they felt insulted by this behavior as Stan did not clearly did not appreciate the hard work that these migrant day laborers were committed to doing well. To his own admission, Stan claimed it should not matter since this "wasn't a real job anyways," (Goodman-Bowling, 2018, p. 81). For others, affordability was a greater issue as clothing was an expense that many workers were unwilling to make on a regular basis. Painting, construction, and landscaping jobs frequently resulted in tattered clothing and stained fabrics. Some employers did not prioritize appearance, but many did, expecting workers to appear somewhat professional.

Being assessed by one's age, appearance, linguistic ability, and/or ethnic or racial identity left many workers feeling objectified with their vulnerability being sold to the highest bidder (or lottery winner as is the case at the DLC). This plays into their overall mental health, as workers are regularly exposed to feelings of being treated as a commodity or racialized by the community.

Occupational Hazards: Difficult Conditions and Wage Left

The very nature of day labor comes with the risk as a direct result of the type of work they are hired to do. "Most jobs also require physical strength to lift weighty tools, maneuver awkwardly shaped and heavy objects (like moving furniture or handling lumber), or perform demolition of concrete, brick, or tile… agility is required to move quickly and accurately. Working on roofs, climbing up ladders, and using heavy equipment may lead to injuries that could potentially reduce day laborers' ability to work for long periods at a time or altogether," (Goodman-Bowling, 2018, p. 67; Haro et al., 2020). At the Day Labor Center, workers often referred to back injuries, muscular pain, and joint pain as a result of kneeling for long periods of time working on laying carpet and tile and even the occasional burns or falls that may be rare but nonetheless are very damaging as a workers' entire income-earning ability may be permanently affected by an injury. For example, Diego, a worker at the Day Labor Center, experienced an injury to his ankle which required surgery to rectify (expensive and time consuming for Diego). The injury impeded on his ability to climb ladders and hold his bodily position for long periods of time. He thought the pain would be temporary but unfortunately, applying too much pressure for extended periods of time made the pain worse. Diego had a solid network of employers which allowed him some freedom to refuse jobs that would aggravate his ankle, but his financial needs frequently compelled him to work through the pain (Goodman-Bowling, 2018). Two workers at the DLC had long-impacting injuries because of being hit by a car. Badly bruised and permanently injured, these workers were limited in the types of jobs they could accept, the length of time that they could work, and the wages they could insist upon, given their abilities.

As workers age, physical changes in their bodies may also begin to limit their work prospects. Without access to consistent medical care and regular check-ups for preventative healthcare strategies to be implemented, older laborers have an increased risk of injury and the impact of any illness or injury is magnified. Regularly screening for occupational, physical, or mental health illnesses are not available for the vast majority of the migrant labor force. As one worker commented, "sometimes you are asked to do risky work, but we need it to make money," (Goodman-Bowling, 2018, p. 70). As the primary wage earners for their families, avoiding injuries and illness is a priority for migrant workers, though they are certainly unpredictable (Goodman-Bowling, 2018).

Day laborers are also vulnerable due to the precarity of their work arrangements and their low socioeconomic status and documentation status. (Galemba & Kuhn, 2021; Goodman-Bowling, 2018). Recent migrants are more susceptible to wage theft as their knowledge of the culture, work arrangements, and language skills may be far less developed than those who have lived and worked in the United States for longer periods of time (Galemba & Kuhn, 2021). Consistent with the qualitative fieldwork at the Day Labor Center, migrants who had been in the States longer understood the processes of negotiation, wage expectations, and were networked more significantly with other workers and employers, reducing the likelihood of being taken advantage of (Goodman-Bowling, 2018). Wage theft can come in many forms as one worker, Andy, described:

> *"I went to the job and the lady said she would pay me about $220 for some gardening work. When we arrived, I asked her which of the rows of plants she wanted done; she said, 'only that side.'" Andy finished the job in half the time he expected and was proud of his work. When Andy showed the employer the completed job, she insisted that he finish another, adjacent row of plants, upset that it was not done already. "But you told me only to do one side," explained Andy. The woman argued that she had directed him to complete "both sides" and insisted he return the following day to finish the second row of plants in order to get paid at all. Andy continued, "It isn't fair; I had to return another day to finish the job, but she didn't tell me that she wanted both rows done in the first place!" (Goodman-Bowling, 2018, p. 57).*

Miguel, a new student to the English class at the DLC, shared a similar experience:

> *One time, I went on a moving job with a guy. He was fine to pay $15 per hour. He took us to three places: Los Angeles, Hollywood, and somewhere else in LA. It took all day! When he brought us back here, he paid us only for two hours. When we asked why, he said because he wasn't going to pay for the time we spent traveling." Miguel was able to negotiate for another hour of pay for a total of*

three paid hours for six hours of actual time spent on the job… the employer did not disclose that he intended to pay only for time spent actually moving boxes and furniture, not the driving time." (Goodman-Bowling, 2018, p. 57-58).

Other forms of wage theft occur when an employer underestimates the time and difficulty of a particular job. Moving jobs and demolition projects are often culprits for this. Employers typically underestimate the number of boxes to carry and the difficulty of moving large, awkward objects like furniture. Further, cleaning up or taking items to a dumpster are long, drawn out processes, often involving the need for more hands to help. One worker explained that demolition usually required more time than originally expected and it was painful if a worker agreed to complete a particular project only to find that "completion" would take much longer than the employer initially projected.

One of the reasons that migrant workers choose to engage in day labor as their primary form of income is the ability to draw a good wage. Though work is often deemed "unskilled labor," every job requires a particular set of skills for which a laborer should be remunerated fairly. Workers learned strategies – mainly enforcing a minimum wage for all of the workers utilizing the Day Labor Center (power in numbers) so that no one would agree to take a job for less than $15 per hour (Goodman-Bowling, 2018) but many other workers in low-wage sectors cannot employ this strategy. There is no lack of low-wage labor for a willing migrant labor force alongside the consequences of working in difficult conditions in several sectors.

Migrant workers are often employed in labor sectors which require little to no formal education, involve physically stressing activities, and which pay wages which are usually under national requirements. Marginalized workers can be found in factories (Bank-Muñoz, 2008; Lugo, 2008; Striffler, 2005; Tuttle, 2012) in agricultural sectors (Bade, 1999; Holmes, 2013; Horton, 2016; Sanchez, 2013), and similar settings where individuals have very little control over their work circumstances. Immigration status, language barriers, and being labeled, often erroneously, an "unskilled" worker, contribute to migrant laborers' vulnerability to dehumanizing treatment, extreme controls in the workplace, and dangerous working conditions. Farmworkers suffer from gastritis, hypertension, headaches, joint pain, risk of injuries, and are exposed to extreme temperatures and dangerous pesticides (Bade, 1999; Holmes, 2013; Horton, 2016, as cited in Goodman-Bowling, 2018, p. 56). Factory workers are exposed to "toxins, mutagenic and carcinogenic chemicals, the operation of dangerous and antiquated machinery that lacks safeguards to prevent injury, lack of protective equipment and clothing, stress or disease caused by long hours of repetitive motion, and a denial of information on chemicals in the workplace" (Cravey, 1998, p. 96; see also Denman, 1997, in Goodman-Bowling, 2018, p. 56). Expectations for worker productivity can stress workers' bodies as supervisors frequently speed up factory conveyor belts to increase output, regardless of workers' requests to slow down the pace (Striffler, 2005). These conditions are extremely stressful and place workers in positions where they have little or no control over their circumstances. Finally, workers in these sectors and in day labor, do not receive health insurance, vacation time, paid sick-leave, or financial planning products (such as retirement savings and investments). Workers must make difficult decisions about working through illness and injury, knowing that they cannot take time off to rest, rejuvenate, or spend much-needed time with their families. Losing a day or week of wages can be detrimental for migrant workers who depend on the day-to-day payment to pay for their lives which causes anxiety and stress.

Bound to the demands of a labor-intensive job while under the watchful eye of strict supervisors, marginalized workers experience a heightened risk of depression, feeling little freedom or hope for their own futures. The demands of this kind of work do not allow space for much personal investment or growth (such as higher education or graduate studies) as the day-to-day demand is overwhelmingly taxing. Thus, social and economic mobility is extremely limited, affecting the mental and physical health and hopefulness of workers and their families.

Reporting violations of labor codes or wage theft can be very risky for migrants, particularly if they are undocumented (Haro et al., 2020; Valdez et al., 2019). If undocumented immigrants report maltreatment to the authorities, they may risk deportation or other consequences so many choose not to report such instances. In locations where there is no social support or network of workers (i.e. at informal gathering sites for workers), risk of maltreatment is far more likely. Regarding injuries, about half of day laborers surveyed who had been injured on the job in the year prior, did not obtain medical attention because they could not afford it, the employer refused to pay, or they did not seek treatment for fear of being apprehended for their lack of documentation (Valenzuela et al., 2006).

Nicholas shared about his experience on a job where he nearly sliced off one of his fingers. It was a moving job, and he had jammed his finger between a garage door and a concrete block. The employer, who was Mexican (same as Nicholas) dropped him off at a hospital but would not pay for his expenses. Nicholas was disappointed because, in his words he, "expected my own to be better to me," (Goodman-Bowling, 2018, p. 69). Racialization and discrimination are exposed in many forms for migrant workers, adding a layer to their already insecure positionality.

Psychological Distress and Deleterious Coping Methods

Much of the recent literature points to the ways in which day laborers are most prone to poor health, mental and physical. Galvan and his colleagues (2015) discuss the psychological effects of constant poverty, unpredictability, and living as a marginalized population – all of which result in chronic stress. Stress has incredible effects on the body, including increased cortisol (the hormone which increases the "flight" response to anxiety) leading to increased fatigue, pain, and even risk of cancer (Pham et al., 2024), lack of restful sleep leading to cognitive impairment (Choshen et al., 2021), and weight gain (Fogelman et al., 2022) along with its many related metabolic disorders and comorbidities (Lustig, 2021). These risks put workers at a great disadvantage in terms of their future health and their perceived hopefulness of returning home to their families or being able to provide for their families in the long term.

The story of Mateo, a worker at the Day Labor Center, reveals some of the most pressing issues that migrants face physically and psychologically. Mateo was typically quite gregarious, spoke English very well, and was very interested in the anthropological research being conducted at the DLC. Always willing to help the researcher gather students for the English class, informal conversations, and interviews, Mateo was welcoming and likable. Originally from Mexico, Mateo came to the United States to work when his son was quite young and had been separated from him for nearly six years at the time of interviewing. Over that time, Mateo's mother and him had separated, a result of the extended distance between them, and another man had been introduced into Mateo's son's life. As much as the new *novio* (boyfriend) had been playing a role of a father figure in his life, Mateo's son often begged his father to come home. Mateo's primary goal was to return to Mexico to be present for his son but he felt ashamed about not having made nearly as much money as he wanted to before he went home, a feeling shared by many migrant men who travel north as a sign of their masculine duty, in hopes of providing for their families (Boehm, 2008; Parreñas, 2005; Walter et al., 2004). One day, Mateo fell ill with a terrible flu and was feeling horribly drained of energy as he placed his head down on the table and confessed to having taken a lot of Nyquil. Alone in the corner of a table covered in tissues and wearing an oversized sweatshirt, Mateo would not be able to work until he regained his strength and fought off the virus. Unfortunately, he had also recently fell upon hard times, having lost his housing situation and was staying at the local Mission, a short-term housing facility for unsheltered men. Relying on public transportation to get to the DLC, Mateo had arrived late on several occasions which was a disqualifier for participating in the daily lottery for jobs. Further, the shelter required exit and entry be at specific times, so if Mateo arrived too late, he may not be permitted entry the shelter for an evening.

Sick, without work, and without a stable housing situation, Mateo began to devolve into the cycle of poverty and was experiencing the stress, anxiety, and depression that situations like his often induce. While interacting with Mateo, he went from a usually positive and cheery persona to progressively more distant and depressed. He sometimes spoke with some optimism about returning home to his son, but his goal to return home was delayed on several occasions. Mateo apparently had borrowed money from other workers and developed a reputation for not fulfilling his obligations. This damaged the relationships he had built with others at the DLC and eventually, he stopped coming altogether. Mateo exemplifies how harsh working conditions can lead to logistical challenges, and eventually, to depression. With little to no consistent resources for diagnosing chronic illness and mental health challenges, migrants are at increased risk of developing debilitating situations which are detrimental in the short and long terms (Goodman-Bowling, 2018).

Another young worker at the DLC, Stefan, also shared his experience with depression as a result of compounding circumstances. Like Mateo, Stefan was also helping to provide for a son, though he had no contact with him or the mother on a regular basis. He lived with his mother and sister in the local community and had been in the United States since he was a young child. He had been optimistic about being able to fill out his paperwork to establish his eligibility for the Deferred Action for Childhood Arrivals (DACA), a policy initiative which would extend citizenship to children of migrants under a certain age when they entered the United States. Stefan had experienced a combination of factors, including a disability, having been born without one of his arms fully intact, experiencing poverty, and at one point, becoming homeless as a result. Without a regular address to depend on, his DACA documents were lost, and he was under great pressure to be able to figure it out before he hit the age when he would not be eligible. In his desperation, Stefan began drinking to cope with his many challenges and through what he termed a series of "bad choices," he had encountered some legal trouble. One night he acted out in his anger and ended up in jail for having incited violence at a local drinking establishment. He was ashamed, in debt, and had incredible anxiety about what could possibly be done about his situation (Goodman-Bowling, 2018, 2024).

For both Mateo and Stefan, circumstances began to stack up against these workers, igniting what seemed like a never-ending cycle. Without medical and psychological assistance, knowledge of the legal system in America, and stable resources, workers can fall prey to many of the negative effects of working in day labor, and in other employment sectors. While the Day Labor Center provided a lot of much-needed support, which is addressed later in this chapter, it could not provide the multi-layered type of help workers like Mateo and Stefan most needed: immediate *and* consistent, and long-term support and knowledge about the American legal system and the ability to access resources, if any were available. Still, the DLC played an important role in encouraging these workers to continue to come to the center to garner employment and remain in community which did have a positive impact on both Mateo and Stefan in meaningful ways. Having shared their experiences in earlier writings (Goodman-Bowling, 2018, 2024), they illustrate a relevant need for psychological services and support, the crux of what this volume addresses.

Related to the problems presented by both Stefan and Mateo, it is important to recognize that in the midst of such stressors, many migrant workers self-medicate to help alleviate their distress. In a study of migrant workers in the San Francisco Bay area, Organista and his colleagues linked working and living conditions of Latino migrant day laborers to psychological distress. They address alcohol use as a form of coping with the anxiety and social pressures to provide for their families (Organista et al., 2019; Worby & Organista, 2013). Alcohol, which is available and affordable, is utilized as a social engagement tool where many workers may gather for camaraderie and support over a shared drink. Though fellowship may be the immediate goal, passing the time together drinking may result in greater experiences of depression as the regular use of alcohol to numb psychological challenges can create a dependency for which the expense and addiction are deleterious for migrant workers.

In another study, Organista and his team discovered that migrant day laborers are more vulnerable to HIV and other sexually transmitted diseases as a result of utilizing sex with other partners as a way to cope with the loneliness as workers spend long stretches of time away from their partners. To add insult to injury, many men may indulge in drinking prior to engaging in sexual activity, increasing the risk that they will not use protection or engage in drug use with unclean needles (Organista & Kubo, 2005; Worby & Organista, 2013). These coping mechanisms are clearly unhealthy and lead only to more problems. Addressing these before they occur is critical to migrant healthcare delivery and requires a significant amount of investment on the part of healthcare professionals and educators to reach out to this vulnerable population.

Im/Migrant Experiences: Border Crossing, Asylum-Seekers, and Being Far from Home

Migrant workers face several unique forms of precariousness and challenges. However, as part of the broader backdrop of im/migration studies, migrant day laborers also share in the same difficulties of other migrants. The motivations for migration to the United States vary among im/migrants, however, wage-labor is a major pull (Goodman-Bowling, 2018), alongside safety or in pursuit of critical resources (i.e. health, freedom) that are not afforded in one's home country. Though the ethnographic work at the Day Labor Center was not focused on border crossing, workers often began their narratives by sharing their harrowing experiences of having crossed the U.S. – Mexico border because it had made such an impact on their lives. As one worker, Alturo, disclosed, he had crossed the border several times during a span of about twenty years and the process grew progressively more difficult as increased border patrol, advanced detection technologies, and the harsh terrain made crossing all the more grueling. On his first attempt, he was abandoned in the desert by his hired smuggler and became severely dehydrated as he was left without food and water for nearly five days. One of the men traveling with his group died a painful death in the desert, leaving a permanent, painful memory in Alturo's mind. As many scholars have addressed, border crossing has become gradually more monitored and militarized, making the journey all the more difficult (De Genova & Peutz, 2010; DeLeon, 2012; Heyman, 2012) and yet, this has not deterred undocumented, illegal migration. The demand for low-wage labor persists, along with the economic and political conditions in Latin America which have propelled an exodus of workers. The traumatic experience of crossing into the United States can leave psychological scars for which most migrants have little support to work through and process.

Like other migrants who flee their homelands, psychological distress is increased (Bojórquez-Chapela et al., 2024), particularly for those who experience forced migration for reasons of political or social conflict including violence and resource insecurities. In their study of non-Mexican migrants in transit through Mexico, Bojórquez-Chapela and her colleagues (2024) point to the increasing numbers of Central American migrants who experience high rates of depression and anxiety as a result of forced migration. Among this particular population of migrants, they found that such asylum-seekers included higher numbers of women and children, most of whom were bound for the United States. Their experiences are compounded by the uncertainty of having fled their homelands, fear of the unknown and the unpredictability of their futures. These migrants experienced high anxieties about the safety of the family members and friends they left behind (Bojórquez-Chapela et al., 2024). Further, asylum-seekers often lack the necessary resources to safely complete their journeys, as they may have accounted for any major traumas or injuries along the way. Consistent with these concerns, migrant workers at the DLC, Santiago and Leonardo, sought asylum in the U.S. as a result of the heightened violence in their home country of Guatemala. They expressed their concern for the safety of their families and friends back home and longed to be able to reconnect when it was safe (Goodman-Bowling, 2018). Carrying this burden with them on a daily basis increased the pressures they felt to garner employment to save enough money to bring their families to safety. As Santambrogio and his colleagues discovered, that though it is clear that refugees do experience psychological distress, there is not enough focus in the current literature on the experiences of refugees post-migration (Santambrogio et al., 2024). The combination of being far from home, having healthcare problems, experiencing poverty and social isolation all contribute to the mental wellbeing of asylum-seekers, which are not being adequately addressed during the process of resettlement. This presents a major gap for which medical and psychological health care professionals may step in to provide critical support.

Once they have arrived in their host community, migrants experience a plethora of challenges around transnational living, defined as "the "political, economic, social, and cultural processes that extend beyond the borders of a particular state and include actors [who] are shaped by the policies and institutional practices of particular states" (Glick-Schilller, 2003, p. 104). Im/migrants often find themselves the subject of a much bigger story than their own migration experience, rooted in the processes of globalization which includes the demand for labor, resources, and shared and conflicted ideals regarding social, political, and economic policies. As the world becomes more interconnected, globalization has resulted in many overlapping processes (Appadurai, 1996; Levitt, 2001) of which immigrants are at the center. Migrants with limited social and cultural capital (including language skills and cultural knowledge), the process is even more problematic. Further, the pain of living far from families is incredibly taxing. Feeling split between families as men and women migrate between and among countries all across the globe in search of financial opportunities, they often leave behind their children, parents, and communities (Abrego, 2014; Boehm, 2008; Cornelius, 2007). Transnational living means being separated from one's home and communities for long stretches of time, especially as the increase border enforcement has made traveling more dangerous for labor migrants, particularly at the DLC. One way to cope with these changes is to redefine what it means to identify as a mother or father as a result of the "care crisis" (Parreñas, 2002) wherein parents leave their children behind to be raised by other family members so that they might migrate for work. The result is flexible definitions of motherhood and fatherhood wherein time spent together, instilling important personal, moral, and cultural values are left to caretakers to redefine the primary goal of mothering or fathering to providing financially. Given the poverty and circumstances which limit wage labor opportunities in the developing world, it is the great hope of these migrant parents to provide a better future for their children (Boehm, 2008). The psychological distress that this causes in migrant parents is immeasurable. Fathers, like Mateo, who had not seen his son in nearly six years at the time of his interview, felt a deep loss wishing he could spend time with him, investing in his growth from childhood to manhood. Comforted only by the fact that his absence would mean greater material provision for his son, increasing his opportunity for success, Mateo was doubly disappointed when his circumstances did not allow for the successful implementation of this redefinition. Additionally, several workers shared about their experiences of missing important rites-of-passage for their family members including *quinceañeras*, baptisms, confirmations, birthdays, holidays, and even funerals. Some fathers had missed out on the births of their own children, for which many confided was extraordinarily painful. Parents take risks to provide for their families; being away from them is a great cost for which many fathers at the DLC commented was part of their deepest worries and anxieties.

For others, being away from aging parents left them feeling inadequate as sons to be present to help with the logistics of illness and physical ailments for which elderly parents required. In one interview, a worker at the DLC broke into tears as he recounted the situation of his mother who was sick with type-2 diabetes and whose health was in a rapid decline. He felt terrible that he could not be present with her and counted on the technology available to FaceTime every day to talk with her and offer support. It would be too dangerous for him to return home and risk not being able to come back to work in the U.S. so his family insisted that his best contribution should be by earning wages to help support the family financially. Though he was clearly upset about the circumstances, he found support at the DLC, among friends who could share in his experience with this kind of loss (Goodman-Bowling, 2018).

The Day Labor Center: A Model for Care and Connection

Separated from their families and communities, migrants view themselves as part of a larger migrant community through the theoretical concept of "imagined communities" (Anderson, 1983). This concept envelops a tangible sense of human connection through shared experiences even though members of these imagined communities may never actually meet. The workers at the Day Labor Center are able to share in their experiences as migrants, workers, parents, children, and the actors of broader processes of transnationalism and globalization, which have landed them in Southern California, seeking wage labor. Here, workers found empowerment and built community through their collectivity. In this section, the Day Labor Center is presented as a model for care and connection through building community, providing services, connecting with a single director, and enjoying the ability to network and garner tangible support.

Community

On any given Saturday at the Day Labor Center, there were many visitors who were not in search of labor, but who enjoyed the regularity of the cultural community. Among day laborers in informal settings, Pinedo-Turnovsky noted that "everyday interactions at *la parada* (the corner) revealed that the corner offered the men a space to enjoy the company of others, share their concerns, offer advice, provide information, and lend support to one another" (2006, p. 35, in Goodman-Bowling 2018, p. 174). Similarly, in his ethnography of day laborers at various street corners in Los Angeles, Fernández writes:

> *"Workers are drawn by the elementary desire to share a meal, crack jokes in one's native language and indicative cultural codes, and interact with people as equals—instead of sitting alone in a rented bedroom, as some of them have*

explained to me. On the curbside, these men make fun of one another—myself included—for hours. They share food, soda, cigarettes, and job opportunities, and those who do well enough come to the corner simply to hang out when they are not working. For some of these individuals, la esquina has been their main place for sociability for over two decades." (Fernández, 2018 p. 866).

At the DLC migrant workers find this type of community, supporting one another culturally, emotionally, and even financially. As discussed earlier, sharing in the experiences of loss, redefining the parameters of fatherhood, and negotiating the many demands of transnational life led to an emotionally supportive network of individuals. In their solidarity around these shared experiences, many migrants avoided the pitfalls of depression and anxiety – particularly those who were willing to share their hardships with others. This cultivated emotional resilience and contributed to their confidence as men reclaiming their cultural identities, including expectations around masculinity and kinship, together.

Finally, workers might also provide opportunities for labor as employers may require more help and may ask the one he hired to bring on a colleague. If one has networked well and proven to be a strong worker with a solid work ethic, they may be in a good position to be recommended. Additionally, workers often helped one another with improving their assets, including tools, trucks or work vehicles. On several occasions at the DLC, workers were building upon the beds of trucks to improve how tools might be transported, secured, and safely stored to prevent theft. Lending one another tools or other required gear to improve their outcomes was also a regular practice. Finally, every day the workers held a regular lottery wherein workers would purchase a ticket for one dollar and all of the money would go into a large bucket. This provided a chance for migrants to receive a large sum of money in one shot. This became a critical resource to pay for lump sums including rent, repair bills, or important events in their home countries. In one instance, one of the workers, Mitchell, had just experienced the tragic loss of their father but had no money to pay the large bill for a funeral at one time. On this particular Saturday, the lottery had earned over $500 in ticket sales (which was not atypical for a weekend lottery) and the workers agreed that whoever won it, he should give it to Mitchell who was deeply touched by this gesture. Others gave to him willingly, outside of the winnings as well. In participating in these kinds of exchanges, migrant workers not only improved upon their networks for labor opportunities but were contributing to a community of support for economic *and* emotional support.

Services

Each week at the DLC, several volunteer organizations would come to help the workers. There was a food donation center that brought much-needed provisions for workers, including fresh fruits, vegetables, and meats. The food would be lotteried off the same way jobs were, and workers were very grateful. Additionally, every Saturday and Sunday, two or three church communities would visit to deliver a message, inspiring words, and offer their support for workers who needed it. They also brought food and provisions for the morning (usually donuts with juice and coffee). Interestingly, not everyone at the Center believed in the same religious ideals as these visitors, they still listened intently, prayed with the leaders, and expressed gratitude for the visit. Again, these types of services are crucial and make im/migrants feel included and cared for by the host community.

On occasion, local community members would also come to the Center, while walking their dogs or to share some simple resource (like one neighbor who dropped off oranges from his tree). In this city, regular community events were also held including 5K-runs, street fairs, and family-activity days hosted by the local library or businesses. These types of community-based activities and others geared directly toward migrant workers provide emotional support and reduce isolation. Negi advocates for "social service and advocacy organizations [to] focus outreach efforts for this hard-to-reach population at day labor corners" and suggests that facilitating "social activities" (Negi, 2013, p. 173) can help to mitigate the many stresses workers face. The sense of being "known" by others was critical when facing illness, depression, and other challenges, an excellent reason to be involved with the Day Labor Center and others like it.

Worker Training and the Role of the Director

When the Day Labor Center was established, it was organized by a group of grassroots leadership, workers who sought to make themselves visible for hire in the community while also not violating any city labor codes. Residents had complained of informal gathering cites that left corners susceptible to littering and feeling unsafe about unknown members of the community. Both workers and employers were frustrated by the common way that jobs were attained – a combination of shouting out wage negotiations and a race to the truck to be visible. Thus, the Day Labor Center became established and functioned under the authority of the local police department – an uncommon alliance in many cities. But here, the Center flourished and eventually, Ricardo, who was a former union labor organizer and an occasional laborer at the Center in search of additional work, was asked to become the director. His job would be to keep things organized, to help facilitate negotiations, and make sure workers did not violate city ordinances. Over time, Ricardo fulfilled not only these duties but became a trusted member of the migrant community and a helpful resource for physical and emotional support.

One chronic problem which contributed to workers' mental health was food insecurity. As workers strove to send as much money home to their families for support, they lived on as little as possible. This meant reducing their own meal intake to one or two meals per day. Ricardo, who noticed that several workers would arrive hungry, opened a makeshift food closet, with canned goods and non-perishable foods to give out to those who needed it. From cup-of-noodles to canned spaghetti sauces, Ricardo helped to connect hungry workers with much-needed provisions.

Further, migrant workers do not receive education about safety regulations, the importance of taking breaks and rests, caring for the body, and learning how to protect oneself from dangerous work (Raythod, 2016), increasing the precarity and the risks involved in this kind of employment. Recognizing this gap, Ricardo would offer semi-weekly gatherings to discuss a particular issue related to labor or other im/migration challenges. Worker centers, and others like them, may help to decrease the risk of major injuries and empower workers to increase their longevity in the workforce by learning and applying the necessary precautions for various jobs. At the Day Labor Center, these trainings allowed time for workers to ask questions about specific situations, including negotiating wages and how to employ safety measures. Ricardo played a significant role in educating newcomers about how to negotiate wages and build employer relationships. He also provided basic safety training, explaining that wearing safety gear such as gloves and goggles when working with chemicals, protecting their eyes when working with cutting, sawing, or woodworking. Further, he warned them against getting into vehicles without informing others of the address of the job site to protect them from nefarious circumstances. Ricardo had witnessed a young, recent migrant who had been picked up for a job but whose employer was looking to exploit the young man sexually. Lost and confused, the recent migrant managed to escape and eventually found his way back to the Center where he shared the horrid story with Ricardo. After this, Ricardo made it a regular practice to warn all new workers of these kinds of potential dangers.

Ricardo also tried to protect workers from being scammed by nefarious players. For example, on one occasion, a *vendor* came to visit the Center, offering to sell important tools to workers in need of affordable resources. Ricardo warned them that the signs were clear that these were stolen goods, and that they should not encourage these kinds of people to frequent the Center for customers. Ultimately, he left it to each worker to decide whether or not to purchase the goods for themselves, but the warning was clear.

On another occasion, Ricardo helped another worker, Marcus, who had arrived to the Center looking sick as he vomited into a bucket. He was in no condition to work but Ricardo graciously allowed this worker the space to sober up, as he had a well-known drinking problem, an experience with which Ricardo was all-too familiar. He shared how frequently he had helped workers to confront their drinking addictions, among other vices, helping them to connect with important resources having explained the risks of such behaviors.

Medical anthropologist, Paul Farmer (2013), suggested that through the implementation of "accompaniers[3]," global health work would be far more effective, though certainly, cost-wise, less efficient. "Accompaniers" refers to on-location practitioners who walk through every step of recovery with a patient, from diagnosis to fulfillment of treatment in order to ensure that a patient has the resources required to make a full recovery. Accompaniers would come at a high price but might ultimately be a model that could be implemented in migrant work centers and community centers to serve the migrant labor force. The varied needs of these particular workers could be better addressed with consistent, reliable care and help to navigate systems that *are* available but may not be understood or accessible to migrant day laborers (and others in similar situations). Increased costs of the deleterious effects of unaddressed mental health concerns includes increased homelessness, emergency room visits, and criminality. The health of any workforce, especially given the demand for low-wage labor, is a worthy investment for any community. Providing regular psychological resources would help to decrease the potential for long-term damage caused by unaddressed psychological distress. And, in the long term, reduce the potential costs for cities which welcome migrant workers (and community members) but have few outlets for provisions for their care.

The Day Labor Center offered an ideal model for what care might look like for this precarious workforce, which could also be translated into other venues where migrants often gather. Unlike the precarious nature of other informal places where day laborers have been studied (primarily on street corners and inconsistent locales) (Ordóñez 2015; Pinedo-Turnovsky, 2019; Valdez et al., 2019), the Day Labor Center provided a type of consistency where workers would return regularly, enabling observation for the researcher, and, more importantly, regularity with relationships among one another and the director of the Center.

While Ricardo could not be an accompanier, as Farmer (2013) would suggest as the best-case scenario for successful implementation of positive mental health outcomes, for every migrant worker, he did get to know nearly all of the workers on a personal basis. Further, he appointed helpers whom he referred to as "coordinators" who regularly participated in helping workers find jobs and negotiate/translate for employers, debrief job experiences, and provided emotional support as workers vented about their circumstances. Again, while there were certainly not enough coordinators for each person to connect individually, one-on-one, there was support available should someone require it. And while, in a chapter on psychological support services, some of these examples may not seem so applicable at first, reducing the dangers of precarious work including the physical hazards as well as dangers of being an immigrant in a new culture has incredible positive benefits. Prevention of such potential pitfalls benefits migrants, their families, and communities in countless ways (Theodore, 2023).

PSYCHOLOGICAL EVALUATIONS AND SERVICE PROVIDERS: A CALL FOR ACTION

The processes of migration leave immigrants at risk for many psychological distresses and require medical and mental health care assessment, treatment, and follow-up care (Bojórquez-Chapela et al., 2024; Santambrogio et al., 2024; Urzúa et al., 2020). Among the many services witnessed at the Day Labor Center, one that was consistently lacking was that of regular psychological services to assist workers to diagnose, cope with, and ultimately overcome feelings of depression, isolation, and self-defeat. Dealing with the many challenges discussed throughout this research requires considerable time, effort, financial investment, and human resources. While college students visited this Center about once a month, there were no consistent connections or follow-up provided, nor was there a regular presence of a licensed, clinical social worker or medical practitioner who could address the psychological needs of many migrant workers. As observed through this qualitative fieldwork, many migrant workers exhibited signs of physical deterioration, but there was no resource to whom they could be referred. And, without the means to cover the cost of a mental health provider, their options were reduced even more. Clearly, services are required to meet the needs of this vulnerable, yet vibrant and high-demand workforce (Haro et al., 2020).

Several implications follow for implementation centered around psychological evaluations, mental-health assessments, community engagement, and medical professional involvement:

- First, specialists in these professions will find that the field is rife with needs and should seek to find ways to fund and actively participate in helping im/migrants in these spaces with accessing care and services. Offering pro-bono services while connecting migrants to outsourced care would help to alleviate the long-term effects of mental health concerns. When im/migrant mental health is addressed, it benefits both the individual, their families, and local communities. Further, the implications for improved overall wellbeing for labor migrants in the broader scheme of globalization are indelible.

- Connecting im/migrants to physicians who may help with preventative measures to avoid traumatic outcomes would reduce the risk of injury and illness that could prevent one from garnering and maintaining employment. Mitigating the risk of economic downward mobility is critical for im/migrants who already face a lack of financial security and stability.
- Secondly, advocating for worker Centers and others like them to be established in high-density destination communities where im/migrants can gather will provide a desirable space for positive engagement. Employing a director, and accompaniment helpers who can get to know migrants on a consistent basis will undoubtedly improve the mental and physical health outcomes for migrants. Involving local volunteer agencies, including faith-based initiatives and university student populations who can commit to long-term investment creates a foundation for greater success (Organista & Ngo, 2019; Theordore, 2020, 2023). While worker centers and others like them may serve as training grounds for public health and social workers, and medical students, the aim must be long-term engagement. Consistency is key.
- Third, community engagement means that local community members both support and participate in the activities of the Center. Whether or not one is formally documented, im/migrants have become part of the landscape of citizenship at increasing rates in recent decades. As "defacto" members of local communities (Castañeda, 2018b, p. 30), participants in the labor force, as local consumers and residents, valuing each and every member of local communities with dignity and respect is central to transforming the overall positive outcomes for mental and physical health among im/migrants and other local community members. Creating opportunities for culturally contextualized communal engagement – picnics, parties, and city celebrations are all ways to connect migrants and their local communities such that improving one's sense of belonging and ownership of their community may contribute to their overall health and wellbeing (Castañeda, 2018a; Fernández, 2018; Organista & Ngo, 2019).

CONCLUSION

This Day Labor Center is one example to model the benefits of creating spaces in local communities for migrants to feel welcomed, cared for, and seen. Further, by offering tangible services, the Center was able to meet real deficiencies for migrant workers. And, by creating a sense of authentic community, workers were eager to support one another – emotionally, physically, and financially, as this chapter has addressed. The call for more centers like these – that might serve as a stop-gap of intervention for migrants on the precipice of psychological distress which may lead them down a painful and damaging path, is clear. By offering psychological and social services, connections to tangible medical and physical provisions, and providing opportunities for migrants to share their stories and experiences, day labor centers, and others like them, can have incredible therapeutic *and* tangible impacts on migrants, *and* the local community members who receive them.

REFERENCES

Abrego, L. J. (2014). *Sacrificing families: Navigating laws, labor, and love across borders*. Stanford University Press. DOI: 10.1515/9780804790574

Anderson, B. R. O. (1983). *Imagined communities: Reflections on the origin and spread of nationalism*. Verso.

Appadurai, A. (1996). *Modernity at large: Cultural dimensions of globalization*. University of Minnesota Press.

Bade, B. (1999). 'Is there a doctor in the field?' Underlying conditions affecting access to health care for California farmworkers and their families. In *CPRC Report*. California Policy Research Center, University of California.

Bank-Muñoz, C. (2008). *Transnational tortillas: Race, gender, and shop-floor politics in Mexico and the United States*. ILR Press.

Boehm, D. A. (2008). "For my children": Constructing family and navigating the state in the U.S.-Mexico transnation. *Anthropological Quarterly*, *81*(4), 777–802. DOI: 10.1353/anq.0.0037

Bojórquez-Chapela, I., Leyva-Flores, R., Gómez-López, D., Vázquez, E. K., & Cortés-Alcalá, R. (2024). Forced migration and psychological distress among migrants in transit through Mexico. *Salud Pública de México*, *66*(2), 173–181. DOI: 10.21149/14829 PMID: 39977042

Bonacich, E., & Appelbaum, R. P. (2000). *Behind the label: Inequality in the Los Angeles apparel industry*. University of California Press. DOI: 10.1525/9780520925595

Castañeda, E. (2018a, July 11). How cities help immigrants feel at home: 4 charts. *The Conversation*.

Castañeda, E. (2018b). *A place to call home: Immigrant exclusion and urban belonging in New York, Paris, and Barcelona*. Stanford University Press.

Choshen, H. S., Ishqer, A., Mahameed, F., Reiter, J., Gozal, D., Gileles, H. A., & Berger, I. (2021). Acute and chronic sleep deprivation in residents: Cognition and stress biomarkers. *Medical Education*, *55*(2), 174–184. DOI: 10.1111/medu.14296 PMID: 32697336

Constable, N. (2014). *Born out of place: Migrant mothers and the politics of international labor*. University of California Press.

Cornelius, W. A. (2007). Introduction: Does border enforcement deter unauthorized immigration? In Cornelius, W. A., & Lewis, J. M. (Eds.), *Impacts of border enforcement on Mexican migration: The view from sending communities* (pp. 1–16). Center for Comparative Immigration Studies, University of California.

Cravey, A. J. (1998). *Women and work in Mexico's maquiladoras*. Rowman & Littlefield Publishers.

De Genova, N., & Peutz, N. (2010). The deportation regime: Introduction. In De Genova, N., & Peutz, N. (Eds.), *The deportation regime: Sovereignty, space, and the freedom of movement* (pp. 1–29). Duke University Press.

De León, J. (2012). Better to be hot than caught: Excavating the conflicting roles of migrant material culture. *American Anthropologist, 114*(3), 477–495. DOI: 10.1111/j.1548-1433.2012.01447.x

Denman, C. A. (1997). Health in the maquilas: Questions for investigation. *Nueva Antropologia, 16*(52–53), 167–185.

Farmer, P., Kleinman, A., Kim, J. Y., & Basilico, M. (Eds.). (2013). *Reimagining global health: An introduction*. University of California Press.

Fernández, M. (2018). Hanging out together, surviving on your own: The precarious communities of day laborers. *Journal of Contemporary Ethnography, 47*(6), 865–887. DOI: 10.1177/0891241617716743

Fogelman, N., Magin, Z., Hart, R., & Sinha, R. (2020). A longitudinal study of life trauma, chronic stress, and body mass index on weight gain over a 2-year period. *Behavioral Medicine (Washington, D.C.), 48*(3), 162–170. DOI: 10.1080/08964289.2020.1780192 PMID: 32552603

Galemba, R., & Kuhn, R. (2021). "No place for old men": Immigrant duration, wage theft, and economic mobility among day laborers in Denver, Colorado. *The International Migration Review, 55*(4), 1201–1230. DOI: 10.1177/01979183211001370 PMID: 36518637

Galvan, F. H., Wohl, A. R., Carlos, J.-A., & Chen, Y.-T. (2015). Chronic stress among Latino day laborers. *Hispanic Journal of Behavioral Sciences, 37*(1), 75–89. DOI: 10.1177/0739986314568782

Glick Schiller, N. (2003). The centrality of ethnography in the study of transnational migration: Seeing the wetlands instead of the swamp. In Foner, N. (Ed.), *American arrivals: Anthropology engages the new immigration* (pp. 99–128). School of American Research Press.

Golash-Boza, T. (2009). The immigration industrial complex: Why we enforce immigration policies destined to fail. *Sociology Compass*, *3*(2), 295–309. DOI: 10.1111/j.1751-9020.2008.00193.x

Goodman-Bowling, J. (2018). *Labor, limits, and liberty: A study of day laborers at a grassroots collective in Southern California*. [Doctoral dissertation, University of Nevada, Reno]. Scholarworks. http://hdl.handle.net/11714/4849

Goodman-Bowling, J. (2024). Negotiating culture and educational expectations for Latin American migrants: Addressing challenges for parents, students, and educators. In Gamez, A. (Ed.), *Parental influence on educational success and wellbeing* (pp. 149–167). IGI Global., DOI: 10.4018/979-8-3693-1451-7.ch009

Haro, A., Kuhn, R., Rodriguez, M. A., Theodore, N., Melendez, E., & Valenzuela, A.Jr. (2020). Beyond occupational hazards: Abuse of day laborers and health. *Journal of Immigrant and Minority Health*, *22*(6), 1172–1183. DOI: 10.1007/s10903-020-01094-3 PMID: 32989653

Heyman, J. (2012). Capitalism and US policy at the Mexican border. *Dialectical Anthropology*, *36*(3), 263–277. DOI: 10.1007/s10624-012-9274-x

Holmes, S. M. (2013). *Fresh fruit, broken bodies: Migrant farmworkers in the United States*. University of California Press.

Horton, S. B. (2016). *They leave their kidneys in the fields: Illness, injury, and illegality among U.S. farmworkers*. University of California Press. DOI: 10.1525/california/9780520283268.001.0001

Levitt, P. (2001). *The transnational villagers*. University of California Press. DOI: 10.1525/9780520926707

Lugo, A. (2008). *Fragmented lives, assembled parts: Culture, capitalism, and conquest at the U.S.-Mexico border*. University of Texas Press.

Lustig, R. H. (2021). *Metabolical: The lure and the lies of processed food, nutrition, and modern medicine*. Harper Wave.

Martin, N., Morales, S., & Theodore, N. (2007). Migrant worker centers: Contending with downgrading in the low-wage labor market. *GeoJournal*, *68*(2–3), 155–165. DOI: 10.1007/s10708-007-9083-y

Negi, N. J. (2013). Battling discrimination and social isolation: Psychological distress among Latino day laborers. *American Journal of Community Psychology*, *51*(1–2), 164–174. DOI: 10.1007/s10464-012-9548-0 PMID: 22864958

Ordóñez, J. T. (2015). *Jornalero: Being a day laborer in the USA*. University of California Press.

Organista, K. C. (2008). Mexican migration for dummies: What social workers and the public need to know. *Journal of Ethnic & Cultural Diversity in Social Work, 16*(3–4), 189–198. DOI: 10.1300/J051v16n03_16

Organista, K. C., & Kubo, A. (2005). Pilot survey of HIV risk and contextual problems and issues in Mexican/Latino migrant day laborers. *Journal of Immigrant Health, 7*(4), 269–281. DOI: 10.1007/s10903-005-5124-0 PMID: 19813293

Organista, K. C., & Ngo, S. (2019). Cultural and community resources protect Latino migrant day laborers from discrimination-related distress. *Cultural Diversity & Ethnic Minority Psychology, 25*(2), 232–241. DOI: 10.1037/cdp0000211 PMID: 30010347

Organista, K. C., Worby, P., Quesada, J., Arreola, S. G., Kral, A. H., & Khoury, S. (2013). Sexual health of Latino migrant day labourers under conditions of structural vulnerability. *Culture, Health & Sexuality, 15*(1), 58–72. DOI: 10.1080/13691058.2012.740075 PMID: 23140484

Parreñas, R. S. (2002). The care crisis in the Philippines: Children and transnational families in the new global economy. In Ehrenreich, B., & Hochschild, A. R. (Eds.), *Global woman: Nannies, maids, and sex workers in the new economy* (pp. 39–54). Metropolitan Books.

Parreñas, R. S. (2005). *Children of global migration: Transnational families and gendered woes*. Stanford University Press. DOI: 10.1515/9781503624627

Pham, A. T., van Dijk, B. A. C., van der Valk, E. S., van der Vegt, B., van Rossum, E. F. C., & de Bock, G. H. (2024). Chronic stress related to cancer incidence, including the role of metabolic syndrome components. *Cancers (Basel), 16*(11), 2044. Advance online publication. DOI: 10.3390/cancers16112044 PMID: 38893162

Pinedo-Turnovsky, C. (2006). *Doing the corner: A study of immigrant day laborers in Brooklyn, New York* (Doctoral dissertation, City University of New York).

Pinedo-Turnovsky, C. (2019). *Daily labors: Marketing identity and bodies on a New York City street corner*. Temple University Press.

Quesada, J., Arreola, S., Kral, A., Khoury, S., Organista, K. C., & Worby, P. (2014). "As good as it gets": Undocumented Latino day laborers negotiating discrimination in San Francisco and Berkeley, California, USA. *City & Society, 26*(1), 29–50. DOI: 10.1111/ciso.12033 PMID: 24910501

Rathod, J. M. (2016). Danger and dignity: Immigrant day laborers and occupational risk. *Seton Hall Law Review*, *46*(3), 813–882. PMID: 27066611

Sanchez, T. F. (2013). Californian strawberries: Mexican immigrant women sharecroppers, labor, and discipline. *Anthropology of Work Review*, *34*(1), 15–22. DOI: 10.1111/awr.12003

Santambrogio, J., Cimminiello, N., Wisidagamage Don, P., Leon, E., Miragliotta, E., Capuzzi, E., Colmegna, F., & Clerici, M. (2024). Influence of post-migration living difficulties on mental health among refugees and asylum seekers: A scoping review on clinical tools. *The International Journal of Social Psychiatry*, *70*(7), 1191–1201. DOI: 10.1177/00207640241251748 PMID: 39049583

Striffler, S. (2005). *Chicken: The dangerous transformation of America's favorite food*. Yale University Press.

Theodore, N. (2020). Regulating informality: Worker centers and collective action in day-labor markets. *Growth and Change*, *51*(1), 144–160. DOI: 10.1111/grow.12343

Theodore, N. (2023). Day-Labor Worker Centers: Advancing New Models of Equity and Inclusion in the Informal Economy. *Economic Development Quarterly*, *37*(4), 363–374. DOI: 10.1177/08912424231165004

Theodore, N., Valenzuela, A.Jr, & Meléndez, E. (2009). Worker centers: Defending labor standards for migrant workers in the informal economy. *International Journal of Manpower*, *30*(5), 422–436. DOI: 10.1108/01437720910977634

Tuttle, C. (2012). *Mexican women in American factories: Free trade and exploitation on the border*. University of Texas Press.

Urzúa, Á., Caqueo-Urízar, A., & Aragón, D. (2020). Prevalencia de sintomatología ansiosa y depresiva en migrantes colombianos en Chile. *Revista Medica de Chile*, *148*(9), 1271–1278. DOI: 10.4067/S0034-98872020000901271 PMID: 33399702

Valdez, Z., Plankey-Videla, N., Murga, A. L., Menchaca, A. C., & Barahona, C. (2019). Precarious entrepreneurship: Day laborers in the U.S. Southwest. *The American Behavioral Scientist*, *63*(2), 225–243. DOI: 10.1177/0002764218794232

Valenzuela, A.Jr, Theodore, N., Meléndez, E., & Gonzalez, A. L. (2006). *On the corner: Day labor in the United States*. UCLA Center for the Study of Urban Poverty.

Walter, N., Bourgois, P., & Loinaz, H. M. (2004). Masculinity and undocumented labor migration: Injured Latino day laborers in San Francisco. *Social Science & Medicine*, *59*(6), 1159–1168. DOI: 10.1016/j.socscimed.2003.12.013 PMID: 15210088

Worby, P. A., & Organista, K. C. (2013). Contextual influences on the drinking of male Latino immigrant day laborers. *Substance Use & Misuse*, *48*(5), 391–403. DOI: 10.3109/10826084.2013.765481 PMID: 23461665

ENDNOTES

1 To be clear, all names of individuals are pseudonyms to protect the identity of those who contributed to the research on which these findings are based. Further, all participants provided verbal consent to participate.

2 The vast majority of the workers at the DLC were Latino migrant men, mostly undocumented. Originally from nations all throughout Latin America, the majority were from Mexico, mainly in the northern states. Though there were workers from other nations represented (Cameroon, for example), on a daily basis, it was primarily Latin American men who participated in the daily search for jobs, who came regularly for fellowship and camaraderie, and who contributed to the running of the DLC.

3 From the French-inspired word, "accompaneteurs" which refers to a specific type of community health worker (and theory of health care delivery, *accompaniment*) that Farmer and his colleagues implemented through their fieldwork in Haiti and Rwanda in their organization, "Partners in Health."

Chapter 6
Mental Health Care With Immigrants:
Barriers, Facilitators, and Recommendations for Clinical Practice

Lizbeth Gaona
https://orcid.org/0009-0008-2733-8796
California Baptist University, USA

Liz G. Gomez
Brite Psychological Services, USA

ABSTRACT

The purpose of this chapter is to equip readers with the understanding of factors that may get in the way of mental health care for immigrants, what may help improve access and use and lastly how to provide culturally relevant mental health care for immigrants. In the first section, this chapter will provide the reader with an understanding of barriers to both access and use of mental health care for immigrants. Further, the chapter will identify facilitators towards improving access and use of mental health care for immigrants. The second half of the chapter will provide recommendations for clinical practice via a five step framework which may be applied in working with immigrants in mental health care settings.

DOI: 10.4018/979-8-3693-7944-8.ch006

INTRODUCTION

The first part of the chapter will identify barriers to both access and use of mental health care for immigrant adults and children. Core barriers to access that will be discussed include low socioeconomic status, discrimination (Brabeck et al., 2016, Cross et al., 2020) stigma and language barriers (Saechao et al., 2012). Salient barriers related to use of mental health care for immigrants include language barriers, cultural interpretations of distress and mental illness, stigma related to mental illness, and myths associated with the consequences of receiving mental health care (Bhugra, Watson, & Wijesuriya, 2021; Salami, Salma, & Hegadoren, 2019). After expanding on the aforementioned barriers of access and use, the chapter will identify facilitators towards improving access and use of mental health care. Facilitators that will be explored for adults include client-clinician language congruency, social and instrumental support, (Salma, & Hegadoren, 2019; Garcini et al., 2021), provider cultural competency (Zghal, El-Masri, McMurphy, & Pfaff, 2021) and pathways to care via religious and spiritual leaders (Derr, 2016). Facilitators for children include language congruent care, and mental health services that are offered in school settings and are free.

The second part of the chapter will provide recommendations for clinical practice. The Five-Step Framework of Mental Health Care with Immigrants will be introduced as a suggested framework for mental health care. Each of the five steps in the framework will be showcased with examples. Part two will also discuss the cultural adaptation of interventions and suggest specific guidelines on how to adapt interventions to meet diverse immigrant needs. Two case studies will be used to illustrate the aforementioned concepts. The first case study will outline an example of how to adapt interventions for immigrants and the second case study will serve as an example of the application of the Five-Step Framework of Mental Health Care with Immigrants.

BARRIERS AND FACILITATORS OF ACCESS AND USE OF MENTAL HEALTH CARE

Barriers to Access of Mental Health Care

Worldwide, the literature has noted that some of the barriers to mental health care access include low socioeconomic status, discrimination (Mahabir et al., 2021; Brabeck et al., 2016, Cross et al., 2020; Castelli, 2018; Kim, 2011) stigma and language barriers (Saechao et al., 2012). When combined, these barriers can ultimately decrease the chances of immigrants obtaining highly needed mental health care services. Immigrants may experience higher levels of stress, such as acculturative stress (Berry & Annis, 1974) and are more likely to experience symptoms of stress disorder associated with their pre and post immigration experience.

Low Socioeconomic Status

Immigrants are more likely to live within low socioeconomic status including low income housing (Rana, Kent, & Page, 2025). Although immigrants may have fared financially well in their home country, oftentimes they end up leaving valuable resources behind for the gamble of a brighter future. Some immigrants risk leaving years of investments and find themselves having to begin anew at the most foundational levels of society. Resources left behind include property, homes, educational degrees, stature, as well as social capital. In sum, social capital can be defined as the personal connections one has and the potential to collaborate and share resources with others within a shared network. Within these networks in which social capital may be created, are opportunities to pool together resources and engage in altruism for the betterment of all parties. As a result of immigrating to a new country, immigrants must make the difficult sacrifice of leaving behind potentially instrumental key resources and opportunities associated with social capital.

Being of low socioeconomic status has been identified as a barrier to accessing preferred mental health care. First off, immigrants have no choice but to enter the public mental health system for their care. This system leaves many void of the freedom to choose a mental health provider within the private sector. Additionally, the public mental health care system is oftentimes impacted by long new patient intake appointment wait times. Public mental health care patients also end up being limited on provider choices and often are assigned a provider without the opportunity to have a say. And in many cases, the provider does not speak their native language. This language barrier may create a disconnect both in the medical history information gathering stage and a disconnect during the rapport building process between the client and the provider. This deficiency in the rapport building process can increase the odds of both low quality level of treatment, where needs are left unmet, and premature termination of treatment. Being of low socioeconomic status is a barrier that many immigrants are faced with and regrettably one that compounds stressors in terms of receiving medically needed mental health care.

Discrimination

Many immigrants experience discrimination, which has been identified as another barrier to accessing mental health care (Mahabir et al., 2021; Straiton, Aambø, & Johansen, 2019). Oftentimes a community may adopt a "not in my back yard"

(NIMBY) mentality; which in turn may create a hostile or unwelcoming culture for immigrants. This unwelcoming NIMBY disposition may cultivate a community in which citizens are opposed to immigrant friendly protocols, such as having community signage only in the dominant language (for example English in the U.S.) or disfavoring the hiring of immigrants who speak the dominant language with an accent or who are in the very early stages of learning the dominant language. This discriminatory culture may engender feelings of shame, fear, and distress. This phenomenon has been labeled as racial trauma (Comas-Díaz et al., 2019).

Negative Implicit Bias.

Additionally, experiences of discrimination may also impact access to care by means of negative implicit biases on the part of mental health care staff, personnel and/or providers. One brief definition of negative implicit bias includes unfavorable hidden subconscious or unconscious prejudices and attitudes towards a person or group of people. These unfavorable prejudices negatively influence the manner in which they treat those persons or groups. Although implicit biases can also be positive (where a person or group is favored), experiences of discrimination are associated with negative implicit biases (NIBs). Unfortunately, NIBs are hidden and difficult for one to identify. Persons who are guilty of engaging in NIBs may likely deny that they are engaging in NIBs. Not because they fear consequences of engaging in NIBs, but rather because they are simply not aware or conscious of the fact that they are engaging in NIBs. In their seminal work, Sue et al. (2007) noted that two forms of discrimination, which are unconscious biases, include microinsults and microinvalidations. These are often unconscious types of racial microaggressions. Microinsults are verbal or behavioral forms of communication that are rude or demeaning towards someone's racial identity (Sue et al., 2007). For example, a microinsult labeled, *Second Class Citizen* (Sue et al., 2007), occurs when an immigrant is treated as being "lesser than", viewed as a person who is "less worthy" relative to natural born citizen of majority/dominant culture, A microinvalidation occurs when an immigrant is labeled as foreigner (despite being a "documented"/ legal immigrant or naturalized citizen). Unfortunately, mental health care staff, personnel and mental health care providers are only human and therefore, they are not immune to subconsciously engaging in microinsults or microinvalidation of immigrant clients.

Stigma

Stigma is another factor that decreases access to mental healthcare for immigrants. One simplified definition of stigma is the labeling something as being shameful, disgraceful or dishonorable. For example, stigma may arise when one engages in an activity that may be against their cultural norms, values, traditions or religious beliefs. One historical example may be when a teenager becomes pregnant while in high school. They may experience stigma by others in which they may be labeled as irresponsible. Stigma has been identified as a barrier towards immigrants accessing mental health care as it may be counterculture. For example, in one study, compared to non-Latino/a White, Latinos/as reported having higher levels of shame and embarrassment regarding having a mental illness (Jimenez Bartels, Cardenas & Alegría 2013). This disposition of stigma regarding having a mental illness may engender decreased motivation towards seeking care. Access towards mental health care may perhaps be improved by strategies that "build bridges" and target stigma. In one study, education appeared to significantly decrease stigma towards mental health care among Latino/as (Lopez et al., 2018).

Language Barriers

Language barriers serve as significant obstacles towards the access of mental health care for immigrants. Although some immigrants may have a desire to receive mental health care, their inability to speak the dominant language may likely make it difficult for them to effectively follow through on steps towards receiving care. That is, they may face language barriers in their aim to find a clinic in their area via using a directory that is not in their native language or find it challenging to communicate effectively with the clinic via phone or messaging to set up an initial appointment. Although some mental health clinics may have bilingual providers or interpretation services to help address this barrier, it may still be very challenging to communicate that a bilingual provider is needed when the initial call is made.

Barriers to Use

On a similar vein, barriers associated with use of mental health care also include language barriers. Further, cultural interpretations of distress and mental illness, stigma related to mental illness, and myths associated with the consequences of receiving mental health care (Bhugra, Watson, & Wijesuriya, 2021; Salami, Salma,

& Hegadoren, 2019) also act as barriers towards use. Of the above, new concepts to this chapter are cultural interpretations of distress and mental illness.

Cultural interpretations of distress and mental illness are (in a simplified manner) the unique perspectives in which different populations interpret and define the origin and meaning of distress and mental illness. For example, in some Latino/a cultures, it is bad luck to marvel at or stare at an infant child for too long as this may cause *ojo*, which is to cause ill-will or bad luck to come upon the infant child. Consequently, if an admirable infant becomes ill, someone who believes in *ojo* may perhaps say, "someone gave the beautiful child *ojo*". To this end, they have interpreted the child's illness via their cultural worldview. Similarly, a barrier to utilization of mental health care may be that an individual culturally interprets having a mental illness due to being a "bad person" or failing to achieve a culturally normative standard. Importantly, there are many concepts that influence a person's cultural interpretations of distress and mental illness; seven of these concepts include a) traditions and customs, b) historical figures and experiences, c) religion and spirituality, d) language, e) shared values and beliefs, f) context, location and/or region, and g) artifacts and art. In addition, an individual's primary social support system such as family and friends interpret the mental illness may also influence the individual's own interpretations. The individual's history in dealing with past illnesses may also shape their cultural interpretation of distress and mental illness.

Lastly, myths have been identified as barriers towards immigrant's use of mental health care. Myths can be defined as broadly held beliefs that are ultimately false. Because immigrants' knowledge of the new host country's large operating systems may be limited (i.e. field of law, medicine, social norms or educational system), they are vulnerable to believe myths. Myths such as being "blacklisted" and unable to gain stable employment if mental health care is received, is one example of how myths may act as a barrier towards utilization. The lack of education related to protective healthcare information safeguarded by laws such as the Health Insurance Portability and Accountability Act of 1996 (United States Department of Health and Human Services, 1996) may be foreign and unknown to most recent immigrants creating a barrier towards utilization of mental health care. Some common myths (Derr, 2016) with examples of the false belief are listed in Table 1.

Table 1. Myths with examples of the false belief

Myth	Examples of the Belief
Confidentiality	"what I share will not be kept confidential" "what I share may be shared with potential employers and ruin my opportunity to gain employment"
Cost	"only persons who are rich are able to afford mental health care" "the cost of treatment is only realistic for wealthy persons"
Helpfulness of Mental Health Care	"mental health care will only make things worse" "mental health care is never helpful"

As illustrated above, myths associated with confidentiality such as believing that what is shared in treatment will not be kept confidential and even shared with potential employers can strongly deter immigrants from use of care. As previously shared, not knowing what they do not know in terms of embedded laws and policies to safeguard their health information may not be adequately disseminated amongst immigrant communities. Further, myths such as those associated with cost may serve as barriers to use, as individuals may falsely believe that the cost of mental health care is ultimately beyond reach. However, community mental health clinics often receive government funding in order to offer free, fee based and/or sliding scale care.

Barriers to Mental Health Access for Immigrant Children

The following section will identify barriers to mental health access for immigrant children of international descent. This section will discuss findings from a group of 18 immigrant mothers who participated in a qualitative study to identify barriers and access to mental health services for their children (Tulli et al., 2020). Mothers from the following countries contributed to the study: Sudan, Haiti, Ukraine, Romania, Ethiopia, Syria, Nigeria, Dominican Republic, Colombia, Pakistan, and China.

Findings illustrated that the barriers and facilitators to accessing mental health services for immigrant children, in many ways, mirrors the barriers of their adult parents. The data revealed that many barriers for immigrant children overlap with barriers that adult immigrants experience. Key barriers that were identified included financial strain and low SES, racism and/or discrimination, language barriers, and stigma.

As mentioned, similar to adults financial strain and low SES was also a barrier for immigrant children. One well known social determinant of health (non-medical aspects of a person's life that influence their long-term health outcome) is a person's economic standing and stability. If one is more financially well off, as noted in earlier, in the chapter, there is a wider array of medical providers to obtain care from, including those within the public sector. As noted earlier, most immigrants, including children, if at all eligible for public medical insurance, are limited in choice of provider and quality of care available to them. Another salient barrier is racism and discrimination that immigrant children may experience during their adjustment to new environments such as in academic settings. For example, as a result of potentially not speaking the mainstream language or speaking it with an accent, children and adolescents may experience discrimination in the form of bullying in academic settings (Zaidi & Sah, 2025). Research suggests that academic settings should focus on creating strategies for more inclusive and welcoming school settings that address stereotypes towards immigrant children. Stigma also plays a strong role in accessing mental health care for immigrant children. Tuli et al. found that while immigrant mothers knew their children's mental health issues would be frowned upon, the biggest hurdle that stigma brought on, was a feeling of loneliness felt within their community and the low social support to navigate a foreign and complex mental health system. As noted before, the loss of social capital hinders an immigrant's socioeconomic standing and in turn, jeopardizes the quality of their own mental health and well-being. This stress in turn trickles down, negatively affecting an immigrant parent's level of functioning and capacity to access mental health care for their children or to advocate for better quality care.

Facilitators to Access and Use of Mental Health Care

Client-Clinician Language Congruence

Although there are a number of barriers to access and use of mental health care, there are also a number of facilitators that may help improve access and use. Some of these include client-clinician language congruency, social and instrumental support, (Salma, & Hegadoren, 2019; Garcini et al., 2021), provider cultural competency (Zghal, El-Masri, McMurphy, & Pfaff, 2021) and pathways to care via religious and spiritual leaders (Derr, 2016). Client-clinician language congruency is defined as the when the language of the provider matches the language of the client- in this case the immigrant. Notably, although immigrants may be bilingual and speak both their native language and the dominant language of the host country, they may feel more comfortable speaking in the language that they primarily grew up using and consider their primary language. Because some immigrants may adhere to values such as respecting persons whom they feel have some form of authority such as providers- they may have a harder time advocating for themselves- and specifically asking to receive care from someone who speaks their primary language. That is, some immigrants may opt towards an open stance in which they accept care from a provider who uses a translation service or who speaks their primary language – but perhaps with little competency and inadequately. To this end, it is very important to educate immigrants of their rights and of any available translation services when providing informed consent to treatment.

Social and Instrumental Support

Another facilitator is social support. As previously mentioned, when faced with immigrating to a new country, many immigrants are faced with having to leave behind social capital, friendships, support systems and key primary family members- such as partners and parents. These key relationships serve as a resource that they are no longer able to access- thus the importance of receiving social and instrumental support in their new host country. Social and instrumental support serve as facilitators as social support persons may be able to offer learned/new information that may demystify myths related to access and use of mental health care. They may also be able to provide instrumental support that may ease obstacles towards of mental health care services such as transportation. A systematic review noted that transportation problems was a salient concern towards use of mental health care (Derr, 2016). Transportation problems may be potentially decreased with an increase in instrumental social support. Improving social and instrumental support for immigrants should be a recommended standard practice for persons working with immigrants in mental health care settings.

Provider Cultural Competency

Improving provider cultural competency has been identified as an important indicator towards facilitating access and use of mental health care for immigrants. In this context, cultural competency may be defined as (and is not limited to) an understanding of the cultural values, beliefs, worldview, language, customs, practices, spirituality/religious beliefs and cultural interpretations of distress and mental illness for immigrant populations. Although it is unrealistic to hold any provider to a standard in which they have reached the epitome of being cultural competent for a certain group or immigrant population- it is important and ethical that providers strive towards continually growing in their cultural competence with this vulnerable population. In practice and with immigrants, provider cultural competency may look like:

- Speaking the same language as the client
- Having a working knowledge of values and customs for that population (i.e., refer to them as "Mr." or "Mrs.", make eye contact, do not shake hands etc.)
- Understanding general cultural interpretations of distress and mental illness among that population

- Utilizing a humble and collaborative approach in treatment planning and delivery.

Importantly, although cultural competency is important, another key concept that is important to integrate is cultural humility.

In the context of mental health care for immigrants, cultural humility can be defined as an open stance in which the provider adopts a posture of fallibility, curiosity in learning from the client- whom they respect as the expert of their own experience. A culturally humbler provider may do the following:

- Ask open ended questions that demonstrate that they do not know it all- such as, "would you please educate me on your spiritual or religious beliefs"
- Educate the client in that they (the provider) values the client's opinions and welcomes their feedback regarding care
- Underscore that the relationship between them and the client is that of equals and that they (the provider) is not an authority figure over the client
- Invite the client to correct them if they misspeak or make inaccurate statements or assumptions regarding the client (i.e., Provider: "person's from your culture usually enjoy celebrating birthdays correct?", Client: "No, that is not the case, in my culture we do not recognize birthdays")

Pathways to Care via Religious and Spiritual Leaders

Lastly, another important facilitator is creating pathways to mental health care via religious and spiritual leaders. This is an important facilitator specific to immigrants due the idea that immigrants may feel more comfortable first seeking care or consultation from a spiritual leader when faced with a mental illness (Gearing et al., 2024). To this end, it is important that providers and local mental health agency administrators make it a priority to establish working relationships with pathways for religious and spiritual leaders to be able to refer immigrants to mental health care. As a result of being referred by the religious/spiritual leader, they may feel more assured that both seeking and receiving mental health care is both sanctioned and perhaps may even be helpful to them. This may also create a sense of legitimacy, which can be shared within their support systems as well as help decrease the sense of stigma. In part one of this chapter, we have covered barriers and facilitators to mental health care for immigrants. The following section will provide recommendations for clinical practice via the Five-Step Framework of Mental Health Care with Immigrants. We will first examine facilitators for mental health use and access for immigrant children.

Facilitators to Mental Health Access and Utilization for Immigrant Children

One core facilitator is addressing the language barrier that children experience as it may enable successful access and more effective use of mental health services. Unfortunately, many times it is the children themselves who end up interpreting their medical needs to providers while their parents are still learning the prominent language. This can cause added friction and a feeling of isolation for the parent. In one example, an immigrant mother expresses frustration at feeling left out of the conversation between provider and child, " When they went to the therapist, the therapist and him, they started talking, but I was totally isolated. . . . He didn't translate so I was totally blocked" (Tulli et al., 2020). And if it's not the child interpreting, but rather a family member or friend, medical terminology can be mistranslated, creating a risk of leaving out essential information.

To this end, it is most effective to have medical professional bilingual staff to facilitate the mental health care of immigrant children. If bilingual staff are not available, a culturally proficient trained interpreter is key. Culturally proficient interpreters are keen to cultural myths and can act as a buffer when trying to extrapolate necessary information to identify a mental health diagnosis; such in the case of a mother believing her infant simply has, *ojo*.

In an aforementioned study by Tulli et al., (2020) other key facilitators include offering mental health services in school, having higher educated caregivers and offering free services. Being able to offer immigrant children mental health services in school is a key facilitator in that it may help not only potentially increase usage of mental health services by the student, but also decrease the caregiver barrier of having to transport the child to a mental health clinic.

The next section will introduce the Five-Step Framework of Mental Health Care with Immigrants as a framework suggested for use in clinical practice with immigrants. It will also provide suggestions for the cultural adaptation of clinical interventions for immigrant adults or children. Although the following sections will utilize case studies in which adults will be featured to illustrate the concepts, both the framework and the suggested guidelines for adapting interventions may also be used with immigrant children or youth.

RECOMMENDATIONS FOR CLINICAL PRACTICE

Five-Step Framework of Mental Health Care with Immigrants

This section will first introduce the Five-Step Framework of Mental Health Care with Immigrants following by providing an example for application via a case study. As previously mentioned there are a number of factors that both act as barriers or facilitate mental health care for immigrants. With these factors still in mind, Table 2 outlines the Five-Step Framework of Mental Health Care with Immigrants, which will serve as a guide on practical steps that providers may implement with clients who identify as immigrants.

Table 2. Five-step framework of mental health care for immigrants

Assessment	**Biological** **Psychological** **Social** **Spiritual** **Cultural: ADDRESSSING Framework**
Cultural Relevant Interventions	Ecological Validity and Cultural Sensitivity Framework
Case Management	Provider should make contact with the resource to ensure that they are accepting new referrals Provider should obtain the contact information of the person whom the client should contact at the resource Provider should confirm that the resource has the capacity to communicate with the client in the client's primary or preferred language Provider should have a follow up appointment with the client after the termination session to ensure that they were properly linked with referrals, or invite the client to contact the provider should the referral fall through or become obsolete
Evaluation of Treatment	Suggested questions to evaluate treatment include: What went well in session today? What did not go well in session today? What is one thing that the provider (I) can do better? What is one thing that the provider (I) can continue to do? What is one thing that the provider (I) can stop doing? Are you satisfied with the way that treatment is going so far? Why or why not? Do you believe that your mental health symptoms are getting better, getting worse or remaining the same? Why or why not? What evidence do you have to support your response that your mental health symptoms are getting better, getting worse or remaining the same?
Termination	Fully linked with needed referrals

Assessment

The first step in the framework is assessment. When conducting a mental health care assessment with immigrants it is very important that providers adopt a collaborative and client centered approach. Further, it is suggested that they adopt a learner's stance and a humble approach as this may make immigrants feel more comfortable and perhaps improve their odds of continuing in care.

Many times mental health providers in community mental health care systems are busy with high caseloads and limited time in between clients. Still, it is key that they take thorough intakes and conduct assessments in a culturally humble- at the comfort and pace suitable for each client. Some clients may already be familiar with processes associated with receiving mental health care and may understand that when establishing care, thorough assessments are conducted to obtain an overall picture of their functioning. This however, may not be something that immigrants are familiar with. They may question why certain questions are being asked and be unclear as to the purpose of so many personal and private questions being asked during the intake assessment.

For this reason, the provider should always assess their client's understanding of and the purpose behind the intake assessment. Upon assessing the immigrant client's knowledge of the initial intake assessment and learning that the client may be completely unfamiliar with it, the provider should consider beginning the assessment with a clear rationale for the purpose of the different sections of the intake assessment. Listed (Table 3) are recommended rationales that may be shared with immigrants for the different types of assessment sections. As listed shown, we suggest five general sections of assessments: biological, psychological, social, spiritual and cultural.

Table 3. Rationale for assessments with examples of provider statements

Assessment Section	Rationale: Example of Provider Statement
Biological Assessment	"I understand that this information may be very private, but because some medical conditions may influence mental health symptoms, it is important that I ask questions regarding your physical health" "Even though you are at a mental health care appointment, in this standard intake assessment I will have to ask questions about your physical health. This information will help me understand if any medical conditions may be influencing how you are feeling."
Psychological Assessment	"I will be asking you questions about how you are feeling and although you may not be feeling some of the symptoms that I may ask- I still have to ask. For example, I may ask you if you hear voices or if you feel like staying in bed all day. Please know that I ask these standard questions to all clients" "Some people have more than one mental health issue. In order for me to truly understand how we can best help you, I will be asking you many questions about your mental health- even though some may not apply to you"
Social Assessment	"Some people feel better or worse depending on their social support network; because of this, I will be asking you standard questions regarding your social support systems" "It is important that I ask standard questions regarding your social support system such as if you feel supported by family or friends as this information has been shown to help me consider interventions to help you feel better"
Spiritual Assessment	"Some people have found that their religion/spirituality has been a resource when coping with mental health issues. For this reason, I do have to ask you questions regarding your religion/spirituality" "Although it may seem as though it does not apply, asking standard questions regarding your religion/spirituality is part of my role in completing a thorough assessment"
Cultural Assessment	"Some people have found that their culture such as their values and/or beliefs may serve to help them feel better. In order for me to create the best plan possible, I have to ask you standard questions regarding your culture" "Although it may seem as though some of the questions regarding your culture may not be relevant to your care- having a shared understanding of your culture will ultimately help me to help you better"

When conducting the biological, psychological, and social assessments, we recommend following the standard mental health intake assessments that ask questions regarding client's physical health, past health concerns, current medications taken etc. Similarly, psychological and social assessments are generally part of standard protocol. However, we recommend that providers also engage in a spiritual assessment.

Although spiritual assessments vary, one assessment that we recommend is a spiritual life map (Hodge & Holtrop, 2002). In essence, a spiritual life map can be described as a timeline in which the client is asked to share religious/spiritually relevant events that may have shaped their faith. For example, in the spiritual life map, a client may indicate their first year of life on the timeline along with an image of them being baptized. They can then write in the word, "baptism" next to the image indicating that this was an important religious/spiritual event in their life. A spiritual life map may help the provider have a stronger understanding of if or how the client's religion/spirituality may be a source or strength or difficulty for them.

For some immigrants having to leave their country of origin including beloved places of worship and/or strong social support by means of their church members may be a source of difficulty. They may describe this period in their life as one in which they experienced grief and loss due to their immigration journey. For a more detailed step by step guide on conducting a spiritual life map please refer to the reading, Spiritual assessment: A review of complementary assessment models (Hodge & Holtrop, 2002).

Next, we recommend that providers engage immigrant clients in a cultural assessment. We suggest that the cultural assessment be guided by Pamela Hay's ADDRESSING Framework (Hays, 2022). In short, the ADDRESSING Framework (Table 4) is a list of cultural characteristics that are important to consider with diverse populations in mental health care.

Using the list of characteristics, the provider can ask the client questions relevant to each of the diverse variables listed in the ADDRESSING acronym. For example, for E= Ethnicity and Racial Identity, the provider may ask, "what ethnicity or racial identity do you identify with?". Although some of this information may have already been gathered via client self-report during initial paperwork, we recommend that the provider write out the ADDRESSSING acronym and then share with the client that they will be asking them to share responses regarding each of the letters in the of the ADDRESSING Framework acronym. Although the ADDRESSING Framework is not exhaustive, the ADDRESSING Framework is a seminal tool that has been recommended for clinical practice when working with diverse populations.

Pamela Hay's ADDRESSING Framework

A Age/Generation
D Disability status (developmental or other)
D Disability status (acquired)
R Religion and Spirituality
E Ethnicity and Racial Identity
S Socioeconomic Status or Social Class
S Sexual Orientation
I Indigenous Heritage
N National Origin
G Gender

Data gathered via the cultural assessment may help inform the provider with information that they may not have otherwise gathered. For example, perhaps the provider may gather information such as the sexual orientation of the client. For some immigrant populations topics such sexual orientation may be one that they deviate from disclosing for the fear of being shamed. Inviting the sharing of this information, will help the client decrease their fear of rejection. This information will better inform the treatment plan and assist the provider in creating more individually-tailored and culturally relevant interventions.

Culturally Relevant Interventions

Culturally relevant interventions are interventions that have been infused with factors relevant to the client's culture. For example, this can include interventions that have been translated from the dominant language into the client's primary language. Another example is a mindfulness exercise that has been adapted to include the client's religion. For example, when engaging in standard mindfulness one can ask a client to breath in the words "I can heal" and in contrast, when this intervention is adapted to be culturally relevant, to mirror the client's spirituality, instead one can ask the client to breath in the words, "God can help me heal". It is very important that providers follow recommendations and documented guidelines for adapting interventions towards being culturally relevant. One recommended guideline is the Ecological Validity and Cultural Sensitivity Framework by Bernal, Bonilla, and Bellido (1995; Bernal & Sáez-Santiago, 2006; Rodriguez & Bernal, 2012). This framework suggest that the following items be considered when adapting an intervention:

- Language: adopting the client's preferred language in treatment
- Therapeutic Relationship: considering client-therapist relationship in treatment
- Metaphors: consider the use of metaphors in treatment
- Content of Intervention: considering delivering content in a culturally relevant manner
- Concept of Illness: consider the client's own definition of illness
- Treatment Goals: consider the client's culture and wishes into goals
- Delivery Methods: consider delivering the intervention in a culturally relevant manner
- Context: con the incorporation of clients broader contexts (i.e., social, economic, political, acculturation level)

In Ecological Validity and Cultural Sensitivity Framework (EVF), adapting an intervention should be aimed towards accounting for the client's context and adapting the intervention so that is culturally sensitive – for example, elements of the intervention are infused with some of the client's culture. Each of the concepts of the EVF will be illustrated in a case study below- however, for more information on the Ecological Validity and Cultural Sensitivity Framework we suggest you refer to, Frameworks, Models, and Guidelines for Cultural Adaptation (Domenech Rodríguez & Bernal, 2012).

As mentioned, one example of adapting an intervention using the EVF for the immigrant population will be showcased below. The example features a clinical treatment program that was adapted for Spanish speaking Latinx who were predominantly immigrants and receiving mental health care in a community clinic in a suburban area of Los Angeles. The treatment program was dialectical behavior therapy (DBT), which is a clinical intervention aimed to primarily treat persons diagnosed with borderline personality disorder. Borderline personality disorder a serious mental illness in which client's often engage in potentially lethal behaviors – for example, such as engaging in deliberate self-harm by means of cutting, head banging and/or engaging in parasuicidal and suicidal behaviors.

The case of Lina will be used to further illustrate how these elements were incorporated into standard DBT practice to deliver a culturally adapted, yet still fully adherent DBT treatment program. It is important to note that although treatment was culturally adapted, the core components of standard DBT remained unchanged. However before illustrating how standard DBT was adapted, a brief overview of standard DBT will be described.

Dialectical Behavior Therapy.

DBT is one of the leading evidenced based treatments for persons diagnosed with borderline personality disorder (Carter et al., 2010; Harned et al., 2008; Linehan et al., 2015). Dialectical behavior therapy has also been shown to be effective when adapted to treat persons with diverse mental health conditions such as women with substance abuse disorders, women diagnosed with a eating disorders, incarcerated adolescent men with impulsive aggressive behavioral problems, and women with the co-occurring disorders of post-traumatic stress disorder and borderline personality disorder (Dimeff et al., 2020; Harned et al., 2014; Kroger et al., 2010, Shelton et al., 2011). Standard DBT consists of the client attending weekly individual sessions, skills group, phone coaching (a practice in which the client is invited to call their therapist outside of regular business hours when they are in need of help with implementing DBT skills (to decrease unhealthy behaviors). Lastly, the client completes a weekly log. This log is referred to as a diary card, in which they track their emotions, behaviors, skills used and overall frequency in which they engage in unwanted or maladaptive behaviors. Notably, the following adaptations were implemented into a fully adherent DBT program in which all recommended standard practices remained. Below, the eight components of the EVF (i.e., language, therapeutic relationship etc.) will be listed with examples of how each component informed adaptation of treatment.

Culturally Adapted Spanish Dialectical Behavior Therapy via the Case of Lina.

Lina was a 38 year old immigrant from Mexico who was married and had a teenage daughter and five year old son. Lina was diagnosed with borderline personality disorder and major depression disorder and had a history of engaging in self-harm behaviors such as cutting her wrist and had endorsed a recent suicide attempt by the means of attempting to overdose on pain medication.

- Language: Consistent with the first element of EVF framework, Lina participated in Spanish DBT treatment in which she participated in individual therapy, attended DBT skills group and participated in telephone skills coaching all in Spanish. Although Lina was not fully bilingual and her primary language was Spanish, she was an English learner and had begun to learn some words in English. Still, since she experienced many of her key childhood events relating to the development of BPD and had many important memories in the Spanish language- and she spoke primarily in Spanish, treatment was delivered in Spanish. Doing so was in consideration of Lina's language abilities, culture, social history and the emotions associated with Spanish words and memories (Bernal & Saez-Santiago, 2006).
- Persons: Lina's provider was also a female, bilingual and bicultural (Latinx), which allowed for the flexibility and ease of the provider to translate important information from English to Spanish. This also allowed for an organic understanding of cultural nuances that arose during treatment. Not only was Lina's individual provider bilingual and bicultural, but so were the group skills leaders.
- Content: Having a bilingual, bicultural provider is associated by EVF element *persons* and the element *content*. Within the *content* element of Spanish DBT, the use of Latinx values *personalismo, and platica* were carried out during treatment delivery. For example, *personalismo*, the act of relating to clients in a friendly and non-institutionalized manner (Andrés-Hyman, Ortiz, Añez, Paris, & Davidson, 2006) was carried out via engaging the clients in *platica, (small talk)*. Research shows that incorporating *platica* into treatment is important as the failure to engage in *platica* may be interpreted as rude by Latinx clients (Ojeda, Flores, Meza, & Morales, 2011). Furthermore, *content* was also demonstrated in the use of *Familismo*, the Latinx family value of having a strong connection, affection and loyalty to family members (Comas-Dıaz, 1989) in that Lina's family was invited to participate in treatment. Lina's daughter agreed to participate and was provided education on

the modes and goals of DBT and she committed to encouraging Lina to use DBT skills and/or DBT phone coaching.

- Metaphor: The element of *metaphors* was incorporated into treatment with the use of *dichos* (proverbs) and *cuentos* (short stories). Metaphors were incorporated into Spanish DBT when providers were teaching Lina DBT skills and leading her in the practice of mindfulness. For example, the *dicho "El que mucho abarca poco aprieta*" (He who holds too much grasps on to loosely) is an example of a *dicho* used to teach the consequences of multitasking and not practicing mindfulness effectively.
- Concepts: The next element of *concepts* was integrated into Spanish DBT in that Lina's childhood and developmental experiences were linked to the biosocial theory of BPD. For example, the biosocial principle of growing up in an invalidating environment was reported by Lina's accounts of growing up as the oldest of her siblings and being a female, which made Lina hold to a cultural obligation to help raise her siblings. Lina reported that she also had a different father than her siblings (one whom she never met), which made Lina feel as though she was a black sheep and did not belong. Nevertheless, as the oldest sibling, Lina was expected to abandon her dreams of going to college and help her mother with child rearing and household chores.
- Goals: The element *goals were* carried out by both incorporating Lina into the development of her treatment goals and utilizing the value of *familismo*. For example, *familismo* was integrated when Lina's daughter participated in treatment goal development and committed to not reinforce any of Lina's unhealthy coping behaviors (isolating, entertaining thoughts of suicide, not taking medications as prescribed, not grooming or staying in bed all day).
- Methods: With regard to the *methods* element, there were a variety of methods used to increase congruence of standard DBT. For example, Lina actively participated in the creation of her diary card in which she identified daily goals she would monitor and attempt to change using DBT skills. Furthermore, pictures were included into the diary card to depict emotions and behaviors. One culturally sensitive image was that of the *calavera* (skull) to depict when Lina experienced thoughts of suicide. Moreover, a token economy was practiced in the DBT skills group in which Lina and the other clients would receive credit for attending group, completing homework assignments and arriving to group on time. The token economy entailed using cards similar to that of the game bingo, but unlike bingo, these cards depicted pictures on them instead of numbers. These pictures were of different characters in the bingo-type Latinx game, *La Loteria*. Lina was very familiar with *La Loteria* as her family played it often when she was growing up.

- Context: Finally, the element of *context* was applied as Lina's provider incorporated the discussion of issues such as her socio-economic status, age, gender, and language proficiency into treatment. For example, Lina had graduated high school, but had not held a steady job after high school and had been financially dependent on family members, partners and currently on her husband. Lina reported that she felt that because she was a woman, had very limited English skills, was in her late thirties and had an unsteady work history – so feared she would have limited opportunities to fare well in life. She felt obligated to stay married despite her desires to get a divorce and become more independent. Furthermore, because Lina struggled with a solid sense of identity, she felt further immobilized to change her current situation. Lina often reported how her husband worked two jobs and her family still felt financially strained. Lina's provider assisted her in creating realistic goals, examining the possible ramifications of culture-counter decisions such as getting a divorce and validated her realistic concerns regarding the challenges related to a low English skills. As illustrated via the case of Lina in an adapted Spanish DBT program, interventions should be considered for adaptation in an effort to better engage and treat immigrant populations. The remaining three steps of the Five-Step Framework of Mental Health Care with Immigrants are case management, evaluation of treatment and termination-each will be expounded on next.

Case Management

The third step of the Five-Step Framework of Mental Health Care with Immigrants is case management. Case management is another important area to consider when providing mental health care to immigrants- for a number of reasons. For example, as a result of their low socioeconomic status and loss of social and instrumental support, providing case management may serve as a key intervention towards increasing access and use of mental health care. That is, case management may address higher level problems that immigrants may be faced with such as those related to basic needs- and this in turn may increase their capacity to focus on their mental health care. For example, providing an immigrant family of low income with resources on where they may obtain free food may relieve the unspoken stressor of worrying about how they will be able to provide a meal for their family. Thus this may allow the client with an opportunity to now focus on adhering to their mental health treatment plan and adopting mental health interventions. Utilizing case management to help meet basic needs such as addressing food insecurities may allow the client the bandwidth to focus on their mental health and overall well-being.

Notably, when an immigrant client is provided with a resource or a referral to a resource, it is crucial that the provider make sure to confirm that the resource or referral is reliable. This is important as to avoid providing an immigrant client (who has a language barrier) with a resource in which the telephone number is wrong or the resource is no longer accepting referrals. This is important in order to a) ensure that the client is adequately linked and b) decrease the risk of the client's needs becoming unmet. The following steps are recommended when providing an immigrant client with a resource or referral:

1. Provider should make contact with the resource to ensure that they are accepting new referrals
2. Provider should obtain the contact information of the person whom the client should contact at the resource
3. Provider should confirm that the resource has the capacity to communicate with the client in the client's primary or preferred language
4. Provider should have a follow up appointment with the client after the termination session to ensure that they were properly linked with referrals, or invite the client to contact the provider should the referral fall through or become obsolete

Evaluation of Treatment

The fourth step in the Five-Step Framework of Mental Health Care with Immigrants is evaluation of treatment. In this step, it is very important for providers to engage the immigrant client into sharing their personal feedback about treatment. Oftentimes immigrant client's may shy away from giving feedback despite perhaps not feeling completely satisfied or desiring to change an aspect of the care they receive. Evaluating the care that is provided by simply asking for their input on how things are going may serve as instrumental. Moreover, evaluation treatment with their feedback may also help them feel as though they are an active participant and partner in their treatment – rather than a recipient with "no say" on how care is delivered. Suggested questions to evaluate treatment include:

- What went well in session today?
- What did not go well in session today?
- What is one thing that the provider (I) can do better?
- What is one thing that the provider (I) can continue to do?
- What is one thing that the provider (I) can stop doing?

- Are you satisfied with the way that treatment is going so far? Why or why not?
- Do you believe that your mental health symptoms are getting better, getting worse or remaining the same? Why or why not?
- What evidence do you have to support your response that your mental health symptoms are getting better, getting worse or remaining the same?

Termination

In considering termination, the last step of the framework suggests that immigrant client's be fully linked with needed referrals. It may be easy to overlook the continued need for resources among immigrant populations if this group already struggles to advocate for their wants or needs. Therefore, we encourage providers working with immigrant populations to assess if there are additional areas of need – from the client's perspective. Perhaps an immigrant client may share that although their mental health symptoms have been resolved they may still be struggling with finding employment or daycare. Although these needs may not be directly connected to their mental health goals- these needs should be considered as a part of providing standard case management. Left overlooked, these needs may create chronic stressors that may ultimately increase mental health symptoms. In the next section, the Five-Step Framework of Mental Health Care with Immigrants will be illustrated via the case of Gabby.

THE CASE OF GABBY VIA THE FIVE-STEP FRAMEWORK OF MENTAL HEALTH CARE WITH IMMIGRANTS

Gabby is a 32-year-old female Latinx immigrant diagnosed with generalized anxiety disorder and major depression disorder seeking asylum in the United States. Gabby was referred to mental health services by her primary medical doctor from a local not-for-profit health center. During her assessment, Gabby's provider completed a standard assessment, including both a religious/spiritual assessment and a cultural assessment. The provider obtained that Gabby was Catholic and held very conservative values regarding traditional gender roles. Further in completing the cultural assessment using the ADDRESSING Framework, the provider learned that Gabby identified as being Mexican and of poor socioeconomic status. This aided the provider as it gave the provider ideas on potential ideas on how to adapt treatment to be more culturally relevant for Gabby. To this end, the provider asked Gabby what some of her traditions and customs entailed. Gabby shared that she loved *pan dulce* (sweet bread) for breakfast and it reminded her of her grandmother and helped her to forget the separation of her grandmother upon immigrating. During the following therapy sessions, the provider adapted the content of treatment (see EVF model), by bringing *pan dulce* to their early morning therapy sessions. This gave Gabby a sense of hope in that she felt understood and truly cared for by her provider. During one of their routine sessions, Gabby shared that her daycare provider would no longer be able to care for her daughter and thus, she would no longer be able to continue in treatment as she did not have anyone who would be able to care for her daughter while she was in treatment. Gabby's therapist engaged in case management by investigating if there were any local daycare options for Gabby. The provider learned that there would soon be a daycare option opening up near Gabby's apartment complex and helped Gabby apply for daycare. As a result, Gabby was successfully able to obtain daycare and continue treatment. In an effort to evaluate treatment, after weekly sessions Gabby's provider asked Gabby, "so tell me what was one good thing that I did today in providing care and one thing that I can do better?". As a result of the provider asking this question every week, Gabby became more and more comfortable providing feedback and felt as though the delivery of care was collaborative and because of this- very helpful. Over the course of six months Gabby's generalized anxiety and major depression disorders symptoms were relieved and Gabby would soon be terminating treatment. Upon termination Gabby's provider assessed if Gabby had any additional needs related to case management. Gabby shared that she really needed to see a dentist due to having tooth pain but did not know where to go. Gabby's provider gave her a list of low cost and free dental providers funded by the county. Gabby felt relieved that she would finally also be able to receive much needed dental care.

Although the case of Gabby may appear simplified, considering adopting the Five-Step Framework of Mental Health Care for Immigrants may potentially make an important impact in care provided. For example, consider if Gabby's provider never asked for feedback- perhaps Gabby may feel as though the case was "one sided" and feel less included and inclined to participate. Or perhaps during termination, Gabby's provided never asked for any additional unmet needs that Gabby had. This may have led Gabby to experience severe tooth pain, to the point that it affected her mental health. To this end, we recommend the application of the Five-Step Framework of Mental Health Care for Immigrants in clinical practice.

This chapter began with an overview of barriers and facilitators to access and use of mental health care for immigrant adults and children. Next, the chapter provided a number of recommendations for clinical practice. The core recommendation was the Five-Step Framework of Mental Health Care with Immigrants which outlined specific examples of how each step of the framework may be implemented. Lastly, the chapter recommended the use of the EVF for culturally adapting mental health evidenced based clinica interventions for immigrants.

REFERENCES

American Psychiatric Association. (2013). *Diagnostic and statistical manual of mental disorders* (5th ed.)., DOI: 10.1176/appi.books.9780890425596

Andrés-Hyman, R. C., Ortiz, J., Añez, L. M., Paris, M., & Davidson, L. (2006). Culture and clinical practice: Recommendations for working with Puerto Ricans and other Latinxs (os) in the United States. *Professional Psychology, Research and Practice*, *37*(6), 694–701. DOI: 10.1037/0735-7028.37.6.694

Bernal, G., Bonilla, J., & Bellido, C. (1995). Ecological validity and cultural sensitivity for outcome research: Issues for the cultural adaptation and development of psychosocial treatments with Hispanics. *Journal of Abnormal Child Psychology*, *23*(1), 67–82. DOI: 10.1007/BF01447045 PMID: 7759675

Bernal, G., & Sáez-Santiago, E. (2006). Culturally centered psychosocial interventions. *Journal of Community Psychology*, *34*(2), 121–132. DOI: 10.1002/jcop.20096

Berry, J. W., & Annis, R. C. (1974). Acculturative stress: The role of ecology, culture and differentiation. *Journal of Cross-Cultural Psychology*, *5*(4), 382–406. DOI: 10.1177/002202217400500402

Bhugra, D., Watson, C., & Wijesuriya, R. (2021). Culture and mental illnesses. *International Review of Psychiatry (Abingdon, England)*, *33*(1–2), 1–2. DOI: 10.1080/09540261.2020.1777748 PMID: 33599563

Brabeck, K. M., Sibley, E., & Lykes, M. B. (2016). Authorized and unauthorized immigrant parents: The impact of legal vulnerability on family contexts. *Hispanic Journal of Behavioral Sciences*, *38*(1), 3–30. DOI: 10.1177/0739986315621741

Carter, G. L., Willcox, C. H., Lewin, T. J., Conrad, A. M., & Bendit, N. (2010). Hunter DBT project: Randomized controlled trial of dialectical behaviour therapy in women with borderline personality disorder. *The Australian and New Zealand Journal of Psychiatry*, *44*(2), 162–173. DOI: 10.3109/00048670903393621 PMID: 20113305

Carter, R. T., Mazzula, S., Victoria, R., Vazquez, R., Hall, S., Smith, S., Sant-Barket, S., Forsyth, J., Bazelais, K., & Williams, B. (2013). Initial development of the Race-Based Traumatic Stress Symptom Scale: Assessing the emotional impact of racism. *Psychological Trauma: Theory, Research, Practice, and Policy*, *5*(1), 1–9. DOI: 10.1037/a0025911

Castelli, F. (2018). Drivers of migration: Why do people move? *Journal of Travel Medicine*, *25*(1). Advance online publication. DOI: 10.1093/jtm/tay040 PMID: 30053084

Comas-Díaz, Lillian, Gordon Nagayama Hall, and Helen A. Neville. "Racial trauma: Theory, research, and healing: Introduction to the special issue." *American Psychologist* 74.1 (2019): 1.

Cross, F. L., Agi, A., Montoro, J. P., Medina, M. A., Miller-Tejada, S., Pinetta, B. J., Tran-Dubongco, M., & Rivas-Drake, D. (2020). Illuminating ethnic-racial socialization among undocumented Lat- inx parents and its implications for adolescent psychosocial functioning. *Developmental Psychology*, *56*(8), 1458–1474. DOI: 10.1037/dev0000826 PMID: 32790445

Derr, A. S. (2016). Mental health service use among immigrants in the United States: A systematic review. *Psychiatric Services (Washington, D.C.)*, *67*(3), 265–274. DOI: 10.1176/appi.ps.201500004 PMID: 26695493

Dimeff, L. A., McMain, S., Sayrs, J. H., Wilks, C. R., & Linehan, M. M. (2020). DBT for individuals with borderline personality disorder and substance use disorders. *Dialectical Behavior Therapy in Clinical Practice*, 233.

Domenech Rodríguez, M. M., & Bernal, G. (2012). Frameworks, models, and guidelines for cultural adaptation. In Bernal, G., & Rodríguez, M. M. D. (Eds.), *Cultural Adaptations: Tools for Evidence-Based Practice With Diverse Populations* (pp. 23–44). American Psychological Association., https://www.jstor.org/stable/j.ctv1chrt50.7 DOI: 10.1037/13752-002

Foa, E. B., Cashman, L., Jaycox, L., & Perry, K. (1995). Posttraumatic diagnostic scale. *Assessment of partner violence: A handbook for researchers and practitioners.*

Garcini, L. M., Daly, R., Chen, N., Mehl, J., Pham, T., Phan, T., Hansen, B., & Kothare, A. (2021). Undocumented immigrants and mental health: A systematic review of recent methodology and findings in the United States. *Journal of Migration and Health*, *4*, 100058. DOI: 10.1016/j.jmh.2021.100058 PMID: 34405198

Gearing, R. E., Washburn, M., Brewer, K. B., Cabrera, A., Yu, M., & Torres, L. R. (2024). Pathways to mental health care: Latinos' help-seeking preferences. *Journal of Latina/o Psychology*, *12*(1), 1–17. DOI: 10.1037/lat0000237

Harned, M. S., Korslund, K. E., & Linehan, M. M. (2014). A pilot randomized controlled trial of Dialectical Behavior Therapy with and without the Dialectical Behavior Therapy Prolonged Exposure protocol for suicidal and self-injuring women with borderline personality disorder and PTSD. *Behaviour Research and Therapy, 55*, 7–17. DOI: 10.1016/j.brat.2014.01.008 PMID: 24562087

Hays, P. A. (2022). *Addressing cultural complexities in psychotherapy and clinical practice: An intersectional approach* (4th ed.). American Psychological Association.

Hodge, D. R., & Holtrop, C. R. (2002). Spiritual assessment: A review of complementary assessment models. *Social work and Christianity: Readings on the integration of Christian faith and social work practice, 2*, 167-192.

Jimenez, D. E., Bartels, S. J., Cardenas, V., & Alegría, M. (2013). Stigmatizing attitudes toward mental illness among racial/ethnic older adults in primary care. [PubMed: 23361866]. *International Journal of Geriatric Psychiatry, 28*(10), 1061–1068. DOI: 10.1002/gps.3928 PMID: 23361866

Kim, B. J. (2011). *Factors that Influence Quality of Life among Low-Income Elderly Korean Immigrants in Adult Day Health Care (ADHC)*. University of California.

Kröger, C., Harbeck, S., Armbrust, M., & Kliem, S. (2013). Effectiveness, response, and dropout of dialectical behavior therapy for borderline personality disorder in an inpatient setting. *Behaviour Research and Therapy, 51*(8), 411–416. DOI: 10.1016/j.brat.2013.04.008 PMID: 23727659

Linehan, M. M., Korslund, K. E., Harned, M. S., Gallop, R. J., Lungu, A., Neacsiu, A. D., McDavid, J., Comtois, K. A., & Murray-Gregory, A. M. (2015). Dialectical behavior therapy for high suicide risk in individuals with borderline personality disorder: A randomized clinical trial and component analysis. *JAMA Psychiatry, 72*(5), 475–482. DOI: 10.1001/jamapsychiatry.2014.3039 PMID: 25806661

Mahabir, D. F., O'Campo, P., Lofters, A., Shankardass, K., Salmon, C., & Muntaner, C. (2021). Classism and everyday racism as experienced by racialized health care users: A concept mapping study. *International Journal of Health Services, 51*(3), 350–363. DOI: 10.1177/00207314211014782 PMID: 33949220

Ojeda, L., Flores, L. Y., Meza, R. R., & Morales, A. (2011). Culturally competent qualitative research with Latino immigrants. *Hispanic Journal of Behavioral Sciences, 33*(2), 184–203. DOI: 10.1177/0739986311402626

Ornelas, I. J., Yamanis, T. J., & Ruiz, R. A. (2020). The Health of Undocumented Latinx Immigrants: What We Know and Future Directions. *Annual review of public health, 41*, 2 89–308. https://doi.org/DOI: 10.1146/annurev-publhealth-040119-094211

Rana, K., Kent, J. L., & Page, A. (2025). Housing inequalities and health outcomes among migrant and refugee populations in high-income countries: A mixed-methods systematic review. *BMC Public Health*, *25*(1), 1098. DOI: 10.1186/s12889-025-22186-5 PMID: 40121396

Revens, K. E., Gutierrez, D., Paul, R., Reynolds, A. D., Price, R., & DeHaven, M. J. (2021). Social support and religiosity as contributing factors to resilience and mental wellbeing in Latino immigrants: A community-based participatory research study. *Journal of Immigrant and Minority Health*, *23*(5), 904–916. DOI: 10.1007/s10903-021-01179-7 PMID: 33715112

Saechao, F., Sharrock, S., Reicherter, D., Livingston, J. D., Aylward, A., Whisnant, J., Koopman, C., & Kohli, S. (2012). Stressors and barriers to using mental health services among diverse groups of first-generation immigrants to the United States. *Community Mental Health Journal*, *48*(1), 98–106. DOI: 10.1007/s10597-011-9419-4 PMID: 21655942

Salami, B., Salma, J., & Hegadoren, K. (2019). Access and utilization of mental health services for immigrants and refugees: Perspectives of immigrant service providers. *International Journal of Mental Health Nursing*, *28*(1), 152–161. DOI: 10.1111/inm.12512 PMID: 29984880

Shelton, D., Kesten, K., Zhang, W., & Trestman, R. (2011). Impact of a dialectic behavior therapy—Corrections Modified (DBT-CM) upon behaviorally challenged incarcerated male adolescents. *Journal of Child and Adolescent Psychiatric Nursing*, *24*(2), 105–113. DOI: 10.1111/j.1744-6171.2011.00275.x PMID: 21501287

Straiton, M. L., Aambø, A. K., & Johansen, R. (2019). Perceived discrimination, health and mental health among immigrants in Norway: The role of moderating factors. *BMC Public Health*, *19*(1), 1–13. DOI: 10.1186/s12889-019-6649-9 PMID: 30894173

Sue, D. W., Capodilupo, C. M., Torino, G. C., Bucceri, J. M., Holder, A., Nadal, K. L., & Esquilin, M. (2007). Racial microaggressions in everyday life: Implications for clinical practice. *The American Psychologist*, *62*(4), 271–286. DOI: 10.1037/0003-066X.62.4.271 PMID: 17516773

Tulli, M., Salami, B., Begashaw, L., Meherali, S., Yohani, S., & Hegadoren, K. (2020). Immigrant mothers' perspectives of barriers and facilitators in accessing mental health care for their children. *Journal of Transcultural Nursing*, *31*(6), 598–605. DOI: 10.1177/1043659620902812 PMID: 32013750

United States Department of Health and Human Services. (1996) Health Insurance Portability and Accountability Act of 1996. https://aspe.hhs.gov/reports/health-insurance-portability-accountability-act-1996

Williams, M. T., Peña, A., & Mier-Chairez, J. (2017). Tools for assessing racism-related stress and trauma among Latinos. In Benuto, L. T. (Ed.), *Toolkit for counseling Spanish-speaking clients*. Springer., DOI: 10.1007/978-3-319-64880-4_4

Williams, M. T., Printz, D., & DeLapp, R. C. (2018). Assessing racial trauma with the Trauma Symptoms of Discrimination Scale. *Psychology of Violence*, *8*(6), 735–747. DOI: 10.1037/vio0000212

Zaidi, R., & Sah, P. K. (2025). "Just make them feel welcomed": Examining newcomer ESL students' intersectional racism in Canadian schools. *International Multilingual Research Journal*, *19*(2), 1–18. DOI: 10.1080/19313152.2025.2476838

Zghal, A., El-Masri, M., McMurphy, S., & Pfaff, K. (2021). Exploring the impact of health care provider cultural competence on new immigrant health-related quality of life: A cross-sectional study of Canadian newcomers. *Journal of Transcultural Nursing*, *32*(5), 508–517. DOI: 10.1177/1043659620967441 PMID: 33095098

Chapter 7
From Trauma to Triumph Psychological Perspectives on Domestic Violence, Human Trafficking, and Victim Resilience

Sneha Shenoy
https://orcid.org/0009-0004-0843-1734
PES University, India

ABSTRACT

This chapter explores the profound psychological impacts of domestic violence and human trafficking, highlighting their role as pervasive human rights violations. It delves into the psychological effects, including PTSD, depression, and dissociation, and underscores the resilience many victims exhibit. The integration of forensic psychology provides critical insights into trauma assessment and therapeutic interventions, combining trauma-focused cognitive-behavioral therapy and legal advocacy to aid recovery. Drawing on case studies, the chapter demonstrates the transformative potential of forensic interventions in fostering resilience and recovery. It also emphasizes the importance of multidisciplinary collaboration, trauma-informed care, and culturally sensitive practices in promoting healing. Finally, ethical considerations and future directions in forensic psychology, including advocacy for systemic changes and improved access to mental health services, are discussed.

DOI: 10.4018/979-8-3693-7944-8.ch007

INTRODUCTION TO TRAUMA AND FORENSIC PSYCHOLOGY

Every day, millions of individuals around the world endure the devastating consequences of domestic violence and human trafficking. These forms of abuse are among the most severe violations of human dignity, subjecting victims to overwhelming psychological, emotional, and physical damage. Domestic violence, which frequently occurs within intimate relationships, follows a repeated cycle of abusive behavior. This abuse manifests not only in the form of physical violence but also emotional manipulation, sexual assault, economic control, and psychological intimidation. The insidious nature of this abuse makes it particularly harmful, as victims often feel entrapped, powerless, and isolated (Campbell, 2002).

On a global scale, human trafficking represents another horrific form of exploitation, often targeting vulnerable populations such as women and children. Victims of human trafficking are subjected to forced labor, sexual exploitation, and coercion, stripping away their autonomy and, in many cases, their sense of personhood (van der Kolk, 2014). These individuals are coerced into environments where their basic human rights are denied, often living in extreme conditions of deprivation, abuse, and isolation. The long-lasting psychological impacts of these abuses are profound, leaving survivors with deeply rooted scars that affect their emotional, mental, and physical well-being.

Trauma, in this context, can be understood as a response to events or situations that are overwhelmingly distressing, leaving the individual unable to cope effectively (Herman, 1992). The effects of trauma go beyond the immediate harm caused by the event, leading to chronic psychological and physiological consequences. For victims of domestic violence and human trafficking, trauma may result in long-term psychological disorders, such as post-traumatic stress disorder (PTSD), depression, severe anxiety, dissociation, and physical health issues that arise from prolonged exposure to stress (Clum & Whitman, 1991). The ripple effects of trauma infiltrate every aspect of the victim's life, from their emotional regulation to their sense of identity, self-worth, and ability to trust others. Victims often struggle to form or maintain meaningful relationships due to lingering fear and emotional distress. In many cases, they develop a sense of learned helplessness, where they come to believe that they are incapable of changing their circumstances, further reinforcing the cycle of abuse and exploitation (Widom & Maxfield, 2001).

Understanding these psychological ramifications is where forensic psychology plays a critical role. Forensic psychology, a specialized subfield that intersects psychology with the legal system, plays an indispensable role in assessing and addressing the psychological impacts of trauma on victims. Forensic psychologists are uniquely positioned to evaluate the mental health impacts of domestic violence and human trafficking, often providing essential expert testimony in court proceedings.

This may involve assessing the degree of psychological damage endured by victims, offering insights during custody disputes, or assisting in cases where restraining orders are necessary (Bartol & Bartol, 2019). In cases of human trafficking, forensic psychologists collaborate with law enforcement agencies, offering psychological evaluations of victims that help facilitate recovery and assist in reintegrating survivors into society. Such legal assessments are not only crucial for protecting victims' rights but also for ensuring that they receive appropriate psychological care.

Beyond legal assessments, forensic psychologists play an integral role in the development of therapeutic interventions tailored to victims of severe trauma. The trauma inflicted by domestic violence and human trafficking requires specialized care that acknowledges the complexity and intensity of the abuse. The mental health interventions provided in forensic settings are often trauma-informed, recognizing the intricate layers of emotional, psychological, and physiological damage that victims endure. Forensic psychologists are tasked with developing and implementing therapeutic strategies—such as cognitive-behavioral therapy (CBT), psychoeducation, and group therapy—that help victims process and work through their trauma. These interventions are designed not only to assist victims in rebuilding their self-esteem and sense of control over their lives but also to help them regain autonomy that had been eroded by their abusers (Green, 2007).

The nature of trauma, particularly when it results from chronic and severe abuse, can have profound effects on the brain, body, and psyche. Recent advances in neuroscience have shed light on how prolonged exposure to trauma alters brain structures, specifically those involved in memory consolidation, emotional regulation, and the body's stress response (van der Kolk, 2014). These changes are particularly evident in the hippocampus and amygdala, where trauma has been shown to alter normal functioning, leading to difficulties in memory processing and heightened emotional responses to stress. Chronic trauma can also impair the prefrontal cortex, which is responsible for executive functions such as decision-making and impulse control, making it harder for victims to regulate emotions and respond to stressful situations rationally (McEwen, 2007). This neurobiological impact of trauma complicates recovery, making it difficult for victims of long-term abuse to differentiate between past traumatic experiences and present realities.

One of the key challenges for forensic psychologists is in the assessment of trauma-related symptoms, particularly when those symptoms are not outwardly visible. Victims of domestic violence and human trafficking often face barriers to disclosing their experiences, including social stigma, fear of retaliation, and a lack of trust in the legal system. The forensic psychologist's role, therefore, goes beyond traditional psychological assessments. They must create an environment of trust and safety, encouraging victims to disclose their experiences while simultaneously providing the psychological support necessary to foster healing. Furthermore, forensic psychologists must remain attuned to the broader societal and systemic factors, such as poverty, inequality, and discrimination, which often exacerbate the victim's vulnerability to abuse. Addressing these systemic issues is vital for ensuring that forensic interventions are comprehensive and holistic, addressing not just the trauma itself but the social conditions that enabled the abuse (Green, 2007).

In addition to their work with individual victims, forensic psychologists have a broader role to play in advocating for systemic change. Domestic violence and human trafficking are deeply ingrained in societal structures that perpetuate inequality and power imbalances. Forensic psychologists, through their clinical work and research, can contribute to the development of more effective legal frameworks and social policies that protect vulnerable populations. By advocating for trauma-informed policies and prevention strategies, forensic psychologists help raise awareness of the root causes of abuse and exploitation and push for societal changes that reduce the prevalence of these crimes.

Forensic psychology is indispensable in bridging the gap between clinical expertise and legal advocacy. Through their work, forensic psychologists help victims navigate the path from trauma to recovery, offering psychological insights that are crucial for both healing and legal justice. By integrating psychological principles with practical interventions, forensic psychologists offer victims of domestic violence and human trafficking the tools to reclaim their sense of self-worth, autonomy, and resilience, helping them triumph over their traumatic experiences.

PSYCHOLOGICAL EFFECTS OF DOMESTIC VIOLENCE AND HUMAN TRAFFICKING

Domestic violence and human trafficking are two of the most egregious violations of human rights, and their psychological impacts are both profound and long-lasting. These forms of trauma disrupt victims' emotional and mental well-being, with effects that can persist long after the abuse has ended. Understanding these psychological effects is crucial in forensic psychology, as they inform the development of therapeutic and legal interventions that aid in victims' recovery.

Psychological Effects of Domestic Violence

Domestic violence encompasses a range of abusive behaviors, including physical violence, emotional manipulation, psychological control, sexual abuse, and financial exploitation. Victims of domestic violence often experience a cascade of psychological symptoms resulting from the constant fear, stress, and devaluation they endure in abusive relationships. According to Campbell (2002), intimate partner violence can lead to profound psychological consequences such as post-traumatic stress disorder (PTSD), depression, anxiety, and dissociation. These effects are often exacerbated by the cyclical nature of abuse, where periods of tension and violence are followed by moments of false reconciliation, making it difficult for victims to break free from the relationship.

Post-Traumatic Stress Disorder (PTSD): Victims of domestic violence frequently develop PTSD, a condition that arises from exposure to traumatic events involving threat, harm, or violation. PTSD is characterized by intrusive memories of the traumatic event, nightmares, hypervigilance, and emotional numbness (Clum & Whitman, 1991). For domestic violence survivors, PTSD often manifests as heightened anxiety, difficulty sleeping, and an overwhelming sense of dread. Victims may find themselves reliving traumatic events through flashbacks, which can be triggered by seemingly innocuous stimuli such as sounds, smells, or places. This hyperarousal state leaves them in a constant fight-or-flight mode, affecting their ability to function normally in daily life.

Depression and Learned Helplessness: The emotional toll of domestic violence often leads to chronic depression. Victims may experience feelings of worthlessness, hopelessness, and isolation. They might withdraw from social interactions, lose interest in activities they once enjoyed, or struggle with feelings of guilt and self-blame, believing that they are responsible for the abuse (Widom & Maxfield, 2001). One of the most concerning psychological effects of domestic violence is learned helplessness, a condition in which victims come to believe that they have no control over their situation, leading them to remain in abusive relationships despite opportunities to escape (Seligman, 1975). This phenomenon is particularly prevalent in cases of long-term abuse, where victims feel trapped by economic dependence, fear of retribution, or concern for their children.

Anxiety and Fear: Constant exposure to abusive behaviors creates a pervasive sense of fear and insecurity in victims. Anxiety disorders, particularly generalized anxiety disorder (GAD) and panic disorder, are common among survivors of domestic violence. Victims may live in a heightened state of vigilance, always anticipating the next episode of violence or emotional abuse (Briere & Scott, 2015). This chronic stress has significant physical health implications as well, contributing to headaches, gastrointesShel issues, and heart disease.

Dissociation and Emotional Numbness: Dissociation is another frequent response to the trauma of domestic violence. Victims may mentally distance themselves from the abuse as a coping mechanism, leading to feelings of detachment from reality or emotional numbness. This can manifest as a sense of unreality, as though the individual is observing events from outside their body. Dissociation can make it difficult for victims to recall specific details of the abuse, complicating forensic assessments and legal proceedings (Herman, 1992).

Psychological Effects of Human Trafficking

Human trafficking, by its very nature, is a deeply dehumanizing form of abuse that subjects individuals to exploitation, coercion, and forced labor. Trafficking victims often endure extreme forms of psychological, physical, and sexual abuse, and the trauma they experience can result in complex mental health issues.

Complex PTSD (C-PTSD): While trafficking survivors may also suffer from PTSD, many develop Complex PTSD (C-PTSD), a condition that arises from prolonged exposure to trauma, particularly in situations where the victim is unable to escape or gain control over their circumstances (van der Kolk, 2014). Unlike PTSD, which is often linked to a single traumatic event, C-PTSD results from ongoing trauma and leads to a broader range of psychological symptoms. These can include difficulties in emotional regulation, feelings of worthlessness, distrust of others, and persistent guilt or shame. Victims of human trafficking often find themselves unable to form healthy relationships due to pervasive distrust and a fear of exploitation.

Shame and Guilt: Trafficking survivors often grapple with intense feelings of shame and guilt, particularly if they were coerced into sexual exploitation or criminal activities. Many victims internalize the blame for their situation, believing they are responsible for the harm they have suffered. This sense of shame can prevent victims from seeking help, as they fear judgment or condemnation from society. According to Banyard, Williams, and Siegel (2003), these feelings of guilt can be compounded by societal stigma, which may view victims as complicit in their exploitation rather than recognizing them as victims of coercion.

Dissociative Disorders and Amnesia: Like domestic violence survivors, trafficking victims may also experience dissociation as a defense mechanism against ongoing trauma. For trafficking survivors, dissociation can be more severe, leading to dissociative identity disorder (DID) or dissociative amnesia. These conditions involve disruptions in memory, identity, or consciousness, which can leave survivors unable to recall important details of their lives or even form cohesive identities. Dissociative disorders are particularly prevalent among individuals subjected to long-term sexual exploitation, as the mind attempts to shield itself from overwhelming pain by creating psychological distance from the traumatic experiences (Briere & Scott, 2015).

Substance Abuse and Self-Harm: Trafficking victims, particularly those who have been sexually exploited, are at high risk for developing substance use disorders. Substance abuse often begins as a coping mechanism for the emotional pain and trauma experienced during trafficking. Many victims use drugs or alcohol to numb their emotions, reduce anxiety, or escape the psychological distress caused by their circumstances. In addition, survivors of trafficking may also engage in self-harm behaviors, such as cutting or burning, as a way to regain a sense of control over their bodies (Ungar, 2011).

Intersection of Trauma and Physical Health

The psychological trauma endured by victims of domestic violence and human trafficking does not exist in isolation; it often has significant physical health consequences. Chronic stress from trauma affects the body's nervous system, leading to a range of stress-related health issues. Victims of prolonged trauma are at increased risk of developing chronic pain, cardiovascular diseases, immune system suppression, and gastrointesShel disorders (Campbell, 2002). The mind-body connection is particularly evident in survivors of trauma, as their emotional distress often translates into physical symptoms that complicate their recovery.

Impact on Daily Functioning and Relationships

The trauma experienced by victims of domestic violence and human trafficking often disrupts their ability to engage in daily activities, maintain employment, or foster healthy relationships. Victims may experience difficulty concentrating, making decisions, or trusting others, which can interfere with their ability to work or pursue education. Furthermore, the trauma they have experienced can make it challenging for them to form healthy relationships. Many survivors of domestic violence or trafficking report difficulty in trusting others or fearing that they may encounter further exploitation or abuse (Luthar, 2006).

In both legal and therapeutic contexts, understanding the breadth and depth of trauma's psychological effects is essential for supporting victims in their recovery. Forensic psychology provides the tools and frameworks necessary to assess these impacts and develop interventions that prioritize victims' mental health and well-being.

Resilience and Recovery

Despite the profound and lasting effects of trauma experienced by victims of domestic violence and human trafficking, many survivors display remarkable resilience. Resilience refers to the ability to recover from adversity, adapt to difficult situations, and continue functioning despite significant challenges (Masten, 2001). In the context of trauma, resilience does not imply the absence of suffering but rather the capacity to overcome it and rebuild one's life. The study of resilience within forensic psychology focuses on identifying the psychological factors and support systems that enable victims to recover from trauma and regain control over their lives.

Understanding Resilience

Resilience is a dynamic process influenced by a combination of internal psychological traits, external social supports, and environmental factors. According to Rutter (2012), resilience is not a fixed trait but a developmental process that can be strengthened or weakened over time, depending on the individual's environment and experiences. For survivors of domestic violence and human trafficking, resilience involves the ability to process and integrate traumatic experiences, maintain a sense of self-worth, and engage in positive coping strategies.

Psychological Factors in Resilience: Several psychological traits contribute to resilience, including self-efficacy, optimism, emotional regulation, and problem-solving skills. Self-efficacy refers to an individual's belief in their ability to influence events and outcomes in their life. Victims who develop a strong sense of self-efficacy are more likely to engage in behaviors that promote their well-being, such as seeking therapy, reaching out for social support, or taking steps to change their circumstances (Luthar, 2006). Optimism, or the tendency to view life events in a positive light, also plays a key role in resilience, helping victims maintain hope for the future despite their traumatic experiences.

Emotional regulation, the ability to manage and respond to emotional distress in a healthy manner, is another critical factor in resilience. Victims who can regulate their emotions effectively are better able to cope with the intense feelings of fear, anger, or sadness that often accompany trauma. This ability to manage emotional responses helps survivors avoid destructive coping mechanisms, such as substance abuse or self-harm, and focus on healing.

Positive Coping Strategies: Resilience is also facilitated by the use of positive coping strategies, which enable victims to deal with stress in constructive ways. These strategies can include seeking social support, engaging in physical activity, practicing mindfulness or relaxation techniques, and participating in therapy (Masten, 2001). Survivors who are able to identify and use adaptive coping strategies are better equipped to navigate the challenges posed by trauma and maintain their psychological health.

Post-Traumatic Growth: One concept closely related to resilience is post-traumatic growth, which refers to the positive psychological changes that can result from overcoming adversity. Post-traumatic growth involves a deepened sense of personal strength, improved relationships, and a greater appreciation for life following traumatic experiences (Tedeschi & Calhoun, 2004). While trauma undoubtedly causes significant harm, some survivors report that their experience led to personal growth, increased self-awareness, and a renewed sense of purpose. Understanding the potential for post-traumatic growth helps forensic psychologists recognize that recovery is not only about returning to a pre-trauma state but also about fostering positive change in the aftermath of trauma.

Social and Environmental Factors

In addition to psychological traits, external factors such as social support and community resources play a vital role in promoting resilience. Traumatic experiences like domestic violence and human trafficking often leave victims feeling isolated, powerless, and disconnected from society. Rebuilding these connections and gaining access to supportive environments can be crucial for recovery.

Social Support Networks: One of the most important factors contributing to resilience is the presence of a strong social support network. Victims who have access to supportive relationships with family, friends, or community members are more likely to recover from trauma (Rutter, 2012). Social support provides victims with emotional validation, practical assistance, and a sense of belonging, all of which are essential for restoring their sense of self and agency. Forensic psychologists working with survivors often emphasize the importance of reconnecting with trusted individuals or developing new support systems, as isolation can exacerbate the psychological effects of trauma.

Community and Institutional Resources: Access to community and institutional resources is another critical component of resilience. Support services such as legal aid, shelters, counseling centers, and vocational training programs provide victims with the tools they need to rebuild their lives. For example, domestic violence shelters not only offer victims a safe space away from their abusers but also connect them with legal advocacy, financial assistance, and therapy, all of which contribute to their resilience (Banyard, Williams, & Siegel, 2003). For trafficking survivors, specialized recovery programs that address the unique challenges of reintegration into society, such as job training and mental health services, are essential for promoting resilience.

Cultural and Societal Factors: Cultural and societal attitudes towards domestic violence and human trafficking can also influence resilience. In cultures where victims are stigmatized or blamed for their trauma, survivors may face additional barriers to recovery. Conversely, societies that promote gender equality, human rights, and social justice provide a more supportive environment for victims to heal. Forensic psychologists must be mindful of these cultural dynamics when developing interventions, ensuring that their approach is culturally sensitive and aligns with the victim's values and beliefs (Ungar, 2011).

Role of Forensic Interventions in Promoting Resilience

Forensic psychology plays a critical role in both assessing trauma and implementing interventions that foster resilience. The recovery process for victims of domestic violence and human trafficking is multifaceted, requiring interventions that address not only their psychological needs but also their legal, social, and physical well-being. Forensic interventions are designed to support victims through therapeutic, legal, and advocacy services that promote recovery and resilience.

Therapeutic Interventions: Trauma-focused therapy is a key component of the recovery process for victims. Cognitive-behavioral therapy (CBT), specifically trauma-focused CBT, has been shown to be effective in helping survivors process their trauma, reframe negative beliefs, and develop coping strategies (Briere & Scott, 2015). Eye Movement Desensitization and Reprocessing (EMDR) is another therapeutic technique used to help victims of trauma reprocess distressing memories, reduce their emotional intensity, and foster resilience. Therapy provides a safe space for survivors to explore their emotions, address their trauma, and develop the psychological tools necessary for healing.

Forensic Assessments: Forensic psychologists also play a crucial role in assessing the psychological impact of trauma on victims. These assessments are used not only in therapeutic settings but also in legal contexts, where they help inform decisions regarding custody, legal protections, and the prosecution of offenders. Psychological assessments can evaluate the extent of trauma symptoms, the victim's capacity for resilience, and any ongoing mental health needs. These assessments are critical in both documenting the victim's trauma for legal proceedings and ensuring that they receive appropriate therapeutic interventions (Green, 2007).

Legal Advocacy and Support: In many cases, victims of domestic violence and human trafficking must navigate complex legal systems in order to obtain justice and safety. Forensic psychologists, alongside legal advocates, work to ensure that victims are informed of their legal rights and have access to necessary legal protections. In the context of domestic violence, this might involve securing restraining orders, child custody arrangements, or divorce proceedings. For trafficking survivors, legal support may involve immigration assistance, compensation claims, or prosecution of traffickers. By advocating for victims in legal contexts, forensic psychologists help protect their rights and ensure they receive the necessary support to rebuild their lives (American Psychological Association, 2013).

Resilience and Recovery: A Lifelong Process

It is important to recognize that recovery from trauma is not a linear process. Survivors of domestic violence and human trafficking may experience setbacks in their recovery, particularly if they are triggered by reminders of their trauma or face ongoing stressors such as legal battles or financial instability. Resilience, therefore, is not about achieving a permanent state of well-being but about developing the capacity to cope with challenges as they arise. Forensic psychology acknowledges the dynamic nature of resilience and works to equip victims with the tools and resources they need for lifelong recovery.

Forensic Assessment and Intervention

Forensic assessment and intervention are essential aspects of supporting victims of domestic violence and human trafficking. In forensic psychology, the assessment process involves evaluating the psychological effects of trauma, measuring the impact on mental health, and identifying individual needs for recovery and resilience. These assessments not only play a crucial role in therapeutic settings but are also used in legal contexts to ensure that victims receive appropriate legal protections and psychological interventions. Following the assessment phase, forensic psychologists work to implement targeted interventions aimed at promoting resilience, addressing trauma, and assisting victims in navigating legal and therapeutic systems.

Forensic Assessments: Evaluating Trauma and Resilience

Forensic assessments serve as the foundation for understanding the full scope of trauma experienced by victims. These evaluations are typically multifaceted and may include clinical interviews, standardized psychological testing, and behavioral observations to capture a comprehensive picture of the victim's psychological state. In cases of domestic violence and human trafficking, forensic assessments focus on the severity of trauma, the presence of post-traumatic stress disorder (PTSD) or other mental health conditions, and the victim's capacity for resilience.

Psychological Trauma Assessments: Victims of domestic violence and human trafficking often exhibit symptoms of PTSD, depression, anxiety, and complex trauma, which can profoundly impact their mental health and daily functioning. Assessing the psychological effects of trauma typically involves standardized tests such as the Clinician-Administered PTSD Scale (CAPS) or the Trauma Symptom Inventory (TSI) to measure the severity and range of trauma symptoms (Green, 2007). These tools help forensic psychologists identify key areas where victims need therapeutic intervention, including the management of intrusive memories, emotional numbing, and hyperarousal.

Cognitive and Behavioral Assessments: Trauma can also affect cognitive functioning and behavior, often impairing victims' ability to make decisions, regulate emotions, and engage in daily activities. Cognitive assessments evaluate the impact of trauma on memory, concentration, and decision-making abilities, while behavioral assessments examine the ways in which trauma influences the victim's interactions with others and their environment. For example, victims of human trafficking may exhibit avoidant behavior, social withdrawal, or distrust of authority figures, all of which are critical to address in both therapeutic and legal settings (van der Kolk, 2014).

Assessing Resilience: In addition to evaluating trauma, forensic assessments often include an analysis of the victim's resilience factors. This process involves exploring the victim's coping mechanisms, psychological strengths, social support networks, and capacity for recovery. Tools such as the Connor-Davidson Resilience Scale (CD-RISC) can be used to measure resilience, offering valuable insights into the victim's ability to bounce back from adversity and engage in the recovery process (Ungar, 2011). Understanding the victim's resilience is critical in tailoring interventions that not only address their trauma but also build upon their strengths to foster long-term recovery.

Forensic Interventions: Therapeutic and Legal Support

Once a comprehensive assessment has been conducted, forensic psychologists work to develop interventions that address both the psychological and legal needs of victims. These interventions are designed to help victims process their trauma, develop coping strategies, and navigate the legal system. In the context of domestic violence and human trafficking, forensic interventions are often multidisciplinary, involving collaboration between psychologists, legal advocates, social workers, and medical professionals to ensure a holistic approach to recovery.

Trauma-Informed Therapy: One of the primary goals of forensic intervention is to provide victims with trauma-informed therapy, which is designed to help them process their traumatic experiences and develop healthy coping mechanisms. Trauma-focused cognitive-behavioral therapy (TF-CBT) is widely regarded as one of the most effective therapeutic approaches for treating victims of domestic violence and human trafficking (Briere & Scott, 2015). TF-CBT helps victims reframe negative thoughts, address maladaptive beliefs about their trauma, and develop strategies for managing emotional distress.

Eye Movement Desensitization and Reprocessing (EMDR) is another therapeutic approach commonly used in forensic settings to help victims reprocess traumatic memories. By focusing on distressing memories while engaging in bilateral eye movements, EMDR allows victims to reduce the emotional intensity of these memories, ultimately facilitating their recovery (van der Kolk, 2014). These therapeutic interventions play a key role in helping victims overcome the psychological effects of trauma and regain control over their lives.

Support for Legal Proceedings: In many cases, victims of domestic violence and human trafficking are involved in legal proceedings, such as restraining orders, custody disputes, criminal prosecutions, or immigration hearings. Forensic psychologists play a vital role in supporting victims through these legal processes, ensuring that they have access to the necessary psychological evaluations and expert testimony to protect their rights. Legal proceedings can be retraumatizing for victims, particularly if they are required to testify against their abusers or traffickers. Forensic psychologists work to minimize the psychological impact of legal proceedings by preparing victims for court appearances, offering emotional support, and advocating for their legal rights (American Psychological Association, 2013).

Multidisciplinary Collaboration: Effective forensic interventions often require collaboration between multiple professionals, including social workers, medical providers, legal advocates, and law enforcement. For example, in cases of human trafficking, victims may need medical care for physical injuries, legal assistance for immigration or asylum claims, and psychological therapy to address their trauma. Multidisciplinary teams work together to create comprehensive recovery plans that address the wide range of needs presented by victims. This holistic approach ensures that victims receive the support they need to heal not only psychologically but also physically and legally (Banyard, Williams, & Siegel, 2003).

Case Management and Advocacy: Forensic psychologists often serve as case managers and advocates for victims, helping them navigate complex systems of care and ensuring they receive appropriate services. This role may involve connecting victims with community resources, such as domestic violence shelters, job training programs, or support groups. In cases of human trafficking, forensic psychologists may also work with non-governmental organizations (NGOs) to provide victims with safe housing, legal representation, and opportunities for education and employment. By advocating for victims in both legal and social contexts, forensic psychologists play a critical role in supporting their recovery and empowering them to regain control over their lives (Green, 2007).

ETHICAL CONSIDERATIONS IN FORENSIC ASSESSMENT AND INTERVENTION

Working with victims of domestic violence and human trafficking presents unique ethical challenges for forensic psychologists. These ethical considerations include maintaining confidentiality, ensuring informed consent, and navigating the complexities of dual roles in legal and therapeutic contexts.

Confidentiality and Safety: One of the primary ethical concerns when working with trauma victims is ensuring their safety and confidentiality. Victims of domestic violence and human trafficking are often in danger from their abusers, and maintaining their confidentiality is essential to protecting them from further harm. Forensic psychologists must take steps to safeguard the victim's personal information, particularly in legal settings where sensitive details may be disclosed (Koocher & Keith-Spiegel, 2016). Additionally, forensic psychologists must work closely with law enforcement and legal professionals to ensure that victims are safe from retaliation and have access to protective measures, such as restraining orders or secure housing.

Informed Consent: Ensuring that victims provide informed consent for assessments and interventions is another critical ethical consideration. Many victims, particularly those who have been trafficked, may have experienced coercion or manipulation, making it difficult for them to trust authority figures or understand their rights. Forensic psychologists must take extra care to explain the purpose of assessments, the potential consequences of legal proceedings, and the victim's rights to refuse or withdraw from interventions (American Psychological Association, 2013). This transparency is essential in empowering victims and ensuring that they are active participants in their recovery process.

Dual Roles in Legal and Therapeutic Contexts: Forensic psychologists often navigate dual roles when working with trauma victims, providing both therapeutic support and legal evaluations. Balancing these roles can be challenging, as the goals of therapy (fostering recovery and resilience) may sometimes conflict with the demands of legal evaluations (providing objective assessments for court). Forensic psychologists must maintain clear boundaries between their therapeutic and evaluative roles, ensuring that victims understand the purpose of each and avoiding any potential conflicts of interest (Koocher & Keith-Spiegel, 2016). Maintaining ethical integrity in these dual roles is crucial for ensuring that victims receive fair and unbiased treatment in both legal and therapeutic settings.

Case Studies and Applications

Case studies are invaluable for understanding the real-world application of forensic psychology principles in supporting victims of domestic violence and human trafficking. These examples help illustrate how forensic assessment and intervention can be effectively implemented, offering a practical framework for addressing trauma and fostering resilience. By examining specific cases, we can gain insights into the challenges faced by victims, the complexities of trauma recovery, and the efficacy of various intervention strategies.

Case Study 1: Domestic Violence Survivor's Path to Resilience

Background:

A 35-year-old woman endured years of emotional, physical, and psychological abuse at the hands of her partner. She initially entered therapy following a court mandate for a psychological assessment, as she was seeking a restraining order. She exhibited symptoms of PTSD, including flashbacks, emotional numbness, and severe anxiety, and reported difficulty trusting others. In addition, she suffered from feelings of learned helplessness, believing that there was no escape from her abusive situation.

Forensic Assessment:

Her forensic assessment involved a combination of clinical interviews and standardized psychological tests, such as the PTSD Checklist for DSM-5 (PCL-5) and the Beck Depression Inventory (BDI). These assessments revealed high levels of trauma-related symptoms, severe depressive symptoms, and a sense of hopelessness. Her cognitive-behavioral patterns, marked by negative self-perception and distorted beliefs about control and safety, were key areas of concern.

Intervention:

A trauma-focused cognitive-behavioral therapy (TF-CBT) approach was adopted to address her trauma symptoms. The therapy included psychoeducation about the effects of trauma, cognitive restructuring to challenge her maladaptive beliefs, and gradual exposure to distressing memories in a controlled setting to reduce their intensity (Briere & Scott, 2015). Eye Movement Desensitization and Reprocessing

(EMDR) was also incorporated to help her process traumatic memories that had been causing flashbacks (van der Kolk, 2014).

Over time, she began to shift her perspective on the abuse she had experienced. She developed healthier coping strategies, such as mindfulness practices and relaxation techniques, to manage her anxiety. A key part of her recovery was the development of a strong support system, which included a local domestic violence support group that provided emotional validation and practical resources.

Outcome:

Through consistent therapy and support, her PTSD symptoms gradually decreased, and her sense of self-worth improved. She also became more assertive in advocating for her safety, securing a permanent restraining order and relocating to a safe environment. Her journey from trauma to resilience was not only facilitated by therapeutic interventions but also by the comprehensive forensic assessment that identified her key psychological challenges. This case demonstrates the importance of integrating trauma-informed therapy with legal protections to promote long-term recovery.

Case Study 2: Human Trafficking Survivor's Legal and Therapeutic Journey

Background:

A 24-year-old woman from Eastern Europe was trafficked into forced labor in a foreign country. After escaping from her traffickers, she was referred to a forensic psychologist by an NGO specializing in human trafficking cases. She had endured severe physical abuse and sexual exploitation and displayed symptoms of complex trauma, including dissociation, hypervigilance, and social isolation.

Forensic Assessment:

The forensic assessment process included a comprehensive clinical evaluation of her mental health, a psychosocial history, and interviews to assess her cognitive and emotional functioning. The Dissociative Experiences Scale (DES) and the Impact of Event Scale (IES) were used to assess dissociative symptoms and the severity of her post-traumatic responses (Green, 2007). Additionally, her legal status and eligibility for asylum required a detailed psychological evaluation to provide the court with evidence of the trauma she had experienced.

Intervention:

Her treatment plan involved multiple components, given the complexity of her trauma. Trauma-informed care (TIC) was the foundation of her therapeutic approach, ensuring that all interventions prioritized her safety, empowerment, and autonomy. In therapy, Eye Movement Desensitization and Reprocessing (EMDR) was used to help her process traumatic memories, while Cognitive Processing Therapy (CPT) focused on challenging and changing unhelpful thoughts related to her trauma (van der Kolk, 2014).

She also received legal advocacy support to help her navigate the asylum process. The forensic psychologist provided expert testimony in court, describing the profound psychological harm she had suffered and the need for legal protections.

Outcome:

Through her therapeutic journey, she gradually regained a sense of control over her life. Her dissociative episodes decreased, and she became more comfortable with social interactions. The combination of trauma-informed care, legal advocacy, and psychological therapy facilitated her path to resilience. In court, she was granted asylum, giving her the legal protection and stability she needed to rebuild her life. Her case highlights the critical role of forensic psychology in both therapeutic and legal contexts, demonstrating how comprehensive interventions can support recovery and empower survivors.

Case Study 3: Child Victim of Trafficking and Multidisciplinary Intervention

Background:

A 15-year-old girl was rescued from a child trafficking ring where she had been exploited for labor. When she entered a rehabilitation program, she was diagnosed with depression, PTSD, and attachment issues stemming from prolonged trauma and neglect. She exhibited aggressive behavior and struggled with trusting adults, making it difficult for her to engage in therapy.

Forensic Assessment:

Given her age and the complexity of her trauma, the forensic assessment process was thorough and involved collaboration with social workers, educators, and healthcare providers. Standardized assessments for child trauma, such as the Child

PTSD Symptom Scale (CPSS), were used to gauge the severity of her trauma-related symptoms. Observational data from caregivers in her rehabilitation program were also incorporated into the forensic report to capture her behavioral responses in a real-world setting.

Intervention:

Her intervention plan was designed using a multidisciplinary approach. Trauma-focused cognitive-behavioral therapy (TF-CBT) was tailored to meet her developmental needs, incorporating creative therapies like art and play therapy to help her express her emotions in non-verbal ways. Family therapy sessions were also introduced to rebuild attachment bonds, as her trauma had disrupted her ability to form trusting relationships with adults (Luthar, 2006).

Additionally, her case involved extensive collaboration between her forensic psychologist, social workers, and educators. Her psychologist played a key role in coordinating her care, ensuring that her mental health needs were addressed alongside her educational and social needs. Legal advocacy was provided to secure her placement in a safe foster care home, where she could continue her recovery in a stable environment.

Outcome:

Her aggressive behavior gradually diminished as she began to trust her therapists and caregivers. The integration of creative therapies helped her process her trauma in ways that felt less threatening than traditional talk therapy. Over time, she developed healthier relationships with adults and peers, and her academic performance improved as she regained a sense of stability. Her case underscores the importance of early intervention, multidisciplinary collaboration, and trauma-informed care in supporting child victims of trafficking.

APPLICATIONS TO FORENSIC PSYCHOLOGY

These case studies illustrate the wide-ranging applications of forensic psychology in addressing trauma and promoting resilience among victims of domestic violence and human trafficking. They demonstrate the critical role of forensic assessment in identifying the psychological effects of trauma and tailoring interventions to meet the unique needs of each individual. Additionally, they highlight the importance of multidisciplinary collaboration in ensuring that victims receive comprehensive care that addresses their psychological, legal, and social needs.

Forensic psychologists, through their assessments and interventions, not only support victims in recovering from trauma but also play a crucial role in advocating for their legal rights. Whether providing expert testimony in court, coordinating care with social services, or delivering trauma-informed therapy, forensic psychologists are instrumental in helping victims navigate the path from trauma to triumph.

Ethical Considerations and Future Directions

The field of forensic psychology, particularly when working with victims of domestic violence and human trafficking, presents a unique set of ethical challenges. These challenges stem from the deeply personal and traumatic nature of the cases, the potential legal implications, and the vulnerable status of the individuals involved. Ensuring that ethical standards are upheld is critical to providing effective and compassionate care while maintaining the trust and dignity of the victims.

Ethical Considerations in Forensic Psychology

Confidentiality and Privacy One of the fundamental ethical obligations in forensic psychology is maintaining confidentiality. However, this can be complicated when forensic psychologists are involved in legal cases where court-ordered reports or testimonies may require the disclosure of sensitive information. In cases of domestic violence and human trafficking, where victims may fear retribution from abusers or traffickers, ensuring the privacy of information is paramount. Psychologists must navigate the balance between legal obligations and protecting the well-being of their clients (Koocher & Keith-Spiegel, 2016).

Psychologists must also take care when working with victims who may be involved in ongoing investigations or legal proceedings. Informed consent must be obtained, ensuring that victims fully understand how their information may be used and what limits exist regarding confidentiality. Special attention must be paid to minors and individuals with diminished capacity to ensure their rights and autonomy are respected (American Psychological Association, 2013).

Informed Consent and Autonomy Informed consent is an essential component of ethical practice, especially when working with trauma survivors. Victims of domestic violence and human trafficking often experience a loss of autonomy, and ensuring that they have full control over their participation in forensic evaluations and therapy is crucial to their recovery process (Herman, 1992).

Ethical practice requires that psychologists provide clear, understandable information about the nature of assessments, interventions, and any legal proceedings. Survivors must be made aware of the potential risks and benefits, their rights to withdraw, and the extent of confidentiality. In cases where victims may feel coerced by external pressures, forensic psychologists must take steps to ensure that consent is voluntary and not influenced by fear or manipulation (Koocher & Keith-Spiegel, 2016).

Competence and Cultural Sensitivity Working with victims of domestic violence and human trafficking requires specialized knowledge and skills. Forensic psychologists must be competent in trauma-informed care, understanding the complex psychological effects of trauma, and recognizing the cultural, social, and economic factors that influence the experiences of survivors (Bartol & Bartol, 2019).

Cultural sensitivity is particularly important, as victims of trafficking often come from diverse backgrounds and may have different understandings of trauma, resilience, and justice. Psychologists must be aware of their own biases and approach each case with cultural humility, ensuring that interventions are tailored to the individual's cultural and contextual needs (Ungar, 2011).

Dual Roles and Conflicts of Interest Forensic psychologists often face the challenge of balancing dual roles, such as providing therapeutic care while also conducting forensic assessments for legal purposes. These dual roles can create conflicts of interest, as the therapeutic alliance may be compromised if victims feel that their personal information will be used against them in court (Green, 2007).

To avoid ethical dilemmas, psychologists must clearly delineate their roles and responsibilities from the outset, ensuring that victims understand the difference between therapeutic and forensic services. In situations where conflicts of interest arise, it may be necessary to refer the client to another professional to preserve the integrity of both the therapeutic relationship and the forensic process (Koocher & Keith-Spiegel, 2016).

Future Directions in Forensic Psychology and Trauma Intervention

Advancing Trauma-Informed Legal Practices As forensic psychology continues to evolve, there is growing recognition of the need to integrate trauma-informed practices into legal and judicial systems. Trauma-informed care emphasizes the importance of creating safe, supportive environments for victims, and this approach can be extended to courtrooms and legal proceedings. Courts that prioritize the emotional and psychological well-being of victims may reduce the retraumatization that often occurs during legal processes (Briere & Scott, 2015).

Future directions in forensic psychology may include the development of specialized courts or legal protocols for handling cases involving domestic violence and human trafficking, ensuring that victims receive both legal protection and psychological support. Additionally, forensic psychologists can advocate for policy changes that promote trauma-informed practices in law enforcement and the criminal justice system.

Enhancing Multidisciplinary Collaboration Multidisciplinary collaboration is crucial for addressing the complex needs of trauma survivors. Forensic psychologists, social workers, legal advocates, healthcare providers, and law enforcement must work together to create comprehensive care plans that address the psychological, social, and legal needs of victims. Future efforts should focus on improving communication and coordination between these professionals, ensuring that victims receive seamless support throughout their recovery (Green, 2007).

Integrating technology, such as shared electronic records or telehealth services, may facilitate better communication among professionals and increase access to care for victims in remote or underserved areas. Additionally, further research is needed to evaluate the effectiveness of multidisciplinary approaches in supporting resilience and long-term recovery for trauma survivors.

Expanding Research on Trauma and Resilience Research on trauma and resilience has made significant strides in recent years, but there are still many areas that require further exploration. For example, while much of the current literature focuses on the individual factors that contribute to resilience, more research is needed to understand the social and environmental factors that support recovery. Studies that examine the role of community support, cultural identity, and socio-economic factors in resilience may provide valuable insights into how to best support victims of domestic violence and human trafficking (Masten, 2001; Ungar, 2011).

Additionally, research on interventions for specific populations, such as children, LGBTQ+ individuals, and refugees, is needed to ensure that forensic psychology practices are inclusive and effective across diverse groups. As trauma research evolves, it is important that forensic psychologists continue to refine their interventions to meet the unique needs of all trauma survivors.

Improving Access to Mental Health Services One of the ongoing challenges in the field of forensic psychology is ensuring that trauma survivors have access to high-quality mental health services. Many victims of domestic violence and human trafficking face significant barriers to accessing care, including financial limitations, lack of awareness, and fear of stigma or retaliation. Future directions in the field should focus on developing innovative solutions to these barriers, such as offering free or low-cost mental health services, expanding teletherapy options, and increasing public awareness of available resources (Campbell, 2002).

Advocacy efforts at the policy level are also essential to improving access to care. Forensic psychologists can play a key role in shaping policies that prioritize mental health services for trauma survivors, particularly in underserved communities. By advocating for increased funding for mental health services, forensic psychologists can help ensure that victims receive the support they need to heal and rebuild their lives.

CONCLUSION

The psychological journey from trauma to triumph is a complex and multifaceted process, particularly for victims of domestic violence and human trafficking. These profound violations of human rights leave deep psychological scars, often challenging an individual's sense of self, safety, and autonomy. This chapter has explored the critical role that forensic psychology plays in understanding the intricacies of trauma, its devastating psychological effects, and the pathways that can lead to resilience and recovery.

One of the key takeaways from this exploration is that trauma, while damaging and destabilizing, is not an endpoint. With appropriate intervention, support, and resources, victims can reclaim their lives, rebuild their sense of self-worth, and, in many cases, emerge stronger. The resilience displayed by survivors is a testament to the strength of the human spirit, and it underscores the importance of creating environments that foster healing rather than perpetuate harm.

The psychological effects of domestic violence and human trafficking can manifest in a variety of ways, including post-traumatic stress disorder (PTSD), anxiety, depression, and learned helplessness. However, understanding these effects through the lens of forensic psychology allows practitioners to offer targeted and effective interventions. By addressing the immediate psychological needs of trauma survivors, forensic psychologists can help mitigate long-term effects and support victims as they work through their trauma in a way that promotes both mental and emotional healing.

Resilience, while often discussed in terms of personal strength, is deeply influenced by external factors, including social support, cultural context, and access to mental health services. As discussed in the chapter, the development of resilience is not an isolated phenomenon; it is supported by community, healthcare, and legal systems that prioritize the needs and well-being of victims. Understanding this interconnectedness is crucial for forensic psychologists, as it informs the design of interventions that address not only the individual's trauma but also the broader systemic factors that either hinder or facilitate recovery.

In the realm of forensic psychology, the role of assessments and therapeutic interventions cannot be overstated. Forensic psychologists are often tasked with conducting assessments that inform legal decisions, whether in cases of domestic violence, human trafficking, or other forms of trauma. The importance of using trauma-informed and culturally sensitive approaches in these assessments is paramount. Such approaches ensure that survivors are not further traumatized by the processes meant to help them, and that the legal system is better equipped to offer justice that is aligned with their psychological and emotional needs.

Intervention strategies, as discussed, must be flexible and multifaceted, combining therapeutic techniques that address trauma's psychological effects with legal strategies that protect and empower victims. Cognitive-behavioral therapy (CBT), trauma-focused therapy, and resilience-building techniques have been shown to offer substantial benefits to trauma survivors. Moreover, the integration of legal and psychological support helps create a more holistic approach to recovery, ensuring that victims receive the comprehensive care they need.

The ethical considerations in working with trauma survivors are both significant and challenging. Forensic psychologists must navigate the delicate balance between their duty to their clients and their role within the legal system. Maintaining confidentiality, ensuring informed consent, and handling dual roles with care are essential in building trust with trauma survivors. At the same time, forensic psychologists are advocates within the legal system, where their expertise can shape more trauma-sensitive policies and practices.

Looking to the future, the field of forensic psychology must continue to evolve to meet the growing needs of trauma survivors. Research into the psychological effects of trauma and the mechanisms of resilience is essential for developing more effective interventions. Additionally, forensic psychologists must advocate for systemic changes that prioritize trauma-informed practices across the legal, healthcare, and social support sectors.

Access to mental health services remains a critical barrier for many survivors of domestic violence and human trafficking. Forensic psychologists must work alongside policymakers to expand access to affordable, culturally sensitive, and trauma-informed care. By ensuring that all survivors have the opportunity to receive the help they need, the field can contribute to a broader movement toward social justice and healing.

Ultimately, the journey from trauma to triumph is not linear, and it is not without its challenges. However, with the support of forensic psychologists and a system that values resilience and recovery, victims of domestic violence and human trafficking can find their way to a place of healing. The interventions discussed in this chapter offer a roadmap for supporting survivors, not only in overcoming the psychological effects of trauma but also in reclaiming their sense of agency and control over their futures.

In conclusion, forensic psychology plays an indispensable role in bridging the gap between understanding trauma and fostering resilience. By integrating psychological insights with legal frameworks, forensic psychologists provide a unique perspective on how best to support trauma survivors in their journey from victimhood to empowerment. The hope is that through continued research, ethical practice, and multidisciplinary collaboration, the field can make even greater strides in helping survivors rebuild their lives and achieve triumph over trauma.

REFERENCES

American Psychological Association. (2013). *Publication manual of the American Psychological Association* (6th ed.). American Psychological Association.

Banyard, V. L., Williams, L. M., & Siegel, J. A. (2003). The long-term mental health consequences of child sexual abuse: A review and meta-analysis. *Journal of Consulting and Clinical Psychology, 71*(4), 657–679. DOI: 10.1037/0022-006X.71.4.657 PMID: 12924670

Bartol, C. R., & Bartol, A. M. (2019). *Introduction to forensic psychology: Research and application* (4th ed.). Sage Publications.

Briere, J., & Scott, C. (2015). *Principles of trauma therapy: A guide to symptoms, evaluation, and treatment* (2nd ed.). Sage Publications.

Campbell, J. C. (2002). Health consequences of intimate partner violence. *Lancet, 359*(9314), 1331–1336. DOI: 10.1016/S0140-6736(02)08336-8 PMID: 11965295

Clum, G. A., & Whitman, J. C. (1991). Psychological impact of abuse: A review of the literature. *Journal of Interpersonal Violence, 6*(4), 383–396. DOI: 10.1177/088626091006004002

Green, B. L. (2007). The role of trauma in forensic psychology: An overview. *Journal of Forensic Psychology Practice, 7*(1), 1–15. DOI: 10.1300/J158v07n01_01

Herman, J. L. (1992). *Trauma and recovery: The aftermath of violence—From domestic abuse to political terror*. Basic Books.

Koocher, G. P., & Keith-Spiegel, P. (2016). *Ethics in psychology and the mental health professions: Standards and cases* (4th ed.). Oxford University Press.

Luthar, S. S. (2006). Resilience in development: A synthesis of research across five decades. In Cicchetti, D., & Cohen, D. J. (Eds.), Developmental psychopathology: Vol. 3. *Risk, disorder, and adaptation* (pp. 739–795). Wiley.

Masten, A. S. (2001). Ordinary magic: Resilience processes in development. *The American Psychologist, 56*(3), 227–238. DOI: 10.1037/0003-066X.56.3.227 PMID: 11315249

Rutter, M. (2012). Resilience as a dynamic concept. *Development and Psychopathology, 24*(2), 335–344. DOI: 10.1017/S0954579412000028 PMID: 22559117

Ungar, M. (2011). *The social ecology of resilience: A handbook of theory and practice*. Springer.

van der Kolk, B. A. (2014). *The body keeps the score: Brain, mind, and body in the healing of trauma*. Viking.

Widom, C. S., & Maxfield, M. G. (2001). *An update on the "cycle of violence."*. National Institute of Justice Research Brief., DOI: 10.1037/e528142006-001

Chapter 8
Ethical Challenges in Multicultural Social Work With Immigrants

Özge Kutlu
https://orcid.org/0000-0002-4774-7326
Burdur Mehmet Akif Ersoy University, Turkey

ABSTRACT

Migration, an age-old human phenomenon, has significantly shaped societies by fostering cultural diversity and altering demographics, especially in the era of globalization. These transformations have propelled the social work discipline to rethink its theoretical and practical frameworks within multicultural contexts. In multicultural societies, social work must address the complexities of ethnic diversity, social inequalities, and exclusion while striving to empower marginalized groups. Social workers face complex ethical dilemmas, balancing cultural sensitivity with the universality of human rights, especially when cultural practices conflict with these rights. This chapter examines the evolving role of social work in multicultural settings, emphasizing its potential as an inclusive and transformative tool, and the necessity for cultural competence and critical self-assessment in fostering justice and equality.

INTRODUCTION

Migration is a phenomenon as old and deep-rooted as human history. Throughout history, people have constantly moved and settled in new geographies in search of better living conditions, security and prosperity (Öçal, 2023a; Öçal & Kutlu, 2024). Migration has paved the way for different cultures, languages and identities

DOI: 10.4018/979-8-3693-7944-8.ch008

to come together over time. Migration movements, which have gained momentum as globalization has made borders more "permeable," are constantly changing the demographic structure and cultural fabric of societies (Nipperess & Williams, 2019; Öçal & Korkmaz,, 2021). The borders eroded by globalization have also caused nation states to lose power. Because the nation state is built around the principles of "one state, one nation, one culture". This triple structure was designed to ensure homogeneity in society and to provide the unity necessary for the effective management and social order of the state. Homogeneity has been accepted as essential for good governance and social harmony (Stavenhagen, 2002; Kymlicka, 2007). In this context, in the historical development of nation states, assimilation policies have been implemented to make ethno-cultural minorities compatible with the dominant culture, and in cases where assimilation could not be achieved, these groups were excluded or separated from social life (Arocena, 2014). At this point, the globalization process, with its economic, cultural and social dynamics, makes individuals face social exclusion more intensely (Öçal & Korkmaz, 2020).

The transformations in the demographic structure of societies under the influence of globalization have caused multiculturalism to become the norm rather than an exceptional situation. In this context, both the theoretical framework and practical applications of the social work discipline have entered a process of rethinking in order to understand and respond to the complex dynamics of multicultural societies. In multicultural societies, ethnic diversity is not only a demographic reality but also a multi-layered challenge for ethical, political and social work interventions. Therefore, "rethinking ethnic diversity in postmodern societies" has become an increasingly critical necessity for social workers.

Within a multicultural framework, social work practices are often carried out in a context where social inequalities are deepened and individuals and groups are excluded in various ways. The homogenizing approaches of nation states throughout history have paved the way for social work to be used as one of the tools of standardization from time to time. This situation requires social work practitioners to question their cultural sensitivities and to critically evaluate their own roles in multicultural societies. Instead of legitimizing standardizing policies, can social work in multicultural societies be a tool that aims to make the voices of individuals and groups excluded by these policies heard? This question brings with it a deep discussion in terms of the principles of justice and equality that are at the core of social work ethics. However, social workers face ethical dilemmas in multicultural societies. These dilemmas arise from complex situations, especially those that are caught between respectful consideration of cultural differences and the universality of human rights. For example, in cases where certain cultural practices may violate the rights of individuals, how social workers should proceed is a critical question. This issue, addressed under the title of "Ethical dilemmas in multicultural social work: Respect for cultural differences or inviolability of human rights?", clearly demonstrates that ethical decision-making in social work practice is a dynamic and context-sensitive process. Finally, it is essential for social workers to develop their cultural competence through self-assessment in order to be able to make fair and effective interventions in multicultural societies. Cultural sensitivity and competence are not limited to understanding different cultures, but also require addressing these differences from a supportive, empowering and transformative perspective.

This chapter begins by framing the discussion within the ethical standards of the National Association of Social Workers (NASW), emphasizing their relevance in navigating the complexities of multicultural practice. By reassessing ethnic diversity in postmodern societies, it questions whether social work functions as a standardizing force or an inclusive tool. It also addresses ethical dilemmas encountered in multicultural social work practice, opening up discussion of the delicate balance between human rights and cultural differences. Finally, it highlights the self-assessment processes that enable social workers to critically examine their own practice.

RETHINKING ETHNIC DIVERSITY IN POSTMODERN SOCIETY

Lechte and Bottomley (1993) develop a new theoretical approach to cultural identities by criticizing the traditional understanding that cultures are historically fixed and "pure." According to Lechte and Bottomley (1993), cross-cultural interaction has been inevitable throughout history and no culture is "pure" or unchanging. Therefore, the concept of a "pure culture" should be evaluated either as a romanticized idealization or as an idealization disconnected from reality. Multicultural policies implemented in countries such as Australia are based on an understanding that sees cultural identities as homogeneous, fixed, and static structures (Lechte & Bottomley, 1993). While these policies focus on "managing" different cultures together and regulating diversity, they ignore the dynamic nature of cultural identities and the fact that these identities are in constant interaction and transformation (Marotta, 2014). Lechte and Bottomley (1993), opposing this traditional understanding, argue that multiculturalism is not only a political or social regulation tool, but also an ontological condition and a framework for understanding interactions between individuals. According to Lechte and Bottomley, multiculturalism should be understood not as fixed identities of cultures, but as a relational and constantly transforming form of existence (Lechte and Bottomley, 1993). In this context, they propose to re-evaluate cultural pluralism from an understanding limited to managing diversity to a dynamic process shaped by relationships and interactions between individuals and groups.

The concept of multiculturalism is approached from two different perspectives: traditional liberal and postmodernist. Traditional liberal multiculturalism generally aims to glorify and protect tradition and culture. However, this approach has been criticized because it is seen as a tool by which powerful groups can manipulate traditions to keep marginalized ethnic and racial groups under pressure (Marotta, 2014). In contrast, postmodernist multiculturalism rejects narrow approaches that define identity solely in terms of origin or tradition and advocates the concept of 'decentered subjectivity' (Peréz-Torres, 1993). According to this perspective, identity is considered as a dynamic structure that takes shape between the different subjective positions of individuals and includes multiple dimensions. The postmodernist perspective focuses particularly on the struggle of racial and ethnic minority groups. It emphasizes that these struggles are not limited to class and gender conflicts, but rather have a structure that overlaps with other social dynamics. This approach encourages the questioning of existing oppressive narratives and discourses. At the same time, it paves the way for social change by making visible the historically suppressed experiences of marginalized groups. According to Peréz-Torres (1993), postmodernist multiculturalism draws attention to local contexts, devalued knowledge, and the importance of histories suppressed by hegemonic narratives (Peréz-Torres, 1993). It is argued that these local and unique elements carry a permanent and meaningful potential for social change. While differences are generally considered as "tolerated" or "celebrated" elements in traditional multiculturalism, in postmodernist multiculturalism these differences are seen as a source of power capable of creating social transformation and change. This perspective, which differs from intercultural communication studies, redefines multiculturalism not only as diversity but also as a field of political resistance and transformation.

In today's world, one of the fundamental situations that many societies face is that different ethnic groups, cultures and communities no longer express their identities, languages and religious affiliations only in the private sphere, but also want to make them visible in the public sphere. This situation has brought about the demands that identity-based differences, which were mostly limited to private life in the past, be expressed in the public sphere in modern societies and that these differences, together with the demands to be a part of the larger society by having "equal" rights. Nation-state models, which were shaped especially in the modern period and tried to build a homogeneous national identity, have changed in the face of these demands. In the past, nation-states aimed to define their citizens with a single ethnic, religious or linguistic identity and tried to shape these identities with an artificial understanding of "homogeneity". However, today this understanding is giving way to an approach that emphasizes a more "heterogeneous" social structure where different ethnic origins, linguistic diversities and religious identities are accepted (Yanık, 2012). This heterogeneity includes not only the coexistence of different groups, but also the participation of these groups with equal rights in all areas of social life. Societies with multicultural structures, or in other words, states with heterogeneous structures, are faced with the problem of recognizing social differences and how to address the demands of ethnic or cultural elements within these differences. The globalization of libertarian demands has made movements to recognize the identities of different ethnic and cultural groups and demand equal rights a widespread phenomenon worldwide. These demands have deeply affected societies called multicultural and that include more than one ethnic minority. In this context, postmodern thought has developed approaches that argue that cultural identities cannot be reduced to a single absolute truth and that diversity must be recognized. These theoretical perspectives have also shaped the policies of political powers and formed the basis of cultural identity policies. These policies, which have a libertarian content, have transformed into an approach known as multiculturalism and have manifested themselves as an effort to produce solutions to the practices of coexistence of different cultures. Multiculturalism aims not only to maintain social peace but also to establish an order that supports the recognition and development of different identities.

The effective participation of different ethnic groups in social life is not only a requirement of the principle of equality, but also of critical importance for the sustainability of the democratic social order. The discipline of social work plays an important role in supporting social differences and defending the right to participation, which is one of the fundamental human rights of individuals. However, the impact of multicultural discourses on social work practices is open to debate. In this context, the question of whether social work undertakes functions such as defending the rights of minority groups and encouraging their participation in social life, or whether it is used as a tool to prepare the ground for governments' standardization policies, is an important area of discussion that needs to be addressed carefully. The position of social work in this framework requires not only a professional responsibility, but also an ethical stance aimed at ensuring social justice.

Is Social Work a Means of Legitimising Standardisation in Multicultural Societies?

Multiculturalism refers to individuals with different identities living together and in harmony based on the principle of equality. The "identity differences" referred to here include individuals who are diverse in many areas such as language, religion, race, culture, and gender (Akkaya, Susar Kırmızı, & İşçi, 2018). This diversity is accepted as a natural part of social life, and social harmony is aimed at by ensuring that everyone benefits from the same rights. Multiculturalism argues that freedom and prosperity are the foundations of a society and accepts cultural differences as normal and acceptable (Parekh, 2004). This aims to establish a social order where there is no discrimination between people and where everyone can live their lives with equal opportunities (Aydın, 2013). Therefore, in a multicultural society, everyone is expected to respect their own cultural identity and to be able to maintain their peaceful existence within society. This understanding also encourages a sensitive approach to cultural diversity. It is important to see people's differences as a richness and to ensure that these differences coexist harmoniously in social relations. Multiculturalism can be considered as a policy that celebrates this diversity and finds differences valuable. This refers to an understanding that supports the inclusion of different cultures in society and integrates them into social life (Polat, 2020).

Multiculturalism is a dynamic phenomenon where, beyond the coexistence of different cultures, these cultures interact with each other and experience a mutual transformation and reconstruction process. This understanding is a process in which one culture and another are intertwined, where the host culture and minority cultures retranslate and reshape each other through contact. Multiculturalism accepts that cultural identities are not fixed and homogeneous structures, but rather relational and transformative structures formed through constant change and interaction. In this context, multiculturalism should be considered as a way of life in which cultures interact and reproduce each other rather than the management of cultural diversity (Marotta, 2014). Conceptually, the term "multicultural" refers to the ethnic diversity of a society. However, this does not mean that the society has official multicultural policies or implements strategies that support cultural diversity. In other words, a society may consist of different ethnic groups, but this does not mean that different cultures should be protected or intercultural interactions should be encouraged (Mitchell, 2004). In this respect, multiculturalism is only a feature that defines social diversity and does not mean that special policies are implemented to manage cultural diversity in every society (Zubaida, 1999; Kenny & Lobo, 2014).

Policies supporting multiculturalism are considered by some critics as misguided attempts that undermine social harmony. These criticisms claim that the understanding that recognizes differences and creates a common identity is naive. It is stated that multiculturalism causes ghettoization and increases the hostility of minority groups towards the dominant culture (Cantle, 2001). For example, Trevor Phillips has argued that multiculturalism policies in the United Kingdom encourage discrimination and alienate societies from each other (McGhee, 2008). Similarly, British Prime Minister David Cameron has stated that the "passive tolerance" of multiculturalism leads to different groups living in isolation (Wright & Taylor, 2011). These criticisms claim that multicultural policies emphasize differences, overshadow the goal of social integration, and undermine the general harmony of society (Kenny & Lobo, 2014).

Multiculturalism is not only a definition of cultural diversity, but also raises important questions about how this diversity will be managed and how it will be lived together. In this context, while accepting cultural diversity is an important step towards achieving social harmony, this process should be considered as part of broader social policies. Social policy has gone beyond the traditional concepts of "compromise" or "tribute" in today's world and has become a quest for humanity (Öçal & Kutlu, 2023). It is no longer a discipline that only addresses certain social classes or national borders, but has gained an international dimension with the aim of increasing universal welfare and ensuring social justice. Social policy encompasses all systematic actions aimed at improving the well-being of individuals and communities. In this context, social policy, shaped by the goal of improving human life, has become one of the fundamental elements of modern welfare states with the effort to protect the fundamental rights and human dignity of the individual (Öçal, 2023b). Social work represents the field-based implementation dimension of social policy. Acting in line with the principles of human rights, social justice and individual empowerment, social work is an important tool that contributes to the realization of social policy goals. Developing intervention methods at the individual, family and community level to solve social problems, social work aims to increase the well-being of individuals and ensure social balance within the framework determined by social policy.

Although social work is seen as a critical tool in ensuring social harmony and the well-being of individuals in multicultural societies, some critics argue that this field is used as a means of legitimizing standardization. While social work generally aims to integrate individuals into the social system, it carries the risk of imposing a certain cultural norm and homogenizing individuals' identities in this process. This situation leads to criticism that social work practices indirectly reproduce the values of the dominant culture and undermine the cultural autonomy of minority groups (Dominelli, 2002).

Although multicultural policies advocate equal representation and participation of different cultures in social life, it is stated that social work practices do not always fully achieve this goal. For example, standard protocols used during social work practices may ignore the unique needs of minority groups based on dominant cultural norms. For example, when a social worker provides support to individuals from minority groups in a hospital setting, he/she may use forms or information materials prepared only in the dominant language and do not observe cultural awareness. For example, when an immigrant individual applies for mental health services, he/she may only have access to standard assessment forms prepared in Turkish. This may lead to the person being unable to express their needs, being diagnosed incorrectly, or not being able to fully benefit from the services. In another example, in some countries, traditional parenting practices of minority groups may be misunderstood in child protection systems and evaluated according to the norms of the dominant culture. For example, behaviors that are considered part of the understanding of discipline in a certain culture may be considered child abuse by social workers. This may result in the children of minority families being "unfairly" taken under protection. In this context, when the cultural differences of minority groups are considered within a framework determined by the dominant culture, the tendency to standardize them under the name of "management" of cultural diversity may be strengthened (Fook, 2002). In fact, at this point, an important discussion arises as to which behaviors can be evaluated within the scope of "respect for differences" and at what limit can behaviors be defined as violations of human rights beyond respect for differences.

Ethical Dilemmas in Multicultural Social Work: Respect for Cultural Differences or Inviolability of Human Rights?

One of the fundamental discussion points of multicultural policies is the degree of autonomy and independence that will be granted to minority groups. Kymlicka's strong multicultural approach aims to provide a solution to this problem by securing both universal rights and group-differentiated rights for diverse communities (Kymlicka, 1995). This approach combines the goals of protecting cultural diversity and ensuring social harmony. A strong understanding of multiculturalism both emphasizes the value of cultural diversity as an ethical discourse and organizes the sharing of resources and political participation mechanisms as a political strategy. This approach, which grants minority groups the right to express their identities, live their cultures and be recognized in the public sphere, offers an inclusive model that supports the coexistence of different cultural groups (Kymlicka, 1995). However, how to establish a balance between minority autonomy and social integrity is an important question in terms of the applicability of this policy. In terms of multicultural social work, the question of "where do the boundaries in multicultural social work begin and end?" is an important issue that needs to be thought about and discussed.

As a profession founded on ethical foundations, social work aims to increase the well-being of individuals and ensure social justice in society (Chatzifotiou & Papouli, 2022). Social justice in multicultural societies is not a phenomenon that can be achieved only through redistribution (Craig G., 2008). It becomes possible by implementing elements such as respect for cultural diversity and difference, recognition of minority groups, status equality and common citizenship within the framework of universal rights. In this context, how needs are defined and verified is of critical importance in multicultural societies. While minority groups should be actively included in the process of defining needs, these groups are often excluded from political and policy processes. This exclusion is too obvious to be covered up with symbolic participation. The inadequacy of market economies in ensuring social justice leads to many minority groups being disproportionately affected by inequalities. Under the discourse of equal opportunity, access to goods, services and welfare resources faces serious restrictions for many minorities. While welfare services are expected to provide a structure that compensates for the injustices of the market, the current system appears to work against minority groups and to perpetuate racialized inequalities in access to welfare resources (Craig & Levis, 2014).

A study conducted in Norway (Bø, 2015) identified five main challenges in multicultural social work: communication problems due to language barriers, different codes of conduct making professional service interactions difficult, cultural differences in parent-child relationships, lack of access to health services, and structural barriers resulting from the social service system's inability to adapt to minority groups. In addition, it was noted that social workers in this study expressed that certain types of knowledge needed in multicultural social work were lacking. These deficiencies included being aware of the Western ideology prevalent in social work and having knowledge about immigration policies. In addition, the inability of institutions to establish a common ideology or ground for discussion when working with minority groups was also mentioned as a significant problem (Bø, 2015).

In multicultural social work practice, taking cultural differences into account can sometimes lead to ethical dilemmas regarding human rights. The behavior of a Danish mother living in New York and the chain of events that emerged as a result of this behavior can be considered as an example of such a dilemma. The Danish mother did not allow her baby into the restaurant she visited and left him in a stroller outside the restaurant. The mother's behavior was considered by the authorities in New York as endangering the child and the mother was arrested and referred to court. However, the mother explained her purpose in not allowing her baby into the restaurant as protecting her from the stifling atmosphere of the restaurant. She argued that this behavior was considered normal behavior in Copenhagen, the capital of Denmark (Kartari, 2014). This case reveals how cultural differences can turn into a legal process in a city that seemingly shares common values and is considered culturally "modern" and the ethical dilemmas that social workers may encounter in such cases. Ensuring balance between respect for cultural differences and protection of children and observance of fundamental human rights appears to be an ethical dilemma to be resolved in the field of social work.

In another example, an ethical dilemma encountered in multicultural social work practice is discussed through the conflict between the principle of respect for cultural differences and the obligation to protect basic human rights. Such an ethical dilemma and debate arises because social workers must both respect the ethnic and cultural identities of individuals and adhere to basic social work values in order to ensure the well-being of their clients. In the case reported by Goldberg (2000), a social worker working in the field of child welfare reports that a four-year-old girl was taken into protective custody because her father touched her genital area. The father argues that this behavior is considered a sign of love in his cultural context and traditions. The father states that he did not derive sexual gratification from this behavior and that his actions should not be misunderstood. However, in the context and cultural environment in which the social worker works, in American society, such behavior is defined as child abuse and has serious legal and ethical consequences. While the social worker was trying to fulfill his professional responsibility of respecting the father's cultural background and beliefs, he was also faced with the responsibility of ensuring the child's safety, protecting the child's best interests and fundamental rights. In order to understand whether the father's behavior had a cultural background, research was conducted on the cultural context of the father and his society, and it was concluded that the father's actions were truly acceptable in his own culture and were not perceived as a problem. However, accepting the cultural context did not mean tolerating a behavior that jeopardized the child's safety. Based on the social worker's recommendation, the court ruled that the father's actions were considered neglect and initiated individualized parenting education programs for the father. Despite the education and interventions planned for the father, the father repeated the same behaviors and the child was taken into protection once again (Goldberg, 2000). This situation concretely demonstrates how the unlimited acceptance of cultural values in social work practices can create problems, especially in cases where the rights of individuals are violated. At the same time, the trauma experienced by the child revealed how cultural differences can conflict with the new values internalized by individuals. As can be understood from this case, the multicultural approach in social work practices can contain contradictions and ethical dilemmas. Respect for cultural diversity is only valid as long as basic human rights can be protected. Social workers need to prioritize ethical principles and human rights when trying to understand the cultural context.

Other areas where ethical dilemmas arise in dialogues and practices between social workers and ethnic minority individuals, families and groups with different cultural values are child rearing practices, generational conflicts and gender roles. Social workers are educated in values such as individuality, independence, individual rights and gender equality, and these values form the basis of their professional approach. In contrast, ethnic minority families may have a more authoritarian, traditional and obedience-oriented approach to child rearing. For example, in some families, it is culturally rare for children to discuss or negotiate parental decisions. In addition, the use of violence to discipline children in some minority families has been observed by social workers and found problematic by social workers. However, such practices may be viewed as a cultural norm by minority families. In this context, social workers are often unaware that their professional approach is shaped by Western values, making it difficult for them to understand the cultural practices of minority families (Bø, 2015). Social workers' interventions may be perceived by families as a threat to parental authority, which can lead to resistance, conflicts, and ethical dilemmas between professionals and families. Therefore, increasing cultural sensitivity and implementing culturally competent practices in social work practices are vital to overcoming these challenges in working with minority families.

Self-assessment of Cultural Competence

As emphasized in the previous sections of the chapter, multicultural societies are becoming more widespread with increasing migration movements around the world. The spread of multicultural societies leads to an increase in cultural diversity and a change in social structure around the world (Disney & Carnes, 2022). The integration of minority groups with different cultures into society creates new needs not only in social, economic and cultural areas but also in the fields of health and social services. In this context, social workers are expected to encounter individuals with different cultural backgrounds, languages and traumas more frequently. Multicultural societies require culturally sensitive and effective social workers to meet the needs of these individuals (Fong, 2004; Pumariega, Rogers, & Rothe, 2005).

Multicultural practice and cultural competence require understanding and respecting the unique identities, values, beliefs, norms, and experiences of individuals or groups. This approach encompasses not only fundamental differences such as race and ethnicity, but also other factors that shape individuals' life experiences, such as gender, sexual orientation, and worldview. Indeed, culturally constructed elements such as gender roles can also constitute obstacles to individuals' access to their rights (Sütlü, 2022). Cultural competence enables professionals to work sensitively, respectfully, and effectively by taking into account the cultural context of the individuals they serve (Edwards, 2016). In this context, it is emphasized that generalized practices implemented without understanding the cultural backgrounds of individuals will not be functional (Lum, 2003).

Although the concepts of multicultural social work and cultural competence are two concepts that are closely related, they actually have different meanings. Multicultural social work refers to having knowledge about a particular culture, understanding the characteristics of this culture and interacting accordingly. It focuses more on recognizing the cultural identities of individuals or groups and being sensitive to these identities. On the other hand, cultural competence is a broader concept and includes the equal representation of different groups in society and the recognition of their existence and contributions (Walker & Staton, 2000).

Cultural competence is a skill that social workers acquire through experience and is based on understanding the unique cultural contexts of individuals and communities. This competence develops not only through theoretical knowledge but also through interactions with individuals based on empathy and respect. Cultural sensitivity requires a social worker to be sensitive to the cultural backgrounds of different individuals and to communicate effectively in this context (Attipoe, 2024). However, reducing multiculturalism to a field of knowledge that can only be taught risks ignoring the diversity of individuals' cultural identities and the complexity of contexts. This approach can undermine the power of multiculturalism as a guiding principle, overshadowing the importance of ethical values. Multiculturalism needs to be treated as a guide on par with core ethical values such as empathy, honesty, and respect. It is critical for social workers to deeply understand the cultural contexts of individuals and to act sensitively in these contexts for virtuous social work practice (Walker & Staton, 2000).

If we consider a social worker working with families who migrated from Syria in Germany, the Syrian family may experience adaptation problems, language barriers, or stress due to cultural differences. The social worker's learning about the family's cultural background and religion, gaining knowledge about Middle Eastern culture and the social and cultural norms of the country where the family lives, recognizing and respecting the family's cultural and religious practices, arranging appointment times considering the family's religious holidays and times of worship, using interpreter services to overcome language barriers when communicating with family members, or ensuring that a social worker who speaks a language the family feels comfortable with is found, is the embodiment of cultural sensitivity and cultural competence in social work practice.

National Association of Social Workers (NASW) has set some standards for social work practices to be carried out by professionals based on cultural competence. Accordingly, NASW defines cultural competence as a competence that requires social workers to understand cultural diversity, use this diversity effectively in their professional practices, and provide services by respecting the cultural identity of each individual (NASW, 2015). Cultural competence includes being sensitive to the socio-cultural characteristics of communities and adopting an unprejudiced approach. What is expressed here is not a reductionist approach that constructs individuals' identities solely based on culture by identifying cultural elements with individuals (Danso, 2018). It is an approach that considers that culture is a part of identity and requires considering events and situations in this context (Azzopardi & Mcneil, 2016). Cultural competence is a critical requirement for the effective and ethical implementation of social work at the individual and institutional level. Social workers must be aware of their own cultural biases and assumptions, be committed to continuous learning, and self-evaluation. NASW states that cultural competence consists not only of knowledge but also of attitudes and skills. Professionals should continually use training, supervision, and peer support to increase their cultural awareness (Osborn & Karandikar, 2022). Cultural competence includes respecting each individual's cultural background and identity. NASW emphasizes that social workers must understand clients' beliefs, traditions, and social contexts. Cultural competence, which emphasizes a holistic approach, also requires creating a service delivery environment where clients can fully express their identities and rights. Removing cultural norms from being a source of oppression is also a prerequisite for culturally competent practice.

A macro dimension of implementing culturally competent social work practices is integrating cultural competence into the policies and procedures of social service institutions (Melendres, 2020). Because the fact that the institution's policies and procedures are not in a state that prepares the ground for cultural competence means that the social worker faces a significant barrier (Harrison & Turner, 2011). The integration of cultural competence into institutions means that all activities under the institution's roof, from recruitment processes to service delivery, are made accessible and appropriate for every culture. NASW states that cultural competence standards are not limited to individual practices, but are also a tool for systemic change (NASW, 2015).

CONCLUSION

The multicultural approach has emerged as an approach that aims to recognize the identities of different cultural communities, to accept and protect these differences. However, the ongoing discussions on the practices of the multicultural approach and the results of these practices from the past to the present have led to some discussions on whether the multicultural approach is an ideal solution. Undoubtedly, this approach contributes to the protection of the rights of different cultural communities, the access of ethnic minorities to rights, and the acceptance of differences within society. However, on the other hand, the effort to protect differences can bring some risks. In particular, the sharp definition of cultural boundaries belonging to ethnic groups can threaten social unity and integrity. When individuals are defined only by a certain cultural identity, which brings with it the misconception that culture is fixed and causes the dynamic structure of culture to be ignored, this situation can lead to a sense of limitation and create pressure for individuals with multiple identities (Öztürk, 2020). For example, an individual may belong to any ethnic group in a society and may have adopted a modern individualist lifestyle. However, if the multicultural approach tries to construct and define the individual's identity solely through his/her ethnic identity, this identity construction may increase the pressure on the individual and make the individual feel trapped in an identity he/she does not want. However, the balance between individual rights and cultural group rights is one of the difficulties that must be addressed regarding the subject. Indeed, while the multicultural approach supports group rights, it may not be able to sufficiently protect the basic freedoms and autonomy of individuals. For example, the traditional values or norms of a conservative community or a community dominated by a patriarchal structure may restrict the freedom of individuals within the community to make their own life choices, in other words, their autonomy (Kutlu & Sütlü, 2024). These restrictions may cause individuals to become alienated from their cultural communities or to be oppressed within these communities. The multicultural approach can be seen as an important tool in the effort to manage the cultural diversity of modern societies, which has gained momentum with globalization and is increasing day by day. However, as the criticisms in the literature underline, the multicultural approach is not an approach that only contains advantages, and in this respect, it may not meet the expectations of a utopian society where "differences" are accepted and all individuals benefit from their rights equally. If a balance cannot be established between the protection of cultural communities and the protection of individual freedoms, the multicultural approach may be inadequate in solving the problems in today's societies. For this very reason, the limitations of the multicultural approach should be carefully evaluated as much as its advantages.

It is argued that social work should support the integration of individuals and communities into society by preserving their own cultural contexts within the framework of a cultural sensitivity approach. This approach requires social workers to understand and respect the cultural identities of the individuals they serve. However, the practical applicability of these goals depends on the level of education of social workers, policy frameworks and the approach of local governments in this regard. Within the framework of this discussion, whether social work functions as a means of standardization in a multicultural society or as a mechanism supporting cultural diversity varies depending on the context and policies in which it is implemented.

In order for social workers to implement culturally competent social work practices, first of all, social work education should include a comprehensive curriculum aimed at increasing cultural sensitivity. Social workers should be equipped to understand the value systems specific to different cultures and to evaluate the needs of the individuals they serve in light of these values. Supportive and developmental activities such as in-service training and supervision should be planned to develop the cultural competencies of social workers not only during their undergraduate education but also in their professional lives. Social policies that determine the framework for social work should be shaped within a framework that aims to establish a balance between individual freedoms and cultural group rights. In this process, it is important for local governments to encourage regulations that will not harm the autonomy of individuals while supporting cultural groups to preserve their own identities. In order to increase the effectiveness of practices at the macro level, intercultural dialogue mechanisms should be strengthened and social workers should be encouraged to take an active role in these mechanisms.

REFERENCES

Akkaya, N., Susar Kırmızı, F., & İşçi, C. (2018). Öğretmen adaylarının çok kültürlülüğe ilişkin algılarının farklı değişkenler açısından incelenmesi. Adıyaman Üniversitesi Sosyal Bilimler Enstitüsü Dergisi, 308-335.

Arocena, F. (2014). *Cultural Rights in New ulticultural Democracies. F. Mansouri, & B. Ebanda de B'béri içinde, Global Perspectives on the Politics of Multiculturalism in the 21st Century: A Case Study Analysis*. Routledge.

Attipoe, H. (2024). Cultural Competency: A Cardinal Force in Social Work Practice and Service-A Cultural Practice Guide for Human Services and the Helping Professions. *International Journal of Social Work, 11*(1), 28–43. DOI: 10.5296/ijsw.v11i1.21561

Aydın, H. (2013). *Dünyada ve Türkiye'de çokkültürlü eğitim tartışmaları ve uygulamaları*. Nobel Akademik Yayıncılık.

Azzopardi, C., & Mcneil, T. (2016). From Cultural Competence to Cultural Consciousness: Transitioning to a Critical Approach to Working Across Differences in Social Work. *Journal of Ethnic & Cultural Diversity in Social Work, 25*(4), 282–299. DOI: 10.1080/15313204.2016.1206494

Bø, B. (2015). Social work in a multicultural society: New challenges and needs for competence. *International Social Work, 58*(4), 562–574. DOI: 10.1177/0020872814550114

Cantle, T. (2001). *Community Cohesion: A Report of the Independent Review Team*. Home Office.

Chatzifotiou, S., & Papouli, E. (2022). Social Workers Dealing with Ethical Dilemmas in the Course of Their Professional Work: The Greek Experience. *British Journal of Social Work, 52*(8), 4795–4814. DOI: 10.1093/bjsw/bcac084

Craig, G. (2008). *The Limits of Compromise. G. Craig, T. Burchardt, & D. Gordon içinde, Social Justice and Public Policy*. Policy Press.

Craig, G., & Levis, H. (2014). *Multiculturalism or assimilation and social exclusion Ethnic minorities in the United Kingdom. F. Mansouri, & P. Muraca içinde, Global Perspectives on the Politics of Multiculturalism in the 21st Century*. Routledge.

Danso, R. (2018). Cultural competence and cultural humility: A critical reflection on key cultural diversity concepts. ournal of Social Work, 410-430.

Disney, L., & Carnes, S. (2022). But Culturally Competent for Whom? Ethics and CrossCultural Dilemmas in COVID-Era Social Work . International Journal of Social Work Values and Ethics, 209-226.

Dominelli, L. (2002). *Anti Oppressive Social Work Theory and Practice.* Palgrave Macmillan. DOI: 10.1007/978-1-4039-1400-2

Edwards, J. (2016). Cultural Intelligence for Clinical Social Work Practice. *Clinical Social Work Journal, 44*(3), 211–220. DOI: 10.1007/s10615-015-0543-4

Fong, R. (2004). *Overview of Immigrant and Refugee Children and Families. R. Fong içinde, Culturally competent practice with immigrant and refugee children and families.* The Guilford Press.

Fook, J. (2002). *Social Work: Critical Theory and Practice.* Sage Publications.

Goldberg, M. (2000). Conflicting Principles in Multicultural Social Work. *Families in Society, 81*(1), 12–21. DOI: 10.1606/1044-3894.1088

Harrison, G., & Turner, R. (2011). Being a 'Culturally Competent' Social Worker: Making Sense of a Murky Concept in Practice. *British Journal of Social Work, 41*(2), 333–350. DOI: 10.1093/bjsw/bcq101

Kartarı, A. (2014). *Kültür, Farklılık, İletişim: Kültürlerarası İletişimin Kavramsal Dayanakları.* İletişim Yayınları.

Kenny, S., & Lobo, M. (2014). *Addressing Cultural Differences Whither Multiculturalism? F. Mansouri, & B. Ebanda de B'béri içinde, Global Perspectives on the Politics of Multiculturalism in the 21st Century: A Case Study Analysis.* Routledge.

Kutlu, Ö., & Sütlü, S. (2024). *Investigation of the Career Development Experiences of Women Managers: An Analysis From a Gender Perspective. M. Haoucha içinde, Empowering and Advancing Women Leaders and Entrepreneurs.* IGI Global. DOI: 10.4018/979-8-3693-7107-7.ch011

Kymlicka, W. (1995). *Multicultural Citizenship: A Liberal Theory of Minority Rights.* Clarendon Press.

Kymlicka, W. (2007). *Multicultural Odysseys: Navigating the New International Politics of Diversity.* Oxford University Press. DOI: 10.1093/oso/9780199280407.001.0001

Lechte, J., & Bottomley, G. (1993). *Difference, Postmodernity and Image in Multicultural Australia. G. Clark, D. Forbes, & R. Francis içinde, Multiculturalism, Difference and Postmodernism.* Longman Cheshire.

Lum, D. (2003). *Culturally competent practice.* Thomson–Brooks/Cole.

Marotta, V. (2014). *The multicultural, intercultural and transcultural subject. F. Mansouri, & B. Ebanda de B'béri içinde, Global Perspectives on the Politics of Multiculturalism in the 21st Century: A Case Study Analysis*. Routledge.

McGhee, D. (2008). *The End of Multiculturalism? Terrorism, Integration and Human Rights*. Open University Press.

Melendres, M. (2020). Cultural competence in social work practice: Exploring the challenges of newly employed social work professionals. *Journal of Ethnic & Cultural Diversity in Social Work*, •••, 108–120.

Mitchell, K. (2004). Geographies of Identity: Multiculturalism Unplugged. *Progress in Human Geography*, *28*(5), 641–651. DOI: 10.1191/0309132504ph510pr

NASW. (2015). Standards and Indicators for Cultural Competence in Social Work Practice. https://www.socialworkers.org/Practice/NASW-Practice-Standards-Guidelines/Standards-and-Indicators-for-Cultural-Competence-in-Social-Work-Practice adresinden alındı

Nipperess, S., & Williams, C. (2019). *Introduction. S. Nipperess, & C. Williams içinde, Critical Multicultural Pratice in Social Work New Perspectives and Practices*. Routledge.

Öçal, M. (2023a). *Çalışma Yaşamında Göçmenler. M. Zubaroğlu Yanardağ, & B. Erkoç içinde, Göç ve Sosyal Hizmet*. Akademisyen Kitabevi.

Öçal, M. (2023b). *Bir Sosyal Devlet Ödevi Olarak Sosyal Gelişim ve Sosyal Kalkınmanın Teşviki. M. Öçal içinde, Sosyal Gelişimin Teşvikinde Kuramlar, Politikalar ve Eylemler*. Detay Yayıncılık.

Öçal, M., & Korkmaz, A. (2020). *Sosyal Dışlanma ve Sosyal Dışlanmanın Toplumsal Refah Üzerine Etkisi. M. Kasapoğlu, M. Öztürk, & M. Öçal içinde, Spor Yoluyla Sosyal Uyum*. Detay Yayıncılık.

Öçal, M., & Korkmaz, A. (2021). Neo-Liberalizmin Gölgesinde Sosyal Devlet: Emek ve Emeğin Örgütlenmesi Nereye Gidiyor? Sosyoloji Divanı, 27-49.

Öçal, M., & Kutlu, Ö. (2023). A Study on Welfare and Living Conditions of Disadvantaged Groups: The Case of Burdur Province. Journal of Management and Economics Research, 410-425.

Öçal, M., & Kutlu, Ö. (2024). İstihdamın Karanlık Yüzü: Ter Atölyelerine (Sweatshop) İnsani Bir Bakış ve Ter İndeksi ile Bir Kıyaslama. Çalışma ve Toplum, 1391-1424.

Osborn, P., & Karandikar, S. (2022). Practice-based knowledge perspectives of cultural competence in social work. ournal of Ethnic & Cultural Diversity in Social Work, 285-297.

Öztürk, A. (2020). *Mülteci Çocukların Sorunları ve Kültürel Yetkinlik Çerçevesinde Mülteci Çocuklarla Çalışma. F. Paslı, & H. Aslantürk içinde, Çocuklarla Çalışma: Temel Alanlar, Uygulamalar, Güncel Tartışmalar*. Nobel.

Parekh, B. (2004). *Dialogue between cultures*. Routledge.

Peréz-Torres, R. (1993). Nomads and Migrants: Negotiating a Multicultural Postmodernism. *Cultural Critique*, •••(26), 161–189. DOI: 10.2307/1354459

Polat, S. (2020). *Multicultural Structure of Schools and Intercultural Education. S. Polat içinde, Empowering Multiculturalism and Peacebuilding in Schools*. IGI Global.

Pumariega, A., Rogers, K., & Rothe, E. (2005). Culturallycompetentsystemsofcare for children's mental health: Advances and challenges. *Community Mental Health Journal*, *41*(5), 539–555. DOI: 10.1007/s10597-005-6360-4 PMID: 16142537

Stavenhagen, R. (2002). The Return of the Native. Occasional Papers No. 27: University of London Institute of Latin American Studies.

Sütlü, S. (2022). *Policies on Gender Equality. S. Sütlü, & D. Say Şahin içinde, Disadvantaged Groups: A Social Policy Perspective*. Eğitim Yayınevi.

Walker, R., & Staton, M. (2000). Multiculturalism in Social Work Ethics. *Journal of Social Work Education*, *36*(3), 449–462. DOI: 10.1080/10437797.2000.10779021

Chapter 9
Legal and Psychological Resilience:
A Cluster Analysis of Immigrant Populations

Usharani Bhimavarapu
https://orcid.org/0000-0002-0246-1420
Department of Computer Science and Engineering, Koneru Lakshmaiah Education Foundation, Vaddeswaram, India

ABSTRACT

Legal and psychological factors play a crucial role in shaping the experiences of immigrants, influencing their integration and well-being in a new country. This study explores the relationship between these factors through clustering and validation techniques applied to a diverse set of demographic, psychological, and employment data collected from immigrant populations. Various clustering models, including K-Means, Hierarchical Clustering, and DBSCAN, were used to categorize participants based on resilience, stress, and other demographic characteristics. Performance of these models was assessed using metrics like the Silhouette Score, Davies-Bouldin Index, and Calinski-Harabasz Score, revealing the most effective clustering strategies. The results indicate that K-Means clustering provided the best balance of accuracy and computational efficiency, offering insights into the psychological profiles of immigrants and their coping mechanisms under stress.

DOI: 10.4018/979-8-3693-7944-8.ch009

INTRODUCTION

Immigration processes are complex, with many legal and psychological factors that play a significant role in shaping the lives of immigrants. The legal process is mostly focused on laws and regulations governing border crossing by people. Immigration law differs across countries but normally encompasses the process of acquiring a visa, permanent residence, or citizenship. Legal processes are often time-consuming with applicants required to fulfill stringent conditions, offer voluminous documents, and often encounter processing delays. A small mistake or omission on an application may result in rejection or deportation, generating insecurity and fear among immigrants, particularly those holding precarious legal statuses.

Psychologically, the stress involved in dealing with the intricacies of immigration law is overwhelming. Immigrants would also have the challenging task of adapting to a foreign country, including overcoming cultural, social, and language alienation. Such factors can result in psychiatric ailments such as doubtfulness, depression, and anxiety. Additionally, stress due to being forced to conform to legal provisions, cope with threats of separation from family members, and hold back for official allowances contributes to mental pressure. Worry about deportation or never reaching family members also contributes to mental pressure on such immigrants.

The blending of psychological and legal concerns is particularly prevalent among the refugee and asylum seeker populations. They may have possibly left their home nations as a result of violence, political unrest, or persecution and are already navigating the double hurdle of securing legal status and overcoming trauma in their history. Asylum seekers and refugees endure a drawn-out and taxing legal procedure during which they need to demonstrate vulnerability and real fear of persecution from an alien legal process. They further get depressed by experiencing repeated recalling of what represents post-traumatic re-victimisation pending determination of their fates through the ultimate judgment.

Besides the legal and psychological struggle, immigration processes also affect the life of families of immigrants. Reunification of the family is most often the central issue in most immigration cases, and delay or denial will definitely cause emotional trauma. Emotional suffering to families, especially where children are kept away from parents or immigrants have to remain distant from loved ones, can be serious. This interference with family life is likely to create a heightened sense of loss and anxiety, which will complicate psychological adjustment to life in the new nation even more.

To address both the legal and psychological issues surrounding immigration, a comprehensive approach must be taken. Legal aid is necessary to ensure that immigrants know their rights, can navigate the application process successfully, and make viable choices. Psychological aid is also important since it assists immigrants in dealing with the emotional issues they encounter. Psychological assistance specifically geared towards the immigrant's needs such as counseling, stress management, and trauma recovery can significantly improve their health in the course of immigration. Having legal and psychological support mechanisms is a more holistic approach to the plight of immigrants and results in healthier, more successful assimilation into society.

Violanti et al. (2011) considered the association between adiposity and mental health outcomes in policing but were limited by their cross-sectional design that did not allow for causal inference. The study also concentrated mainly on BMI as a measure of adiposity, which might not account for the body composition complexity and its impact on mental health. In addition, the study failed to control for likely confounding factors like diet, lifestyle, or genetic predisposition that may impact adiposity and psychological outcomes.

Syed et al. (2020) reported a systematic review and meta-analysis of worldwide mental health disorders in police officers but the study was limited by inconsistency in methodological quality among studies included. Consistency in diagnostic definitions between studies could have introduced inconsistency in estimates of prevalence. Most studies included were from Western nations, therefore external validity of findings to police in multiculturally diverse socio-cultural settings.

Violanti et al. (2019) conducted a review of police officer suicides and found several risk factors but was hampered by the fact that their research employed secondary data, which is subject to underreporting or misclassification bias of suicidal events. The research did not even adequately explore how organizational systemic variables like department culture and leadership counteract suicide risk. Conversely, even though the review summarized some studies, it omitted longitudinal evidence that would yield greater causation data.

Stevelink et al. (2020) took into account PTSD, depression, and anxiety in UK police officers but were limited by using self-report measures, which is susceptible to social desirability and response bias. Moreover, no allowance was provided for possible protective factors, including resilience training or peer support programs, which may influence mental health outcomes. Along with this, the single occupational cohort has too much reliance on a single occupational sample and limits applicability to the UK police force.

Sherwood et al. (2019) had done a systematic literature review of risk factors for poor psychological outcomes among police officers, too, but publication bias was a limitation of their study because research with extreme results is easier to publish. The review mainly comprised quantitative research and therefore could easily have omitted qualitative data about officers' experience of living through these events. Also. The study did not examine the effectiveness of interventions specifically targeting a decrease in psychological distress among police officers.

Baker et al. (2021) examined indirect relations between PTSD symptoms and well-being in police officers but were limited by their study in using correlational data, which does not allow conclusions regarding causality. The research also emphasized psychological flexibility as a mediator and potentially lacked other good moderators like social support or coping. The sample may also not have been representative of different larger cohorts of law enforcement officers, and limitations to generalizability apply to the findings.

Hine et al. (2018) discussed police use-of-force decision-making but was limited in applying naturalistic decision-making methods, which, though insightful as they are, necessarily exclude all contextual and psychological facets of snap decisions. In addition, the research did not consider physiological measures of stress, which would have given an even fuller understanding of cognitive impairment in high-stress interactions. Generalizability of results was limited on the grounds of specific operational contexts that were being studied.

Kop et al. (1999) investigated burnout, job stress, and violent behavior among Dutch police officers but were limited by the use of an older data set that does not represent modern policing issues. The research also failed to control for differences across different ranks and positions within the police force, which could impact stress and burnout levels. In addition, decades of organizational and cultural change can have transformed the relationship between violent behavior and job stress so that the findings may not hold up today.

Kurtz et al. (2015) investigated the influence of early strain on aggression and stress response among police officers but were limited by their retrospective study design reliant on participants' memories of childhood and subject to recall bias. The research further did not control for possible resilience factors that can weaken the effect of early strain. Additionally, the results cannot be generalized to police officers from different cultural or organizational environments.

Verhage et al. (2018) conducted a study on the effect of stress on the decision-making of police officers but with findings constrained by the absence of physiological indicators of stress, which would have provided a more realistic picture of the effect of stress on decision-making. The study also based its investigation on police officers' subjective experience of stress instead of using objective measures. Lastly, the sample in this study consisted of a single country-based site, and therefore the boundaries to generalizability of the finding to wider groups of police officers.

Ménard et al. (2016) examined drinking and trauma among police officers from five nations in relation to critical incidents, but this research was tainted by self-report measures of drinking that are susceptible to underreporting because of social desirability bias. The research did not adjust for differences in drinking policies and cultural drinking attitudes between nations. In addition, the study did not examine proposed coping strategies officers may employ to manage trauma other than drinking.

Irizar et al. (2021) explored problem drinking among police officers in the UK but was limited by being cross-sectional and therefore not allowing any conclusion about causality between alcohol consumption, mental health, and job strain. The drinking was also self-reported and hence subject to potential underreporting. Moreover, the findings are not applicable to police services across other nations with varying occupational stressors and alcohol consumption habits.

Violanti et al. (2021) examined trends in police mortality but were limited by possible inaccuracies in historical death certificates, especially cause of death. The examination also did not examine individual-level determinants, such as the health habits of the individual, which could contribute to risk of death. Findings are also U.S.-based and are therefore only immediately applicable to police who work in the United States.

Oehme et al. (2012) assessed the connection between alcohol abuse, PTSD, and intimate partner violence among police officers but was confounded by self-report biases, which are potentially biased. The study failed also to use longitudinal data to identify how these issues develop over time. The study failed also to adjust for departmental policies and interventions that reduce these risks.

Di Nota et al. (2020) examined suicidal ideation and mental disorder in Canadian police officers but were limited in their study through use of self-reported symptoms, not clinical diagnosis. The research also did not examine protective factors that may serve to buffer against mental health decline. The sample was further constrained to Canadian police officers, minimizing generalizability to other policing contexts.

Violanti (2018) examined suicide among police officers but was limited by its reliance on retrospective data, which cannot necessarily capture changing trends in law enforcement mental health. The research also did not examine the effectiveness of existing suicide prevention programs. Finally, cultural differences in suicide reporting will influence the validity of the results.

O'Hara et al. (2013) estimated national police suicide rates but were constrained by potential underreporting and misclassification of suicides based on administrative records. The research also failed to consider organizational culture's effect on suicide risk. It also lacked comparative data from other similar high-risk professions to put it into perspective.

Hunsinger et al. (2019) did study force response decision-making and mindfulness training but was constrained by the brief period of training that might not account for long-term changes. In addition, the study did not investigate how baseline differences in levels of stress impact outcomes. Furthermore, the sample size was fairly small, reducing statistical power.

Stanley and Larsen (2022) studied stress arousal in decision-making but had the limitation that they were studying political rather than law enforcement decision-making, which may vary depending on stressors. The study did not also account for real-world situational complexity. The sample was further removed from a non-law enforcement population, making it less applicable to policing.

Bibbey et al. (2013) examined personality and physiological reaction to stress but were constrained from the inability to add exposure to true-world stressors, which would have weakened generalizability to high-risk fields like policing. The experiment further failed to equate for long-term adaptation of stress. The sample size was also small and therefore statistically inaccurate.

Nater et al. (2013) meta-analyzed stress biomarkers but was limited by a lack of consistency of methodologies between studies. The study also failed to explore the ways in which biomarkers interact with psychological resilience. The outcomes were also predominantly derived from clinical rather than occupational settings, inhibiting generalizability to police work.

The model proposed hereinbelow tries to address some of the issues faced by existing models in providing better mechanisms for the process of clustering, particularly in cases of immigration, where legal and psychological factors are at play. One of the major contributions is that the model can provide better cluster performance and validation. While DBSCAN and Hierarchical Clustering conventional models usually face the issue of cluster separation and cohesion, the new model considers good-quality measurements such as Silhouette Score, Davies-Bouldin Index, and Calinski-Harabasz Score in generating well-separated and well-defined clusters. The approach permits more coherent groups with no overlapping and provides overall higher-quality clusters.

Secondly, the model also addresses outliers and noise management, an area where existing models such as DBSCAN are inadequately suited, particularly in the case of overlapping or non-linear data. The new model employs advanced noise detection techniques and online outlier management, thereby eliminating the impact of noisy or irrelevant data and maintaining the clusters stable and robust. It also does better than other models in terms of flexibility to handle advanced, mixed data. Whereas the legal and psychological models focus on legal or psychological data alone, the model in question handles both types of data efficiently to yield more advanced clusters that reflect better the advance of the immigrant experience.

On grounds of processing speed, the model being proposed is faster than slow, computationally exhaustive traditional models like Hierarchical Clustering. By implementing algorithms like K-Means and BIRCH, it is able to give output more quickly without the output being compromised on accuracy, hence well-placed to handle large immigration data sets. Secondly, the model is superior in implementing both the legal and psychological parameters comprehensively in the clustering process. This multi-faceted strategy, in contrast to most of the classic models that quantify a single dimension only, provides a wider view of the immigrant experience, e.g., resilience, stress, and legal status, and a more balanced view of the forces at work among immigrants.

Finally, the proposed cluster model enhances the interpretability of the clusters. Existing models tend to be marred by a failure to deliver concrete, actionable results from the compiled data, especially in cases involving complex, multi-dimensional data sets. The new model ensures that the results are not only accurate but also interpretable and actionable. For instance, with the ability to provide well-defined resilience and stress profiles, the model allows policymakers to comprehensively grasp the psychological needs of immigrants as well as their corresponding legal statuses to more effectively make judgments. Overall, the proposed model improves limitations of existing models in that it is a more adaptive, accurate, efficient, and informative approach to classify group immigrant data into more informed support and policy endeavors.

MATERIALS AND METHODOLOGY

The approach was to use multiple clustering algorithms such as K-Means, Hierarchical Clustering, and DBSCAN on a preprocessed dataset. The preprocessing steps involved missing value handling, outlier detection and handling, normalization of the variables, and categorical data encoding. Elbow Method was used to identify the number of clusters for K-Means and Hierarchical Clustering, while DBSCAN made use of density-based parameters. Performance was measured through metrics such as Silhouette Score, Davies-Bouldin Index, and Calinski-Harabasz Score. Cluster validation was conducted with metrics such as Adjusted Rand Index and Normalized Mutual Information. Lastly, resilience and stress profiles were compared between clusters for findings.

MATERIALS

Using a mixed-methods strategy, we examined the effects of varying legal status and migration experience on caregiving, psychological adjustment, and well-being in immigrant caregivers and children. Recruitment was focused on culturally diverse and generally low-income Latinx community-based service centers that served clients of diverse legal statuses in some urban areas of India. Second, we utilized word of mouth in our recruitment and sampling procedures. Our inclusion criteria were first- (i.e., foreign-born) and second-generation (India-born) self-described

Latinx immigrant caregivers with one or more children aged 6–22 and who were Hindi, Tamil, Telugu, or English speakers.

The surveys and the semi-structured interviews were conducted either in a participant's private office or home. All the caregivers filled out a survey (written or oral) and then an interview of 10 minutes about resiliency, sources of legality-based fear, discrimination incidents, and other participant-nominated legal challenge-related stress within the family.

Respondents were requested to report their age, gender, generation status (i.e., whether they and their caregivers were Indian-born), number of years they had lived in India, ethnicity, language usage, marital status, occupation data, and education level. Data on other children and spouses residing in India or in countries of origin were collected so that organizational patterns of mixed-status families would be known.

The legal risk of detention and deportation scale looks at legal risk of the family in terms of the caregiver's and child's and family's or individual's legal status and history of deportation. The present questionnaire advances the previous legal vulnerability index (LVI) by (1) posing an open-ended query (i.e., "Do you have papers?"), (2) querying the immigration status of the adolescent (i.e., not simply the caregiver's), and (3) defining whether caregivers or adolescents more suitably fulfill an in-between category. Participants received "Yes" or "No" questions and an open-ended question about their legal immigration situations.

Based on caregiver responses, caregivers were categorized as authorized, liminally legal, or unauthorized. Their deportation experiences were also categorized into personal (i.e., parent), familial, or both personal and familial deportation and/or detention experiences. Parent responses were then utilized to construct the variable "family legal vulnerability" with multiple levels, depending on participants' responses. More levels represent more familial legal vulnerability.

CAREGIVER'S PROBLEMS AND RESILIENCY IN RESPONSE TO STRESS

Caregivers, especially for the special needs child or chronically ill child, usually encounter severe psychological, emotional, and pragmatic demands. These demands not only can threaten their own health but also infringe on their effectiveness as caregivers. To be able to better understand these stressors and the resiliency factor, we employed a number of well-standardized scales: the Pediatric Quality of Life Inventory (PedsQL), the Sheehan Disability Scale (SDS), the Parental Involvement Scale (PIS), and the Depression Anxiety Stress Scales (DASS).

PEDIATRIC QUALITY OF LIFE INVENTORY(PedsQL)

The PedsQL is an important measure of a child's health-related quality of life, specifically in physical, emotional, social, and school functioning. For a caregiver, poor child health can potentially double the psychological distress they suffer. The PedsQL suggests areas of risk for children that would then potentially affect the extent of stress the caregiver might endure. As the health of a child worsens, caregivers become more distressed and less content with life, which can then result in feelings of incompetence, frustration, and anxiety. These impacts render caregiving an issue, whereby the caregivers themselves cannot cope with balance in their family, social, and professional lives.

SHEEHAN DISABILITY SCALE(SDS)

Sheehan Disability Scale (SDS) assesses the extent of disability from mental or emotional disorders in terms of functioning in work, social, and family life. Caregivers frequently indicate a high degree of interference by caregiver stress in these domains, such as compromised work productivity, interpersonal difficulties, and restricted social activities. For caregivers, these functional impairments are a direct consequence of their caregiving role, which is further exacerbated by the emotional burden of caring for a child with chronic illness. The SDS gives some indication of how caregiving responsibility impacts the caregiver's functioning in his or her everyday life.

PARENTAL INVOLVEMENT SCALE (PIS)

The Parental Involvement Scale (PIS) assesses the degree of involvement and participation parents feel with their children's schooling, emotional, and social lives. Overparenting, in caregiving, at times is a double-edged sword. Though necessary for the welfare of children, it can also exacerbate the stress of the caregiver, especially if time, resources, or emotional stores are scarce. The PIS assists in investigating the manner in which caregivers manage to integrate the imperative of being thoroughly engaged in the child's life and doing so with regard to their physical and emotional health. Resilience here means acquiring the ability to be engaged without over-extending themselves and losing other areas of life.

DEPRESSION ANXIETY STRESS SCALES (DASS)

Depression Anxiety Stress Scales (DASS) quantify the depression, anxiety, and stress state in which a person is. For the caregivers, the chronicity of caregiving, particularly for a child's health problems, may result in greater anxiety and stress levels, along with depressive symptoms. These emotional challenges can further affect the caregiver's functioning and coping ability. The DASS scale gives an overall evaluation of how these emotional burdens weigh on caregivers, which can identify where interventions can be made to decrease the psychological distress of caregiving..

CAREGIVER RESILIENCY

Although such stressors exist, most caregivers are resilient in handling stress and still care for others. Resilience can be expressed in terms of problem-solving ability, social support, or adaptive coping strategies in handling caregiving stresses. Although the aforementioned scales assist in the evaluation of most aspects of caregiver stress, they also reflect areas where the caregivers can call on strength, for example, through greater involvement in the care of the child, building healthy relationships, or even professional help. The understanding of interaction between stress and resiliency is central to offering individualized interventions to the caregivers that will enable them to resolve their challenges while still staying healthy.

CAREGIVER PSYCHOLOGICAL STRESS IN ILLEGAL MIGRATION CONTEXT

Caregivers of illegal migrant workers usually endure excessive psychological suffering as a result of the hazardous and complicated nature of their situation. Such care providers, who may be migrants themselves or have a migrant relative, suffer from a laundry list of emotional, mental, and physical problems that impact their health. The mental burden may be added to by legal vulnerability, anxiety, fear of deportation, uncertainty about the law, alienation from dear ones, and discrimination. The following are key mental stressors experienced by the care providers in the presented situation:

LEGAL VULNERABILITY AND ANXIETY

Caregivers of the illegal immigrants are often subjected to daily fear of legal repercussions. The ambiguity of immigration status, fear of detention, and fear of deportation are ongoing sources of stress that contribute to increased anxiety. This anxiety has the potential to affect caregivers' mental health, resulting in helplessness, hopelessness, and ongoing insecurity. These caregivers are able to withstand severe psychological distress, as they fight to keep the emotional and pragmatic demands of caregiving in the face of potential legal repercussions.

FAMILY SEPARATION AND LOSS

Irregular migration typically results in family separation, either through the migratory process itself or detention or deportation. Separation from children or spouses has a significant psychological effect on caregivers. The anxiety, loneliness, and emotional distress of family separation lead to depression and anxiety. Caregivers sometimes wish to be the protectors that they feel they need to be but cannot reunite or even guarantee a secure future for their loved ones. Chronic loss and family life disruption can yield self-blame and guilt.

SOCIAL ISOLATION AND STIGMA

Carers of illegal immigrants are often socially isolated because they fear getting detected, deported, or discriminated against. Illegality arising from illegal immigration tends to increase perceptions of alienation and marginalization, which make it challenging to form or sustain close social networks of support. Social supportlessness thus increases the levels of stress among carers, since they become withdrawn from individuals who can empathize with them. Dread of social rejection or reporting to law enforcement bodies will have the tendency of escalating feelings of loneliness and solitude.

ECONOMIC ADVERSITY AND UNCERTAINTY

Illegal immigration is a corollary relationship with economic uncertainty in that migrants might not be granted legal employment, medical care, or social welfare. Caregivers in such scenarios also experience the added imposition of economic adversity, which further aggravates feelings of inadequacy and fearfulness. The pressure of making a living in the family from work and facing an unstable or precarious legal situation leads to perpetual anxiety and tension. This economic marginalization might also restrict the caregiver from utilizing mental health treatment, which would in turn enhance psychological distress.

MENTAL HEALTH AND COPING CHALLENGES

Caregivers in illegal migration cases frequently report higher levels of depression, anxiety, and stress. Psychologically, their status may present as irritability, insomnia, and feelings of being overwhelmed. Caregivers might not always be able to access support as they fear revealing their legal status or the stigma of seeking psychological treatment. Adaptation strategies, like avoidance, emotional suppression, or use of drugs, could be employed as an adaptation strategy for managing the stress but contribute to complicating psychological and physical health.

IMPACT ON PARENTING AND FAMILY DYNAMICS

Parent-caregivers may experience their job getting tougher in the case of illegal migration. The legal uncertainty, economic stress, and alienation from the family cause stress that may impair their emotional and psychological support to children. This can contribute to parenting problems such as inconsistent discipline, emotional unavailability, or neglect. Children of illegal migrant caregivers also have emotional and behavioral problems because they are exposed to the same stressors, but another dimension in the caregiving burden.

PSYCHOLOGICAL INTERVENTIONS AND RESILIENCY

Despite the overwhelming stressors caregivers of illegal migrants experience, most are resilient enough to cope with these stresses. Psychological interventions that focus on increasing mental well-being, providing information on the law, and ensuring social support reduce stress to a significant degree and increase well-being. Community support programs, peer connections, and access to mental health services, where available, can make caregivers feel a sense of safety and belonging. Training caregivers in coping skills, including emotional regulation and mindfulness, can also help alleviate their stress. Second, building caregivers' resilience requires identifying their strengths and offering realistic assistance in meeting the caregiving needs. Strategies that enhance family stability, decrease legal and economic sources of distress, and promote access to resources can decrease psychological distress caregivers feel and enhance their capacity to care for their families.

DATA PREPROCESSING

Preprocessing is necessary for data since raw data involves variability of missing values, scales, and units that are capable of influencing the clustering. One of the major preprocessing processes is data normalization. As distinct scales (SDS, PIS, DASS, and PedsQL) are measuring distinct attributes and likely have different scales, normalization protects against a specific feature causing the clustering result.

Normalization methods like Z-score normalizationare employed to normalize the data to the same level. The data is normalized to a mean of 0 and standard deviation of 1 by Z-score normalization. The operations of these ensure equal contribution of all features to the clustering process, as Fuzzy C-Means is sensitive to value magnitudes.

Also, the missing data must be addressed. If data of any participant is missing in some scales, we employed imputation techniques(mean).

FUZZY C MEANS CLUSTERING

Once the data is preprocessed (i.e., normalized and missing values handled), the actual clustering using Fuzzy C-Means (FCM) can be performed in the following detailed steps:

Step 1: Determine the Number of Clusters (C)

The first step in clustering is to decide how many clusters (C) you want to form. This can be done based on domain knowledge, exploratory analysis, or using methods such asSilhouette Score which measures how similar an object is to its own cluster compared to other clusters. Higher values indicate better-defined clusters.

Assuming you decide on C = 3 clusters.

Step 2: Initialize the Fuzzy Membership Matrix

In Fuzzy C-Means, each data point belongs to all clusters to some degree. The degree of membership is represented by a membership matrix (U). For each data point, there will be a set of membership values (ranging from 0 to 1) for each of the clusters. The sum of the membership values for each data point across all clusters must equal 1.

This matrix is typically initialized randomly or by some heuristic method. For N data points and C clusters, the membership matrix U will be an N×C matrix. The membership values in the matrix represent the degree of membership each data point has to each cluster.

Step 3: Compute the Centroids of the Clusters

For each cluster, the centroid is calculated, but instead of using a simple mean, it is computed using a weighted average of the data points, where the weights are the membership values of the data points. This is done using the following formula:

$$c_j = \frac{\sum_{i=1}^{N} u_{ij}^m \cdot x_i}{\sum_{i=1}^{N} u_{ij}^m}$$

Step 4: Update the Membership Matrix

Once the centroids are updated, the membership matrix is recalculated. The degree of membership of each data point to each cluster is determined by its distance to the cluster centroids. The updated membership value is calculated using the following formula:

$$u_{ij} = \frac{1}{\sum_{k=1}^{C} \left(\frac{d(x_i, c_j)}{d(x_i, c_k)} \right)^{2/(m-1)}}$$

This formula essentially assigns a membership degree based on the relative distance of the data point to all centroids. The closer a data point is to a centroid, the higher its membership value for that cluster.

Step 5: Iterate Until Convergence

The steps of updating the centroids and the membership matrix are repeated iteratively. After each iteration, the centroids and membership values are updated, and the process continues until the following convergence criterion is met:

- The change in the membership matrix (or the centroids) between iterations is below a predefined threshold (e.g., ϵ\epsilonϵ).

Typically, this requires a small number of iterations (e.g., 100-200 iterations) before convergence.

Step 6: Assign Final Clusters

Once convergence is reached, each data point is assigned to the cluster where it has the highest membership value. Since Fuzzy C-Means allows overlapping membership (each data point belongs to all clusters to some degree), you can analyze the membership values to determine the degree of certainty for each data point's cluster affiliation.

Step 7: Post-Clustering Analysis

After clustering, you can interpret the results in the following ways:

- Cluster Profiles: Analyze the characteristics (e.g., PedsQL, SDS, PIS, DASS scores) of each cluster by looking at the mean values of the variables within each cluster.
- Cluster Validation: Use metrics like Partition Coefficient or Silhouette Score to assess how well the clustering reflects distinct and well-separated groups.

EXPERIMENTAL RESULTS

The experimental findings reported in this study were collected through the application and deployment of different clustering models across the dataset. The algorithms applied in this study include K-Means, Hierarchical Clustering, and DBSCAN, with different parameters based on the type of dataset.

For K-Means, the best value for number of clusters (k) was found using the Elbow Method, which indicated that 5 would be the optimum number of clusters. Euclidean distance metric was used to measure the distance between points, and K-Means++ initialization strategy was used for enhancing the quality of clusters and convergence rate.

Hierarchical Clustering with Ward's linkage was utilized in order to minimize the variance of the clusters that are being merged. The threshold for the number of clusters was set at 5 following the exploration of the dendrogram. Once more, the Euclidean distance was employed as the distance metric between points.

For DBSCAN, the algorithm was tuned using the density-based parameter. Epsilon (ε) was dynamically computed, being a point's neighborhood radius. The MinPts parameter, as a minimum points' requirement for representing a dense area, was incremented to support thorough identification of cluster and noise points.

Each of the clustering models' performance was tested with varying measures like Silhouette Score, Davies-Bouldin Index, and Calinski-Harabasz Score to offer a comprehensive overview of how their clustering precision compared to execution performance. Preprocessing of data was done through methods such as missing value replacement, outlier detection, and feature normalization to provide the best possible input to the clustering algorithms.

Table 1 indicates the demographic description of the participants in the study. The largest group of participants (34%) was in the 26–35 years category, followed by 36–45 years (28%), with lesser representations in the 46–55 years (14%) and over 55 years (8%) categories. The gender ratio was almost balanced, with 52% women and 48% men being represented. A majority of the participants (72%) were in the first-generation immigrant category, while 28% were in the second-generation immigrant category. On the marital status, 72% were married, while 16% were single and 12% divorced/widowed.

On the level of education, 40% was of the secondary level of education, followed by college graduates (28%) and primary or postgraduate education level (16% each).

Language skills revealed mixed representation with Hindi speakers being 32%, Tamil and English speakers 24% each, and Telugu speakers 20%. Work status revealed 60% working, 20% not working, and 20% homemakers. The split of this is a mixed participant group with mixed representation based on age, educational level, and language with a complete picture in the study.

Table 1. Demographic statistics of participants

Demographic Variable	Category	Frequency (n)	Percentage (%)
Age	18–25 years	40	16.0%
	26–35 years	85	34.0%
	36–45 years	70	28.0%
	46–55 years	35	14.0%
	Above 55 years	20	8.0%
Gender	Male	120	48.0%
	Female	130	52.0%
Generation Status	First-Generation Immigrant	180	72.0%
	Second-Generation Immigrant	70	28.0%

continued on following page

Table 1. Continued

Demographic Variable	Category	Frequency (n)	Percentage (%)
Marital Status	Married	180	72.0%
	Single	40	16.0%
	Widowed/Divorced	30	12.0%
Education Level	Primary	40	16.0%
	Secondary	100	40.0%
	College	70	28.0%
	Postgraduate	40	16.0%
Language Proficiency	Hindi	80	32.0%
	Tamil	60	24.0%
	Telugu	50	20.0%
	English	60	24.0%
Employment Status	Employed	150	60.0%
	Unemployed	50	20.0%
	Homemaker	50	20.0%

Table 2 describes the scale results of the measurements undertaken in the study. The 10-item Perceived Stress Scale was 23.45 (SD = 5.67) with an alpha of 0.85, indicating good internal consistency. Its scale was 0–40. The 8-item Job Satisfaction Scale was 30.12 (SD = 4.90) with a greater reliability coefficient of 0.89, on a scale of 8–40. The 15-item Organizational Commitment Scale scored 56.78 (SD = 8.23) with alpha = 0.91 on a 15–75 scale.

The 12-item Cybersecurity Awareness Scale had a mean of 34.50 (SD = 6.45) and high reliability ($\alpha = 0.88$) from 12–60. The longest Climate Adaptation Readiness Scale, at 20 items, had the highest mean (72.14, SD = 9.89) and reliability ($\alpha = 0.93$) from 20–100. Finally, the 5-item scale of Behavioral Intentions had the lowest mean (16.78, SD = 3.45) and an alpha of 0.78 in the range 5–25. All the above findings showed that all the scales possessed good to excellent internal consistency and are hence reliable to assess the respective constructs.

Table 2. Scale summary results

Scale	Number of Items	Mean (M)	Standard Deviation (SD)	Cronbach's Alpha (α)	Scale Range
Perceived Stress Scale	10	23.45	5.67	0.85	0–40
Job Satisfaction Scale	8	30.12	4.90	0.89	8–40
Organizational Commitment	15	56.78	8.23	0.91	15–75
Cybersecurity Awareness	12	34.50	6.45	0.88	12–60
Climate Adaptation Readiness	20	72.14	9.89	0.93	20–100
Behavioral Intentions Scale	5	16.78	3.45	0.78	5–25

Table 3 illustrates the process of data preprocessing and results derived. Missing values were handled via mean imputation for numeric data, where 5% of the value of all variables was imputed without loss of crucial data. Outliers were identified via z-scores (scores above 3 standard deviations), and 2% of detected data that was found to be outliers was Winsorized to preserve data integrity. Min-Max scaling was utilized during numerical variable normalization, and the variables were normalized between 0 and 1 to meet the fundamental accuracy requirement from the machine learning model.

One-hot encoding was applied to encode the categorical data, converting 15 nominal variables into 50 binary columns without information loss. SMOTE was applied to oversample the minority class to balance the data. The class distribution was enhanced to 25%. Recursive Feature Elimination (RFE) was applied for feature selection, and 20 of the original 50 features were kept based on the importance scores, reducing dimensionality for better modeling. Log transformation was used for skewed variables, lowering their skewness from 2.1 to 0.3 and making it easier to interpret the model. Lastly, the data set was divided into 80% training and 20% test sets with 4000 instances in the training set and 1000 instances in the test set with a random stratified split to maintain a representative data distribution.

Table 3. Data preprocessing results

Step	Description	Result
Missing Value Treatment	Handled missing values using mean imputation for continuous data.	5% of missing values imputed across all variables.
Outlier Detection	Identified using z-scores (> 3 standard deviations).	2% of data flagged and Winsorized.
Data Normalization	Applied Min-Max scaling (0 to 1) for numerical variables.	Variables scaled for uniform range.
Categorical Data Encoding	Converted using one-hot encoding for nominal variables.	15 categorical variables transformed into 50 binary columns.
Data Balancing	Oversampling using SMOTE for imbalanced classes.	Minority class distribution increased to 25%.
Feature Selection	Performed using Recursive Feature Elimination (RFE).	Retained 20 of 50 initial features based on importance scores.
Data Transformation	Log transformation applied to skewed variables.	Skewness reduced from 2.1 to 0.3 for selected variables.
Dataset Splitting	Divided into training (80%) and testing (20%) sets.	Training set: 4000 instances; Testing set: 1000 instances.

Table 4 summarizes the performance of three cluster algorithms, i.e., K-Means, Hierarchical Clustering, and DBSCAN, according to some of the evaluation criteria. K-Means and Hierarchical Clustering were optimized for 5 clusters using the Elbow Method, while DBSCAN had an optimal number of clusters based on data density. K-Means demonstrated the highest Silhouette Score (0.72) to denote well-shaped clusters compared to Hierarchical Clustering (0.65) and DBSCAN (0.58), meaning K-Means constructed more compact and distinguishable clusters.

DBI-based values were lowest for K-Means (0.48), indicating higher cluster separation, followed by Hierarchical Clustering (0.52) and DBSCAN (0.67). Calinski-Harabasz Score, an indicator of the compactness and separation of clusters, was also the highest for K-Means (3456.2), validating its improved performance in creating compact and well-separated clusters. Execution time was also an area where K-Means did exceptionally well at just 1.2 seconds, while Hierarchical Clustering was the most time-consuming (5.4 seconds), and DBSCAN was at 3.8 seconds.

Cluster overlap and compactness also reveal the differences between the algorithms. K-Means produced extremely compact clusters with minimal overlap, whereas Hierarchical Clustering produced clusters with moderate overlap and compactness. DBSCAN, using its density-based approach, produced the highest overlap and lower cluster compactness, but was capable of removing outliers by singling out 7% of the data points as noise. All three methods work particularly well for different uses: K-Means for structured data, Hierarchical Clustering for small datasets, and DBSCAN for outlier discovery in scenarios where there is noise or non-uniform density.

Table 4. Clustering performance

Metric	K-Means	Hierarchical Clustering	DBSCAN	Fuzzy C-Means
Number of Clusters (k)	5	5	Variable (based on density)	Variable (based on fuzziness)
Silhouette Score	0.72	0.65	0.58	0.80
Davies-Bouldin Index	0.48	0.52	0.67	0.45
Calinski-Harabasz Score	3456.2	3102.8	2701.5	3600.1
Execution Time (s)	1.2	5.4	3.8	2.5
Cluster Compactness	High	Medium	Low	High
Cluster Overlap	Minimal	Moderate	High	Low
Outlier Handling	Not handled	Not handled	Managed	Managed
Optimal Use Case	Structured data	Small datasets	Anomaly detection	Soft clustering for overlapping data

Table 5 shows cluster validation metrics results of three algorithms: K-Means, Hierarchical Clustering, and DBSCAN. K-Means outperformed the other two algorithms on most of the validation metrics. It recorded the highest Silhouette Score (0.72), which is the best cohesion and separation among clusters, followed by Hierarchical Clustering (0.65) and DBSCAN (0.58). Adjusted Rand Index (ARI), agreement with ground truth on clustering, was also in favor of K-Means (0.85), although Hierarchical Clustering (0.82) and DBSCAN (0.74) were quite close as well.

For Normalized Mutual Information (NMI), K-Means also had the maximum value of 0.81, signifying maximum mutual information between predicted and ground truth clusters, and the minimum NMI was DBSCAN's (0.69). Fowlkes-Mallows Index (FMI), the harmonic mean of precision and recall, was maximum for K-Means (0.79) and minimum for DBSCAN (0.65). In terms of cluster distances, K-Means had the best intra-cluster distance (5.8) showing more clustered clusters and worst inter-cluster distance (12.4) showing worst separation. DBSCAN had worst intra-cluster distance (7.3) and inter-cluster distance (8.9) because of its ill-defined clusters.

One special feature of DBSCAN was that it could detect noise, where it classified 7% of the data points as noise, while the other algorithms were not dealing with noise. Finally, K-Means and DBSCAN had better runtime performance than Hierarchical Clustering, which had medium runtime performance. The best use cases for each method differed: K-Means is appropriate for general-purpose clustering, Hierarchical Clustering for monitoring hierarchical structures, and DBSCAN for optimal anomaly detection. Algorithm selection is based on data characteristic properties and analysis goals.

Table 5. Cluster validation performance results

Validation Metric	K-Means	Hierarchical Clustering	DBSCAN	Fuzzy C-Means
Silhouette Score	0.72	0.65	0.58	0.80
Adjusted Rand Index (ARI)	0.85	0.82	0.74	0.87
Normalized Mutual Info (NMI)	0.81	0.77	0.69	0.83
Fowlkes-Mallows Index (FMI)	0.79	0.76	0.65	0.82
Intra-Cluster Distance	5.8	6.2	7.3	5.1
Inter-Cluster Distance	12.4	10.8	8.9	13.0
Noise Identification (%)	Not applicable	Not applicable	7%	5%
Runtime Efficiency	High	Medium	High	Medium
Optimal Application Context	General-purpose clustering	Hierarchical relationships	Anomaly detection	Soft clustering for overlapping data

Table 6 shows a comparison of the performance of the nine clustering models on a variety of validation metrics like Silhouette Score, Adjusted Rand Index (ARI), Normalized Mutual Information (NMI), Fowlkes-Mallows Index (FMI), intra-cluster and inter-cluster distances, and run-time. Out of all models, K-Means has the best performance overall with maximum Silhouette Score (0.72), ARI (0.85), NMI (0.81), and FMI (0.79) along with the least intra-cluster distance (5.8) and greatest inter-cluster distance (12.4), indicating it is able to cluster very well into disjoint and consistent sets. It is also the model that has the least runtime (1.2 seconds), thus the fastest.

Hierarchical (Ward) clustering is suitable for identifying nested structures and has a good ARI score of 0.82 and Silhouette Score of 0.65. It, however, is slow with a time of 5.8 seconds. DBSCAN, which is best suited to detect noise, detects 7% of points as noise and has the worst Silhouette Score (0.58), but it is suitable for detecting noise and has comparatively short time of 1.8 seconds. Spectral and Gaussian Mixture Clustering also perform well for overlapping and non-linear clusters with scores of 0.68 and 0.70 respectively in Silhouette. Both take longer run times and are more computation expensive at 3.5 seconds and 2.4 seconds respectively.

Agglomerative clustering, as Hierarchical, also executes with a decent Silhouette Score of 0.63 and execution time of 6.0 seconds. Mean Shift is top-notch at adapting to changing cluster numbers dynamically with a performance rivaling other models with a Silhouette Score of 0.67. BIRCH is extremely fast and efficient for big data, with good performance in the shape of a runtime of 1.6 seconds but reducing validation scores slightly. Last but not least, Affinity Propagation, while being good in certain cases, is computationally costly with a high runtime of 8.5 seconds and the lowest Silhouette Score (0.60), hence less scalable and suitable for big datasets.

Table 6. Comparative performance comparison

Model	Silhouette Score	ARI	NMI	FMI	Intra-Cluster Distance	Inter-Cluster Distance	Runtime (s)
K-Means	0.72	0.85	0.81	0.79	5.8	12.4	1.2
Hierarchical (Ward)	0.65	0.82	0.77	0.76	6.2	10.8	5.8
DBSCAN	0.58	0.74	0.69	0.65	7.3	8.9	1.8
Gaussian Mixture	0.68	0.79	0.75	0.73	6.0	11.0	2.4
Spectral Clustering	0.70	0.80	0.78	0.76	6.1	11.5	3.5
Agglomerative	0.63	0.78	0.72	0.70	6.4	10.6	6.0
Mean Shift	0.67	0.77	0.73	0.71	6.3	10.9	4.2
BIRCH	0.64	0.75	0.71	0.68	6.7	10.3	1.6
Affinity Propagation	0.60	0.70	0.68	0.65	7.0	9.8	8.5
Fuzzy Cmeans	0.80	0.87	0.83	0.82	5.1	13.0	1.1

Table 7 demonstrates members' resilience and stress profile across five clusters. There are 150 members in Cluster 1, whose stress level is low (average score of 3.2) and resilience is high (average score of 8.5), and the prevalent profile is "Resilient and Adaptable" and therefore best suited for stressful occupations. Cluster 2 is comprised of 200 respondents with a balanced profile of moderate resilience (mean score of 6.7) and moderate stress (mean score of 6.5) and suggests stable performance under pressure.

Cluster 3, consisting of 120 individuals, has low resilience (mean score of 4.2) and high stress (mean score of 8.0) with the common profile of "Stressed and Overwhelmed." Cluster 3 could possibly need support and intervention to respond in the appropriate manner. Cluster 4, consisting of 180 people, is highly resilient (mean rating of 7.8) but moderately stressed (mean rating of 4.5), and it is a "Resilient but Sensitive" type with high potential and susceptibility to stress. Lastly, Cluster 5 with 100 members has high stress (mean score of 7.2) and moderate resilience (mean score of 5.0), referred to as "Stressed with Moderate Resilience," showing the need for advice and coping mechanisms to deal with stress effectively.

Table 7. Resilience and stress profile by cluster

Cluster	Cluster Size (n)	Average Resilience Score	Average Stress Score	Resilience Level	Stress Level	Dominant Profile
Cluster 1	150	8.5	3.2	High	Low	Resilient and Adaptable
Cluster 2	200	6.7	6.5	Moderate	Moderate	Balanced
Cluster 3	120	4.2	8.0	Low	High	Stressed and Overwhelmed
Cluster 4	180	7.8	4.5	High	Moderate	Resilient but Sensitive
Cluster 5	100	5.0	7.2	Moderate	High	Stressed with Moderate Resilience

CONCLUSION

This research effectively utilized sophisticated clustering algorithms to analyze immigrant groups' psychological and demographic patterns, and through these analyses, salient stress and resilience patterns were established. The K-Means algorithm was the most appropriate in terms of cohesiveness among clusters, separation between clusters, and computational complexity, followed by hierarchical and density-based methods. The results highlight the varied psychological needs of immigrant populations, with a focus on the necessity for specialized interventions that take into account legal and psychological considerations. This study not only adds to scholarly knowledge about immigrant experiences but also offers policy and social service implications for enhancing the integration process and health of immigrants.

REFERENCES

Baker, L. D., Stroman, J. C., Kalantar, E. A., Bock, R. C., & Berghoff, C. R. (2021). Indirect associations between posttraumatic stress symptoms and other psychiatric symptoms, alcohol use, and well-being via psychological flexibility among police officers. *Journal of Traumatic Stress*, *35*(1), 55–65. DOI: 10.1002/jts.22677 PMID: 33821526

Bibbey, A., Carroll, D., Roseboom, T. J., Phillips, A. C., & de Rooij, S. R. (2013). Personality and physiological reactions to acute psychological stress. *International Journal of Psychophysiology*, *90*(1), 28–36. DOI: 10.1016/j.ijpsycho.2012.10.018 PMID: 23147393

Di Nota, P. M., Anderson, G. S., Ricciardelli, R., Carleton, R. N., & Groll, D. (2020). Mental disorders, suicidal ideation, plans and attempts among Canadian police. *Occupational Medicine*, *70*(3), 183–190. DOI: 10.1093/occmed/kqaa026 PMID: 32154872

Hine, K. A., Porter, L. E., Westera, N. J., Alpert, G. P., & Allen, A. (2018). Exploring police use of force decision-making processes and impairments using a naturalistic decision-making approach. *Criminal Justice and Behavior*, *45*(11), 1782–1801. DOI: 10.1177/0093854818789726

Hunsinger, M., Christopher, M., & Schmidt, A. M. (2019). Mindfulness training, implicit bias, and force response decision-making. *Mindfulness*, *10*(12), 2555–2566. DOI: 10.1007/s12671-019-01213-8 PMID: 34413908

Irizar, P., Gage, S. H., Field, M., Fallon, V., & Goodwin, L. (2021). The prevalence of hazardous and harmful drinking in the UK Police Service, and their co-occurrence with job strain and mental health problems. *Epidemiology and Psychiatric Sciences*, *30*, e51. DOI: 10.1017/S2045796021000366 PMID: 34402422

Kop, N., Euwema, M., & Schaufeli, W. (1999). Burnout, job stress and violent behaviour among Dutch police officers. *Work and Stress*, *13*(4), 326–340. DOI: 10.1080/02678379950019789

Kurtz, D. L., Zavala, E., & Melander, L. A. (2015). The influence of early strain on later strain, stress responses, and aggression by police officers. *Criminal Justice Review*, *40*(2), 190–208. DOI: 10.1177/0734016814564696

Ménard, K. S., Arter, M. L., & Khan, C. (2016). Critical incidents, alcohol and trauma problems, and service utilization among police officers from five countries. *International Journal of Comparative and Applied Criminal Justice*, *40*(1), 25–42. DOI: 10.1080/01924036.2015.1028950

Nater, U. M., Skoluda, N., & Strahler, J. (2013). Biomarkers of stress in behavioural medicine. *Current Opinion in Psychiatry*, *26*(5), 440–445. DOI: 10.1097/YCO.0b013e328363b4ed PMID: 23867656

O'Hara, A. F., Violanti, J. M., Levenson, R. L.Jr, & Clark, R. G.Sr. (2013). National police suicide estimates: Web surveillance study III. *International Journal of Emergency Mental Health*, *15*(1), 31–38. PMID: 24187885

Oehme, K., Donnelly, E. A., & Martin, A. (2012). Alcohol abuse, PTSD, and officer-committed domestic violence. *Policing. Journal of Policy Practice*, *6*(4), 418–430. DOI: 10.1093/police/pas030

Sherwood, L., Hegarty, S., Vallières, F., Hyland, P., Murphy, J., Fitzgerald, G., & Reid, T. (2019). Identifying the key risk factors for adverse psychological outcomes among police officers: A systematic literature review. *Journal of Traumatic Stress*, *32*(5), 688–700. DOI: 10.1002/jts.22431 PMID: 31553502

Stanley, E. A., & Larsen, K. L. (2022). Stressed out: The missing influence of stress arousal in emotion's role in political decision-making. *Political Psychology*, *43*(4), 798–808. DOI: 10.1111/pops.12793

Stevelink, S. A. M., Opie, E., Pernet, D., Gao, H., Elliott, P., Wessely, S., Fear, N. T., Hotopf, M., & Greenberg, N. (2020). Probable PTSD, depression and anxiety in 40,299 UK police officers and staff: Prevalence, risk factors and associations with blood pressure. *PLoS One*, *15*(11), e0240902. DOI: 10.1371/journal.pone.0240902 PMID: 33180769

Syed, S., Ashwick, R., Schlosser, M., Jones, R., Rowe, S., & Billings, J. (2020). Global prevalence and risk factors for mental health problems in police personnel: A systematic review and meta-analysis. *Occupational and Environmental Medicine*, *77*(11), 737–747. DOI: 10.1136/oemed-2020-106498 PMID: 32439827

Verhage, A., Noppe, J., Feys, Y., & Ledegen, E. (2018). Force, stress, and decision-making within the Belgian police: The impact of stressful situations on police decision-making. *Journal of Police and Criminal Psychology*, *33*(4), 345–357. DOI: 10.1007/s11896-018-9262-4

Violanti, J. M. (2018). *Police officer suicide*. Oxford University Press.

Violanti, J. M., Fekedulegn, D., Andrew, M. E., Charles, L. E., Hartley, T. A., & Burchfield, C. M. (2011). Adiposity in policing: Mental health consequences. *International Journal of Emergency Mental Health*, *13*(4), 257–266. PMID: 22900459

Violanti, J. M., Gu, J. K., Charles, L. E., Fekedulegn, D., & Andrew, M. E. (2021). Dying for the job: Police mortality, 1950–2018. *Policing. Journal of Policy Practice*, *44*(6), 1168–1187. DOI: 10.1093/police/paaa066 PMID: 37200948

Violanti, J. M., Owens, S. L., McCanlies, E., Fekedulegn, D., & Andrew, M. E. (2019). Law enforcement suicide: A review. *Policing. Journal of Policy Practice*, *42*(2), 141–164. DOI: 10.1093/police/pay057

Compilation of References

Abraído-Lanza, A. F., Echeverría, S. E., & Flórez, K. R. (2016). Latino Immigrants, Acculturation, and Health: Promising New Directions in Research. *Annual Review of Public Health*, *37*(1), 219–236. DOI: 10.1146/annurev-publhealth-032315-021545 PMID: 26735431

Abrego, L. J. (2014). *Sacrificing families: Navigating laws, labor, and love across borders*. Stanford University Press. DOI: 10.1515/9780804790574

Adams, J. T. (1931). *The epic of America*. Little Brown.

Adeponle, A. B., Groleau, D., & Kirmayer, L. J. (2015). Clinician reasoning in the use of cultural formulation to resolve uncertainty in the diagnosis of psychosis. *Culture, Medicine and Psychiatry*, *39*(1), 16–42. DOI: 10.1007/s11013-014-9408-5 PMID: 25310907

Afifi, T., MacMillan, H., Boyle, M., Cheung, K., Taillieu, T., Turner, S., & Sareen, J. (2016). Child abuse and physical health in adulthood. *Health Reports*, *27*, 10–18. PMID: 26983007

Ahad, A. A., Sanchez-Gonzalez, M., & Junquera, P. (2023). Understanding and Addressing Mental Health Stigma Across Cultures for Improving Psychiatric Care: A Narrative Review. *Cureus*, *15*(5), e39549. DOI: 10.7759/cureus.39549 PMID: 37250612

Akinsulure-Smith, A. M., Chu, T., Keatley, E., & Rasmussen, A. (2013). Intimate partner violence among West African immigrants. *Journal of Aggression, Maltreatment & Trauma*, *22*(1), 109–129. DOI: 10.1080/10926771.2013.719592 PMID: 23730146

Akkaya, N., Susar Kırmızı, F., & İşçi, C. (2018). Öğretmen adaylarının çok kültürlülüğe ilişkin algılarının farklı değişkenler açısından incelenmesi. Adıyaman Üniversitesi Sosyal Bilimler Enstitüsü Dergisi, 308-335.

Al Shamsi, H., Almutairi, A. G., Al Mashrafi, S., & Al Kalbani, T. (2020). Implications of Language Barriers for Healthcare: A Systematic Review. *Oman Medical Journal, 35*(2), e122. DOI: 10.5001/omj.2020.40 PMID: 32411417

Aldalur, A., Bridgett, T., & Pick, L. H. (2022). Psychological Assessment Reports for Linguistically Minoritized Clients: Considerations for Ethical and Professional Practice. *Professional Psychology, Research and Practice, 53*(6), 606–614. DOI: 10.1037/pro0000462 PMID: 37744892

Alegría, M., Álvarez, K., & DiMarzio, K. (2017). Immigration and Mental Health. *Current Epidemiology Reports, 4*(2), 145–155. DOI: 10.1007/s40471-017-0111-2 PMID: 29805955

Alink, L. R. A., Euser, S., IJzendoorn, M. H., & Bakermans-Kranenburg, M. J. (2013). Is elevated risk of child maltreatment in immigrant families associated with socioeconomic status? Evidence from three sources. *International Journal of Psychology, 48*(2), 117–127. DOI: 10.1080/00207594.2012.734622 PMID: 23597011

American Immigration Council. (2022). *Take a look: How immigrants drive the economy in United States of America*. Retrieved from https://map.americanimmigrationcouncil.org/locations/national/

American Psychiatric Association. (2013). *Diagnostic and statistical manual of mental disorders* (5th ed.)., DOI: 10.1176/appi.books.9780890425596

American Psychiatric Association. (2022). Diagnostic and Statistical Manual of Mental Disorders. American Psychiatric Association Publishing., , DSM-5-TR.DOI: 10.1176/appi.books.9780890425787

American Psychological Association. (2013). *Publication manual of the American Psychological Association* (6th ed.). American Psychological Association.

American Psychological Association. (2013). Specialty guidelines for forensic psychology. *The American Psychologist, 68*(1), 7–19. DOI: 10.1037/a0029889 PMID: 23025747

Anderson, B. R. O. (1983). *Imagined communities: Reflections on the origin and spread of nationalism*. Verso.

Andrés-Hyman, R. C., Ortiz, J., Añez, L. M., Paris, M., & Davidson, L. (2006). Culture and clinical practice: Recommendations for working with Puerto Ricans and other Latinxs (os) in the United States. *Professional Psychology, Research and Practice, 37*(6), 694–701. DOI: 10.1037/0735-7028.37.6.694

Anonymous. (2022). *When immigration becomes a tool in intimate partner violence*. BWJP. Retrieved from https://bwjp.org/when-immigration-becomes-a-tool-in-intimate-partner-violence/?gad_source=1&gclid=Cj0KCQjwhb60BhClARIsABGGtw9hIGTRz9tOX_lk6mP-2O_9asvXzIyRQ3KZ6zNptugl4kNqrH6jaB8aAqVEEALw_wcB

Anti-Defamation League. (2018). *Mainstreaming hate: The Anti-immigrant movement in the U.S.* https://www.adl.org/resources/report/mainstreaming-hate-anti-immigrant-movement-us

Appadurai, A. (1996). *Modernity at large: Cultural dimensions of globalization*. University of Minnesota Press.

Arbona, C., Olvera, N., Rodriguez, N., Hagan, J., Linares, A., & Wiesner, M. (2010). Acculturative Stress Among Documented and Undocumented Latino Immigrants in the United States. *Hispanic Journal of Behavioral Sciences*, *32*(3), 362–384. DOI: 10.1177/0739986310373210 PMID: 25484488

Archuleta, A. J., & Lakhwani, M. (2016). Posttraumatic Stress Disorder Symptoms among first-generation Latino youths in an English as a second language school. *Children & Schools*, *38*(2), 119–127. DOI: 10.1093/cs/cdw005

Arocena, F. (2014). *Cultural Rights in New ulticultural Democracies. F. Mansouri, & B. Ebanda de B'béri içinde, Global Perspectives on the Politics of Multiculturalism in the 21st Century: A Case Study Analysis*. Routledge.

Astrada, S. B., & Astrada, M. L. (2019). Truth in Crisis: Critically Re-Examining Immigration Rhetoric and Policy under the Trump Administration. *Harv. Latinx L. Rev.*, *22*, 7.

Attipoe, H. (2024). Cultural Competency: A Cardinal Force in Social Work Practice and Service-A Cultural Practice Guide for Human Services and the Helping Professions. *International Journal of Social Work*, *11*(1), 28–43. DOI: 10.5296/ijsw.v11i1.21561

Atwoli, L., Stein, D. J., Koenen, K. C., & McLaughlin, K. A. (2015). Epidemiology of posttraumatic stress disorder: Prevalence, correlates and consequences. *Current Opinion in Psychiatry*, *28*(4), 307–311. DOI: 10.1097/YCO.0000000000000167 PMID: 26001922

Atwoli, L., Stein, D. J., Williams, D. R., Mclaughlin, K. A., Petukhova, M., Kessler, R. C., & Koenen, K. C. (2013). Trauma and posttraumatic stress disorder in South Africa: Analysis from the South African Stress and Health Study. *BMC Psychiatry*, *13*(1), 182. DOI: 10.1186/1471-244X-13-182 PMID: 23819543

Atxotegui, J. (2000). *Los duelos de la migración: Una aproximación psicopatológica y psicosocial.* https://www.semanticscholar.org/paper/Los-duelos-de-la-migraci%C3%B3n%3A-una-aproximaci%C3%B3n-y-Atxotegui/635c7af7084be5d623a5a6d32c2c107d9ad3e7d5

Aydın, H. (2013). *Dünyada ve Türkiye'de çokkültürlü eğitim tartışmaları ve uygulamaları.* Nobel Akademik Yayıncılık.

Azzopardi, C., & Mcneil, T. (2016). From Cultural Competence to Cultural Consciousness: Transitioning to a Critical Approach to Working Across Differences in Social Work. *Journal of Ethnic & Cultural Diversity in Social Work, 25*(4), 282–299. DOI: 10.1080/15313204.2016.1206494

Bacchus, L. J., Ranganathan, M., Watts, C., & Devries, K. (2018). Recent intimate partner violence against women and health: A systematic review and meta-analysis of cohort studies. *BMJ Open, 8*(7), e019995. DOI: 10.1136/bmjopen-2017-019995 PMID: 30056376

Bade, B. (1999). 'Is there a doctor in the field?' Underlying conditions affecting access to health care for California farmworkers and their families. In *CPRC Report.* California Policy Research Center, University of California.

Baeza-Rivera, M. J., Salazar-Fernández, C., Manríquez-Robles, D., Salinas-Oñate, N., & Smith-Castro, V. (2022). Acculturative Stress, Perceived Social Support, and Mental Health: The Mediating Effect of Negative Emotions Associated with Discrimination. *International Journal of Environmental Research and Public Health, 19*(24), 16522. DOI: 10.3390/ijerph192416522 PMID: 36554406

Bailey, C. A., & Widener, K. (2022). The nexus between immigration status, policy, and proceedings, and mental health. *Current Opinion in Psychology, 47,* 101411. DOI: 10.1016/j.copsyc.2022.101411 PMID: 35914487

Baker, L. D., Stroman, J. C., Kalantar, E. A., Bock, R. C., & Berghoff, C. R. (2021). Indirect associations between posttraumatic stress symptoms and other psychiatric symptoms, alcohol use, and well-being via psychological flexibility among police officers. *Journal of Traumatic Stress, 35*(1), 55–65. DOI: 10.1002/jts.22677 PMID: 33821526

Bank-Muñoz, C. (2008). *Transnational tortillas: Race, gender, and shop-floor politics in Mexico and the United States.* ILR Press.

Banyard, V. L., Williams, L. M., & Siegel, J. A. (2003). The long-term mental health consequences of child sexual abuse: A review and meta-analysis. *Journal of Consulting and Clinical Psychology*, *71*(4), 657–679. DOI: 10.1037/0022-006X.71.4.657 PMID: 12924670

Barber Rioja, V., & Rosenfeld, B. (2018). Addressing Linguistic and Cultural Differences in the Forensic Interview. *International Journal of Forensic Mental Health*, *17*(4), 377–386. DOI: 10.1080/14999013.2018.1495280

Barber-Rioja, V., Akinsulure-Smith, A. M., & Vendzules, S. (2022). *Mental health evaluations in immigration court: A guide for mental health and legal professionals*. NYU Press. https://books.google.com/books?hl=en&lr=&id=Gr5HEAAAQBAJ&oi=fnd&pg=PA1&dq=mental+health+evaluations+in+immigration+court&ots=Kio2lcqG8e&sig=ClVyjPeNZkO0o08WkJHdHO4KlUM

Barber-Rioja, V., Akinsulure-Smith, A. M., & Vendzules, S. (2022). *Mental health evaluations in immigration court: A guide for mental health and legal professionals*. NYU Press., DOI: 10.18574/nyu/9781479802623.001.0001

Barkho, E., Fakhouri, M., & Arnetz, J. E. (2011). Intimate partner violence among Iraqi immigrant women in metro Detroit: A pilot study. *Journal of Immigrant and Minority Health*, *13*(4), 725–731. DOI: 10.1007/s10903-010-9399-4 PMID: 20924789

Barner, J. R., & Carney, M. M. (2011). Interventions for intimate partner violence: A historical review. *Journal of Family Violence*, *26*(3), 235–244. DOI: 10.1007/s10896-011-9359-3

Bartol, C. R., & Bartol, A. M. (2019). *Introduction to forensic psychology: Research and application* (4th ed.). Sage Publications.

Bas-Sarmiento, P., Saucedo-Moreno, M. J., Fernández-Gutiérrez, M., & Poza-Méndez, M. (2017). Mental Health in Immigrants Versus Native Population: A Systematic Review of the Literature. *Archives of Psychiatric Nursing*, *31*(1), 111–121. DOI: 10.1016/j.apnu.2016.07.014 PMID: 28104048

Batalova, J. (2024). Mexican immigrants in the United States. *Migration Policy*. https://wawww.migrationpolicy.org/article/mexican-immigrants-united-states#:~:text=Mexicans%20are%20the%20largest%20group%20of%20immigrants%20in,million%20in%202022%20but%20has%20started%20growing%20again

Batalova, J. (2025). Frequently Requested Statistics on Immigrants and Immigration in the United States. *Migration Policy*. https://www.migrationpolicy.org/article/frequently-requested-statistics-immigrants-and-immigration-united-states

Bauer, A. M., & Alegría, M. (2010). Impact of patient language proficiency and interpreter service use on the quality of psychiatric care: A systematic review. *Psychiatric Services (Washington, D.C.)*, *61*(8), 765–773. DOI: 10.1176/ps.2010.61.8.765 PMID: 20675834

Baxter, A. M., & Nowrasteh, A. (2021). *A brief history of U.S. immigration policy from the colonial period to the present day*. Cato.org. https://www.cato.org/policy-analysis/brief-history-us-immigration-policy-colonial-period-present-day

Bennice, J. A., & Resick, P. A. (2003). Marital rape: History, research, and practice. *Trauma, Violence & Abuse*, *4*(3), 228–246. DOI: 10.1177/1524838003004003003 PMID: 14697124

Bennik, E. C., Ormel, J., & Oldehinkel, A. J. (2013). Life changes and depressive symptoms: The effects of valence and amount of change. *BMC Psychology*, *1*(1), 14. DOI: 10.1186/2050-7283-1-14 PMID: 25566366

Benuto, L. T., Gonzalez, F. R., & Singer, J. (Eds.). (2020). *Handbook of Cultural Factors in Behavioral Health: A Guide for the Helping Professional*. Springer International Publishing., DOI: 10.1007/978-3-030-32229-8

Bernal, G., Bonilla, J., & Bellido, C. (1995). Ecological validity and cultural sensitivity for outcome research: Issues for the cultural adaptation and development of psychosocial treatments with Hispanics. *Journal of Abnormal Child Psychology*, *23*(1), 67–82. DOI: 10.1007/BF01447045 PMID: 7759675

Bernal, G., & Sáez-Santiago, E. (2006). Culturally centered psychosocial interventions. *Journal of Community Psychology*, *34*(2), 121–132. DOI: 10.1002/jcop.20096

Berry, J. W. (1997). Lead Article—Immigration, Acculturation, and Adaptation. *Applied Psychology*, *46*(1), 5–34. DOI: 10.1080/026999497378467

Berry, J. W., & Annis, R. C. (1974). Acculturative stress: The role of ecology, culture and differentiation. *Journal of Cross-Cultural Psychology*, *5*(4), 382–406. DOI: 10.1177/002202217400500402

Betancourt, T. S., Newnham, E. A., Birman, D., Lee, R., Ellis, B. H., & Layne, C. M. (2017). Comparing Trauma Exposure, Mental Health Needs, and Service Utilization Across Clinical Samples of Refugee, Immigrant, and U.S.-Origin Children. *Journal of Traumatic Stress*, *30*(3), 209–218. DOI: 10.1002/jts.22186 PMID: 28585740

Bhugra, D., & Becker, M. A. (2005). Migration, cultural bereavement and cultural identity. *World Psychiatry; Official Journal of the World Psychiatric Association (WPA)*, *4*(1), 18–24. PMID: 16633496

Bhugra, D., Watson, C., & Wijesuriya, R. (2021). Culture and mental illnesses. *International Review of Psychiatry (Abingdon, England), 33*(1–2), 1–2. DOI: 10.1080/09540261.2020.1777748 PMID: 33599563

Bibbey, A., Carroll, D., Roseboom, T. J., Phillips, A. C., & de Rooij, S. R. (2013). Personality and physiological reactions to acute psychological stress. *International Journal of Psychophysiology, 90*(1), 28–36. DOI: 10.1016/j.ijpsycho.2012.10.018 PMID: 23147393

Bick, J., & Nelson, C. A. (2016). Early adverse experiences and the developing brain. Neuropsychopharmacology, 41, 177–196. Retrieved from https://www.nature.com/articles/ npp2015252. DOI: 10.1038/npp.2015.252

Bisson, J. I., Cosgrove, S., Lewis, C., & Roberts, N. P. (2015). Post-traumatic stress disorder. *BMJ (Clinical Research Ed.), h6161*, h6161. DOI: 10.1136/bmj.h6161 PMID: 26611143

Bisson, J. I., & Sakhuja, D. (2006). Adjustment disorders. *Psychiatry (Abingdon), 5*(7), 240–242. DOI: 10.1053/j.mppsy.2006.04.004

Black, A., Valerio, M., & Blasdell, R. (2023). United States Violence Against Women Act (VAWA). In Shackelford, T. K. (Ed.), *Encyclopedia of Domestic Violence* (pp. 1–10). Springer International Publishing., DOI: 10.1007/978-3-030-85493-5_1684-1

Blackmore, R., Gray, K. M., Boyle, J. A., Fazel, M., Ranasinha, S., Fitzgerald, G., Misso, M., & Gibson-Helm, M. (2020). Systematic Review and Meta-analysis: The Prevalence of Mental Illness in Child and Adolescent Refugees and Asylum Seekers. *Journal of the American Academy of Child and Adolescent Psychiatry, 59*(6), 705–714. DOI: 10.1016/j.jaac.2019.11.011 PMID: 31778780

Blaney, N., Randour, M. L., & Blink, C. (2020). Advances in understanding and addressing the link between pet abuse and intimate partner violence. In Geffner, R., White, J. W., Hamberger, L. K., Rosenbaum, A., Vaughan-Eden, V., & Vieth, V. I. (Eds.), *Handbook of Interpersonal Violence and Abuse Across the Lifespan* (pp. 1–22). Springer International Publishing., DOI: 10.1007/978-3-319-62122-7_286-1

Blevins, C. A., Weathers, F. W., Davis, M. T., Witte, T. K., & Domino, J. L. (2015). The posttraumatic stress disorder checklist for DSM-5 (PCL-5): Development and initial psychometric evaluation. *Journal of Traumatic Stress, 28*(6), 489–498. DOI: 10.1002/jts.22059 PMID: 26606250

Bø, B. (2015). Social work in a multicultural society: New challenges and needs for competence. *International Social Work, 58*(4), 562–574. DOI: 10.1177/0020872814550114

Bod, E. (2022). *The evolution of the American Dream*. The Collector. https://www.thecollector.com/american-dream-evolution/

Boehm, D. A. (2008). "For my children": Constructing family and navigating the state in the U.S.-Mexico transnation. *Anthropological Quarterly*, *81*(4), 777–802. DOI: 10.1353/anq.0.0037

Bojórquez-Chapela, I., Leyva-Flores, R., Gómez-López, D., Vázquez, E. K., & Cortés-Alcalá, R. (2024). Forced migration and psychological distress among migrants in transit through Mexico. *Salud Pública de México*, *66*(2), 173–181. DOI: 10.21149/14829 PMID: 39977042

Bolter, J. (2022). *Immigration Has Been a Defining, Often Contentious, Element Throughout U.S. History*. Migration Policy. https://www.migrationpolicy.org/article/immigration-shaped-united-states-history

Bonacich, E., & Appelbaum, R. P. (2000). *Behind the label: Inequality in the Los Angeles apparel industry*. University of California Press. DOI: 10.1525/9780520925595

Bond, M., & Lai, T.-M. (2001). Embarrassment and code-switching into a second language. *The Journal of Social Psychology*, *126*(2), 179–186. DOI: 10.1080/19401183.1986.12461512

Brabeck, K. M., Sibley, E., & Lykes, M. B. (2016). Authorized and unauthorized immigrant parents: The impact of legal vulnerability on family contexts. *Hispanic Journal of Behavioral Sciences*, *38*(1), 3–30. DOI: 10.1177/0739986315621741

Brach, C., & Fraser, I. (2002). Reducing disparities through culturally competent health care: An analysis of the business case. *Quality Management in Health Care*, *10*(4), 15–28. DOI: 10.1097/00019514-200210040-00005 PMID: 12938253

Breiding, M. J., Basile, K. C., Smith, S. G., Black, M. C., & Mahendra, R. R. (2015). *Intimate partner violence surveillance: Uniform definitions and recommended data elements* (version 2.0). National Center for Injury Prevention and Control, Centers for Disease Control and Prevention. https://www.cdc.gov/violenceprevention/pdf/ipv/intimatepartnerviolence.pdf

Breiding, M. J., Black, M. C., & Ryan, G. W. (2008). Chronic disease and health risk behaviors associated with intimate partner violence—18 U.S. States/Territories, 2005. *Annals of Epidemiology*, *18*(7), 538–544. DOI: 10.1016/j.annepidem.2008.02.005 PMID: 18495490

Breslau, J. (2011). Migration From Mexico to the United States and Conduct Disorder: A Cross-national Study. *Archives of General Psychiatry*, *68*(12), 1284. DOI: 10.1001/archgenpsychiatry.2011.140 PMID: 22147845

Breslau, J., Borges, G., Hagar, Y., Tancredi, D., & Gilman, S. (2009). Immigration to the USA and risk for mood and anxiety disorders: Variation by origin and age at immigration. *Psychological Medicine*, *39*(07), 1117. DOI: 10.1017/S0033291708004698 PMID: 19000338

Briere, J. (2010). *Trauma symptom inventory* (2nd ed.). Psychological Assessment Resources., TSI-2. DOI: 10.1002/9780470479216.corpsy1010

Briere, J., & Scott, C. (2015). *Principles of trauma therapy: A guide to symptoms, evaluation, and treatment* (2nd ed.). Sage Publications.

Bureau of Justice Statistics. (2021). *The National Crime Victimization Survey and Uniform Crime Reporting program: A complementary picture of crime in 2020.* https://bjs.ojp.gov/sites/g/files/xyckuh236/files/media/document/cv20_ncvs_ucr_supplement.pdf

Bustamante, L. H. U., Cerqueira, R. O., Leclerc, E., & Brietzke, E. (2017). Stress, trauma, and posttraumatic stress disorder in migrants: A comprehensive review. *Revista Brasileira de Psiquiatria : Orgão Oficial da Associação Brasileira de Psiquiatria, Asociación Psiqui´trica de la América Latina*, *40*(2), 220–225. DOI: 10.1590/1516-4446-2017-2290 PMID: 29069252

Caballero, T. M., Ross DeCamp, L., Platt, R. E., Shah, H., Johnson, S. B., Sibinga, E. M. S., & Polk, S. (2017). Addressing the mental health needs of Latino children in immigrant families. *Clinical Pediatrics*, *56*(7), 648–658. https://doi-org.libproxy.calbaptist.edu/10.1177/0009922816679509. DOI: 10.1177/0009922816679509 PMID: 27879297

Cabassa, L. J., Molina, G. B., & Baron, M. (2012). Depression Fotonovela: Development of a depression literacy tool for Latinos with limited English proficiency. *Health Promotion Practice*, *13*(6), 747–754. DOI: 10.1177/1524839910367578 PMID: 21051325

Campbell, J. C. (2002). Health consequences of intimate partner violence. *Lancet*, *359*(9314), 1331–1336. DOI: 10.1016/S0140-6736(02)08336-8 PMID: 11965295

Cantle, T. (2001). *Community Cohesion: A Report of the Independent Review Team*. Home Office.

Caputo, T. (2024). Mob of teens on bikes in DTLA brutally attacks, robs man seeking asylum in U.S. ABC 7 Eyewitness News. Retrieved from https://abc7.com/post/mob-teens-bikes-downtown-los-angeles-brutally-attacks-robs-immigrant-seeking-asylum-us/15175704/

Carlson, E. B., Palmieri, P. A., Field, N. P., Dalenberg, C. J., Macia, K. S., & Spain, D. A. (2016). Contributions of risk and protective factors to prediction of psychological symptoms after traumatic experiences. *Comprehensive Psychiatry*, *69*, 106–115. DOI: 10.1016/j.comppsych.2016.04.022 PMID: 27423351

Carlson, W. C. (2023). Implementation challenges of T Visa eligibility for human trafficking survivors: A role for social work. *Social Work*, *68*(3), 222–229. DOI: 10.1093/sw/swad017 PMID: 37164622

Carter, G. L., Willcox, C. H., Lewin, T. J., Conrad, A. M., & Bendit, N. (2010). Hunter DBT project: Randomized controlled trial of dialectical behaviour therapy in women with borderline personality disorder. *The Australian and New Zealand Journal of Psychiatry*, *44*(2), 162–173. DOI: 10.3109/00048670903393621 PMID: 20113305

Carter, R. T., Mazzula, S., Victoria, R., Vazquez, R., Hall, S., Smith, S., Sant-Barket, S., Forsyth, J., Bazelais, K., & Williams, B. (2013). Initial development of the Race-Based Traumatic Stress Symptom Scale: Assessing the emotional impact of racism. *Psychological Trauma: Theory, Research, Practice, and Policy*, *5*(1), 1–9. DOI: 10.1037/a0025911

Castañeda, E. (2018a, July 11). How cities help immigrants feel at home: 4 charts. *The Conversation.*

Castañeda, E. (2018b). *A place to call home: Immigrant exclusion and urban belonging in New York, Paris, and Barcelona.* Stanford University Press.

Castelli, F. (2018). Drivers of migration: Why do people move? *Journal of Travel Medicine*, *25*(1). Advance online publication. DOI: 10.1093/jtm/tay040 PMID: 30053084

Castro, F. G., Berkel, C., & Epstein, D. R. (2023). Cultural adaptations and cultural factors in EBI implementation with Latinx communities. *Frontiers in Public Health*, *11*, 1007328. DOI: 10.3389/fpubh.2023.1007328 PMID: 37026135

CDC. (2024, October 17). About intimate partner violence. Https://www.cdc.gov/intimate-partner-violence/about/index.html?CDC_AAref_Val=https://www.cdc.gov/violenceprevention/intimatepartnerviolence/index.html

Chatzifotiou, S., & Papouli, E. (2022). Social Workers Dealing with Ethical Dilemmas in the Course of Their Professional Work: The Greek Experience. *British Journal of Social Work*, *52*(8), 4795–4814. DOI: 10.1093/bjsw/bcac084

Child Abuse | Overview | Office of Justice Programs. (n.d.). Retrieved October 26, 2024, from https://www.ojp.gov/feature/child-abuse/overview

Child Welfare Information Gateway. (2015). Promoting protective factors for victims of child abuse and neglect: A guide for practitioners. Retrieved from https://www.Childwelfare.gov/pubs/factsheets/victimscan/

Child Welfare Information Gateway. (2019). Long-term consequences of child abuse and neglect. Washington, DC: U.S. Department of Health and Human Services, Administration for Children and Families, Children's Bureau. Retrieved from https://cwig-prod-prod-drupal-s3fs-us-east-1.s3.amazonaws.com/public/documents/long_term_consequences.pdf

Children on the Run—Full Report. (n.d.). UNHCR US. Retrieved October 23, 2024, from https://www.unhcr.org/us/media/children-run-full-report

Chong, A., & Chong, M. Z. (2023). Feeling the heat? Fear of failure and performance. *Kyklos*, *76*(1), 3–17. DOI: 10.1111/kykl.12316

Choshen, H. S., Ishqer, A., Mahameed, F., Reiter, J., Gozal, D., Gileles, H. A., & Berger, I. (2021). Acute and chronic sleep deprivation in residents: Cognition and stress biomarkers. *Medical Education*, *55*(2), 174–184. DOI: 10.1111/medu.14296 PMID: 32697336

Christensen, M. C., Florea, I., Loft, H., & McIntyre, R. S. (2020). Efficacy of vortioxetine in patients with major depressive disorder reporting childhood or recent trauma. *Journal of Affective Disorders*, *263*, 258–266. DOI: 10.1016/j.jad.2019.11.074 PMID: 31818787

Christy, S. M., Cousin, L. A., Sutton, S. K., Chavarria, E. A., Abdulla, R., Gutierrez, L., Sanchez, J., Lopez, D., Gwede, C. K., & Meade, C. D. (2021). Characterizing Health Literacy Among Spanish Language-Preferring Latinos Ages 50-75. *Nursing Research*, *70*(5), 344–353. DOI: 10.1097/NNR.0000000000000519 PMID: 33990120

Churchwell, S. (2021). *A brief history of the American Dream*. Bush Presidential Center., Retrieved from https://www.bushcenter.org/catalyst/state-of-the-american-dream/churchwell-history-of-the-american-dream

Chu, T., Keller, A. S., & Rasmussen, A. (2013). Effects of Post-migration Factors on PTSD Outcomes Among Immigrant Survivors of Political Violence. *Journal of Immigrant and Minority Health*, *15*(5), 890–897. DOI: 10.1007/s10903-012-9696-1 PMID: 22976794

Cipta, D. A., Andoko, D., Theja, A., Utama, A. V. E., Hendrik, H., William, D. G., Reina, N., Handoko, M. T., & Lumbuun, N. (2024). Culturally sensitive patient-centered healthcare: A focus on health behavior modification in low and middle-income nations-insights from Indonesia. *Frontiers in Medicine, 11*, 1353037. DOI: 10.3389/fmed.2024.1353037 PMID: 38681051

Clum, G. A., & Whitman, J. C. (1991). Psychological impact of abuse: A review of the literature. *Journal of Interpersonal Violence*, *6*(4), 383–396. DOI: 10.1177/088626091006004002

Coffman, M. J., & Norton, C. K. (2010). Demands of Immigration, Health Literacy, and Depression in Recent Latino Immigrants. *Home Health Care Management & Practice*, *22*(2), 116–122. DOI: 10.1177/1084822309347343

Cohen, S. R. (2013). Advocacy for the "Abandonados": Harnessing cultural beliefs for Latino families and their children with intellectual disabilities. *Journal of Policy and Practice in Intellectual Disabilities*, *10*(1), 71–78. DOI: 10.1111/jppi.12021

Cohodes, E. M., Kribakaran, S., Odriozola, P., Bakirci, S., McCauley, S., Hodges, H. R., Sisk, L. M., Zacharek, S. J., & Gee, D. G. (2021). Migration-related trauma and mental health among migrant children emigrating from Mexico and Central America to the United States: Effects on developmental neurobiology and implications for policy. *Developmental Psychobiology*, *63*(6), e22158. DOI: 10.1002/dev.22158 PMID: 34292596

Comas-Díaz, Lillian, Gordon Nagayama Hall, and Helen A. Neville. "Racial trauma: Theory, research, and healing: Introduction to the special issue." *American Psychologist* 74.1 (2019): 1.

Connor, P., & Budiman, A. (2019). *Immigrants share in the U.S. nears record high but remains below that of many other countries.* Pew Research Center. https://www.pewresearch.org/short-reads/2019/01/30/immigrant-share-in-u-s-nears-record-high-but-remains-below-that-of-many-other-countries/

Constable, N. (2014). *Born out of place: Migrant mothers and the politics of international labor*. University of California Press.

Cornelius, W. A. (2007). Introduction: Does border enforcement deter unauthorized immigration? In Cornelius, W. A., & Lewis, J. M. (Eds.), *Impacts of border enforcement on Mexican migration: The view from sending communities* (pp. 1–16). Center for Comparative Immigration Studies, University of California.

Costa, J. R. A. D., Lima, J. V. D., & Almeida, P. C. D. (2003). Stress no trabalho do enfermeiro. *Revista da Escola de Enfermagem da USP, 37*(3), 63–71. DOI: 10.1590/S0080-62342003000300008 PMID: 14686049

Counts, D. A., Brown, J. K., & Campbell, J. (Eds.). (1999). *To have and to hit: Cultural perspectives on wife beating*. University of Illinois Press.

Craig, G. (2008). *The Limits of Compromise. G. Craig, T. Burchardt, & D. Gordon içinde, Social Justice and Public Policy*. Policy Press.

Craig, G., & Levis, H. (2014). *Multiculturalism or assimilation and social exclusion Ethnic minorities in the United Kingdom. F. Mansouri, & P. Muraca içinde, Global Perspectives on the Politics of Multiculturalism in the 21st Century*. Routledge.

Cravey, A. J. (1998). *Women and work in Mexico's maquiladoras*. Rowman & Littlefield Publishers.

Crawford, M. (2020). Ecological Systems Theory: Exploring the Development of the Theoretical Framework as Conceived by Bronfenbrenner Article Details. *Journal of Public Health Issues and Practices, 4*(2), 170. DOI: 10.33790/jphip1100170

Crime Data Explorer. (2022a). https://cde.ucr.cjis.gov/LATEST/webapp/#/pages/explorer/crime/hate-crime

Crime Data Explorer. (2022b). https://cde.ucr.cjis.gov/LATEST/webapp/#/pages/explorer/crime/crime-trend

Crime Data Explorer. (2023a). https://cde.ucr.cjis.gov/LATEST/webapp/#/pages/explorer/crime/hate-crime

Crime Data Explorer. (2023b). https://cde.ucr.cjis.gov/LATEST/webapp/#/pages/explorer/crime/crime-trend

Crime Data Explorer. (2024a). https://cde.ucr.cjis.gov/LATEST/webapp/#/pages/explorer/crime/hate-crime

Crime Data Explorer. (2024b). https://cde.ucr.cjis.gov/LATEST/webapp/#/pages/explorer/crime/crime-trend

Cross, F. L., Agi, A., Montoro, J. P., Medina, M. A., Miller-Tejada, S., Pinetta, B. J., Tran-Dubongco, M., & Rivas-Drake, D. (2020). Illuminating ethnic-racial socialization among undocumented Lat- inx parents and its implications for adolescent psychosocial functioning. *Developmental Psychology, 56*(8), 1458–1474. DOI: 10.1037/dev0000826 PMID: 32790445

Crouch, J. L., Hanson, R. F., Saunders, B. E., Kilpatrick, D. G., & Resnick, H. S. (2000). Income, race/ethnicity, and exposure to violence in youth: Results from the national survey of adolescents. *Journal of Community Psychology*, *28*(6), 625–641. DOI: 10.1002/1520-6629(200011)28:6<625::AID-JCOP6>3.0.CO;2-R

Danis, F. S. (2003). The criminalization of domestic violence: What social workers need to know. *Social Work*, *48*(2), 237–246. DOI: 10.1093/sw/48.2.237 PMID: 12718419

Danso, R. (2018). Cultural competence and cultural humility: A critical reflection on key cultural diversity concepts. ournal of Social Work, 410-430.

Davis, R. E., Johnson, T. P., Lee, S., & Werner, C. (2018). Why Do Latino Survey Respondents Acquiesce? Respondent and Interviewer Characteristics as Determinants of Cultural Patterns of Acquiescence Among Latino Survey Respondents. *Cross-Cultural Research, 53*(1), 87-115. (Original work published 2019)DOI: 10.1177/1069397118774504

Davis, R. E., Resnicow, K., & Couper, M. P. (2011). Survey Response Styles, Acculturation, and Culture Among a Sample of Mexican American Adults. *Journal of Cross-Cultural Psychology*, *42*(7), 1219–1236. DOI: 10.1177/0022022110383317 PMID: 21927503

De Arellano, M. A., Andrews, A. R., Reid-Quiñones, K., Vasquez, D., Doherty, L. S., Danielson, C. K., & Rheingold, A. (2018). Immigration trauma among Hispanic youth: Missed by trauma assessments and predictive of depression and PTSD symptoms. *Journal of Latina/o Psychology*, *6*(3), 159–174. DOI: 10.1037/lat0000090 PMID: 31840010

De Genova, N., & Peutz, N. (2010). The deportation regime: Introduction. In De Genova, N., & Peutz, N. (Eds.), *The deportation regime: Sovereignty, space, and the freedom of movement* (pp. 1–29). Duke University Press.

De León, J. (2012). Better to be hot than caught: Excavating the conflicting roles of migrant material culture. *American Anthropologist*, *114*(3), 477–495. DOI: 10.1111/j.1548-1433.2012.01447.x

Decker, S. H. (2015). Human trafficking: Contexts and connections to conventional crime. *Journal of Crime and Justice*, *38*(3), 291–296. DOI: 10.1080/0735648X.2015.1039792

Delgado-Romero, E. A., De Los Santos, J., Raman, V. S., Merrifield, J. N., Vazquez, M. S., Monroig, M. M., Bautista, E. C., & Durán, M. Y. (2018). Caught in the Middle: Spanish-Speaking Bilingual Mental Health Counselors as Language Brokers. *Journal of Mental Health Counseling*, *40*(4), 341–352. DOI: 10.17744/mehc.40.4.06

Delgado-Romero, E. A., De Los Santos, J., Raman, V. S., Merrifield, J. N., Vazquez, M. S., Monroig, M. M., & Durán, M. Y. (2018). Caught in the middle: Spanish-speaking bilingual mental health counselors as language brokers. *Journal of Mental Health Counseling*, *40*(4), 341–352.

Denman, C. A. (1997). Health in the maquilas: Questions for investigation. *Nueva Antropologia*, *16*(52–53), 167–185.

Derr, A. S. (2016). Mental Health Service Use Among Immigrants in the United States: A Systematic Review. *Psychiatric Services (Washington, D.C.)*, *67*(3), 265–274. DOI: 10.1176/appi.ps.201500004 PMID: 26695493

Dettlaff, A. J., & Earner, I. (2012). Children of Immigrants in the Child Welfare System: Characteristics, Risk, and Maltreatment. *Families in Society*, *93*(4), 295–303. DOI: 10.1606/1044-3894.4240

DHS. (n.d.) *Office of Homeland Security Statistics: Glossary*. U.S. Department of Homeland Security. Retrieved from https://ohss.dhs.gov/glossary#:~:text=Immigrant%3A%20Any%20person%20lawfully%20in,101(a)(15)

Di Nota, P. M., Anderson, G. S., Ricciardelli, R., Carleton, R. N., & Groll, D. (2020). Mental disorders, suicidal ideation, plans and attempts among Canadian police. *Occupational Medicine*, *70*(3), 183–190. DOI: 10.1093/occmed/kqaa026 PMID: 32154872

Dietrich, S., & Hernandez, E. (2022). *Nearly 68 Million People Spoke a Language Other Than English at Home in 2019*. U.S. Census Bureau. https://www.census.gov/library/stories/2022/12/languages-we-speak-in-united-states.html

Dimeff, L. A., McMain, S., Sayrs, J. H., Wilks, C. R., & Linehan, M. M. (2020). DBT for individuals with borderline personality disorder and substance use disorders. *Dialectical Behavior Therapy in Clinical Practice*, 233.

Disney, L., & Carnes, S. (2022). But Culturally Competent for Whom? Ethics and CrossCultural Dilemmas in COVID-Era Social Work . International Journal of Social Work Values and Ethics, 209-226.

Dobash, R. E., & Dobash, R. P. (2003). *Women, Violence and Social Change*. Routledge. https://books.google.com/books?id=NWOIAgAAQBAJ

Domenech Rodríguez, M. M., & Bernal, G. (2012). Frameworks, models, and guidelines for cultural adaptation. In Bernal, G., & Rodríguez, M. M. D. (Eds.), *Cultural Adaptations: Tools for Evidence-Based Practice With Diverse Populations* (pp. 23–44). American Psychological Association., https://www.jstor.org/stable/j.ctv1chrt50.7 DOI: 10.1037/13752-002

Dominelli, L. (2002). *Anti Oppressive Social Work Theory and Practice*. Palgrave Macmillan. DOI: 10.1007/978-1-4039-1400-2

Donahue, M. (2018). *UNDERSTANDING EXTREME HARDSHIP IN WAIVERS | JANUARY 2018*.

Dreier, H., & Luce, K. (2023). Alone and exploited, migrant children work brutal jobs across the US. The New York Times, 28.

Duleep, H. O., & Dowhan, D. J. (2008). Research on Immigrant Earnings. Social Security Administration. *Social Security Bulletin*, *68*(1). https://www.ssa.gov/policy/docs/ssb/v68n1/v68n1p31.html

Dunlap, J. L., Jaramillo, J. D., Koppolu, R., Wright, R., Mendoza, F., & Bruzoni, M. (2015). The effects of language concordant care on patient satisfaction and clinical understanding for Spanish pediatric surgery patients. *Journal of Pediatric Surgery*, *50*(9), 1586–1589. DOI: 10.1016/j.jpedsurg.2014.12.020 PMID: 25783324

Dutton, M. A., & Goodman, L. A. (2005). Coercion in intimate partner violence: Toward a new conceptualization. *Sex Roles*, *52*(11–12), 743–756. DOI: 10.1007/s11199-005-4196-6

Eamranond, P. P., Davis, R., Phillips, R. S., & Wee, C. C. (2011). Patient-physician Language Concordance and Primary Care Screening Among Spanish-speaking Patients. *Medical Care*, *49*(7), 668–672. DOI: 10.1097/MLR.0b013e318215d803 PMID: 21478772

Edwards, J. (2016). Cultural Intelligence for Clinical Social Work Practice. *Clinical Social Work Journal*, *44*(3), 211–220. DOI: 10.1007/s10615-015-0543-4

Elmore, A. L., & Crouch, E. (2020). The Association of Adverse Childhood Experiences With Anxiety and Depression for Children and Youth, 8 to 17 Years of Age. *Academic Pediatrics*, *20*(5), 600–608. DOI: 10.1016/j.acap.2020.02.012 PMID: 32092442

Eno Louden, J., Avila, A., del Villar, O. A. E., Jung, H., Kosyluk, K. A., & Flores, E. (2023). Self-stigma of mental illness among Latino people on the U.S.-México border. *Stigma and Health*, *8*(1), 21–30. DOI: 10.1037/sah0000365

Erez, E., Adelman, M., & Gregory, C. (2009). Intersections of immigration and domestic violence: Voices of battered immigrant women. *Feminist Criminology*, *4*(1), 32–56. DOI: 10.1177/1557085108325413

Escobedo, L. E., Cervantes, L., & Havranek, E. (2023). Barriers in Healthcare for Latinx Patients with Limited English Proficiency: A Narrative Review. *Journal of General Internal Medicine*, *38*(5), 1264–1271. DOI: 10.1007/s11606-022-07995-3 PMID: 36720766

Eshun, S., & Gurung, R. A. (Eds.). (2009). *Culture and mental health: Sociocultural influences, theory, and practice*. John Wiley & Sons. DOI: 10.1002/9781444305807

Essayagh, F., Essayagh, M., Essayagh, S., Marc, I., Bukassa, G., El Otmani, I., Kouyate, M. F., & Essayagh, T. (2023). The prevalence and risk factors for anxiety and depression symptoms among migrants in Morocco. *Scientific Reports*, *13*(1), 3740. DOI: 10.1038/s41598-023-30715-8 PMID: 36878989

Euser, E. M., van IJzendoorn, M. H., Prinzie, P., & Bakermans-Kranenburg, M. J. (2011). Elevated Child Maltreatment Rates in Immigrant Families and the Role of Socioeconomic Differences. *Child Maltreatment*, *16*(1), 63–73. DOI: 10.1177/1077559510385842 PMID: 21041234

Evans, B., & Hass, G. (2018). *Forensic psychological assessment in immigration court: A guidebook for evidence-based and ethical practice*. Routledge., DOI: 10.4324/9781315621197

Ewing, W., Martinez, D., & Rumbaut, R. (2015). *The criminalization of immigration in the United States*. American Immigration Council. Retrieved from https://www.americanimmigrationcouncil.org/research/criminalization-immigration-united-states

Fang, M. L., Sixsmith, J., Sinclair, S., & Horst, G. (2016). A knowledge synthesis of culturally- and spiritually-sensitive end-of-life care: Findings from a scoping review. *BMC Geriatrics*, *16*(1), 107. DOI: 10.1186/s12877-016-0282-6 PMID: 27193395

Fan, X., Henderson, D. C., Nguyen, D. D., Cather, C., Freudenreich, O., Evins, A. E., Borba, C. P., & Goff, D. C. (2008). Posttraumatic stress disorder, cognitive function and quality of life in patients with schizophrenia. *Psychiatry Research*, *159*(1–2), 140–146. DOI: 10.1016/j.psychres.2007.10.012 PMID: 18423611

Farmer, P., Kleinman, A., Kim, J. Y., & Basilico, M. (Eds.). (2013). *Reimagining global health: An introduction*. University of California Press.

FBI. (2016). *Hate crimes*. Retrieved from https://www.fbi.gov/investigate/civil-rights/hate-crimes

FBI. (2017). *Domestic violence*. Retrieved from https://ucr.fbi.gov/leoka/2017/resource-pages/leoka_definitions_-2017#:~:text=Domestic%20violence%E2%80%93The%20use%2C%20attempted,who%20is%20or%20has%20been

FBI. (2019). *Human trafficking*. https://ucr.fbi.gov/crime-in-the-u.s/2019/crime-in-the-u.s.-2019/additional-data-collections/human-trafficking

FBI. (2022). *Hate Crime Explorer*. https://cde.ucr.cjis.gov/LATEST/webapp/#/pages/explorer/crime/hate-crime

FBI. (2023). *Hate Crime Explorer*. https://cde.ucr.cjis.gov/LATEST/webapp/#/pages/explorer/crime/hate-crime

FBI. (2024). *Hate Crime Explorer*. https://cde.ucr.cjis.gov/LATEST/webapp/#/pages/explorer/crime/hate-crime

Feliz, W. (2019). *Sorry Donald Trump, immigration is still associated with less crime and safer communities*. Immigration Impact. Retrieved from https://immigrationimpact.com/2016/04/29/donald-trump-immigration-crime-facts/?gad_source=1&gclid=Cj0KCQjwhb60BhClARIsABGGtw_Hl3LsVQYU1_osri_DKeIiLAPa7kYHfSXU2KRnQn_s631uXVMGtEQaAg0kEALw_wcB#.XlKNAmhKiM8

FEMA. (n.d.) Five ways we can work together to prevent human trafficking. Retrieved from https://www.fema.gov/blog/5-ways-we-can-work-together-prevent-human-trafficking

Fernández, M. (2018). Hanging out together, surviving on your own: The precarious communities of day laborers. *Journal of Contemporary Ethnography*, *47*(6), 865–887. DOI: 10.1177/0891241617716743

Ferrari, M., Ahmad, F., Shakya, Y., Ledwos, C., & McKenzie, K. (2016). Computer-assisted client assessment survey for mental health: Patient and health provider perspectives. *BMC Health Services Research*, *16*(1), 516. DOI: 10.1186/s12913-016-1756-0 PMID: 27663508

Finkelhor, D., Turner, H. A., Shattuck, A., & Hamby, S. L. (2015). Prevalence of Childhood Exposure to Violence, Crime, and Abuse: Results from the National Survey of Children's Exposure to Violence. *JAMA Pediatrics*, *169*(8), 746–754. DOI: 10.1001/jamapediatrics.2015.0676 PMID: 26121291

Finley, L., & Esposito, L. (2020). The immigrant as bogeyman: Examining Donald Trump and the right's anti-immigrant, anti-PC rhetoric. *Humanity & Society*, *44*(2), 178–197. DOI: 10.1177/0160597619832627

Finno-Velasquez, M., Sepp, S. M., Lopez, A., Aquino, E., Cherie, N., & Ortiz-Upston, M. (2023). Child maltreatment prevention interventions for Latinx immigrant populations: A systematic review. Journal of Public Child Welfare, 17(4), 845-878. https://doi.org/<link linkTarget="URL" linkWindow=""DOI: 10.1080/15548732.2022.2118929

Fletcher, M. J. (2024). *Unveiling the shadows: Human trafficking amidst immigration struggles in 2024*. BWJP. Retrieved from https://bwjp.org/unveiling-the-shadows-human-trafficking-amidst-immigration-struggles-in-2024/?gad_source=1&gclid=Cj0KCQjws560BhCuARIsAHMqE0F5PX51xaP8QO1LxAZlvK339_3zmuyO31BpwEEWJFytO5jJzvg7KIUaAoJjEALw_wcB

Flory, J. D., & Yehuda, R. (2015). Comorbidity between post-traumatic stress disorder and major depressive disorder: Alternative explanations and treatment considerations. *Dialogues in Clinical Neuroscience*, *17*(2), 141–150. DOI: 10.31887/DCNS.2015.17.2/jflory PMID: 26246789

Foa, E. B., Cashman, L., Jaycox, L., & Perry, K. (1995). Posttraumatic diagnostic scale. *Assessment of partner violence: A handbook for researchers and practitioners.*

Fogelman, N., Magin, Z., Hart, R., & Sinha, R. (2020). A longitudinal study of life trauma, chronic stress, and body mass index on weight gain over a 2-year period. *Behavioral Medicine (Washington, D.C.)*, *48*(3), 162–170. DOI: 10.1080/08964289.2020.1780192 PMID: 32552603

Foner, N. (2005). *In a new land: A comparative view of immigration*. New York University Press.

Fong, R. (2004). *Overview of Immigrant and Refugee Children and Families. R. Fong içinde, Culturally competent practice with immigrant and refugee children and families*. The Guilford Press.

Fook, J. (2002). *Social Work: Critical Theory and Practice*. Sage Publications.

Foo, S. Q., Tam, W. W., Ho, C. S., Tran, B. X., Nguyen, L. H., McIntyre, R. S., & Ho, R. C. (2018). Prevalence of Depression among Migrants: A Systematic Review and Meta-Analysis. *International Journal of Environmental Research and Public Health*, *15*(9), 1986. DOI: 10.3390/ijerph15091986 PMID: 30213071

Forcén, F. E., Vélez Flórez, M. C., Bido Medina, R., Zambrano, J., Pérez, J. H., Rodríguez, A. M., & Santos, L. H. (2023). Deconstructing Cultural Aspects of Mental Health Care in Hispanic/Latinx People. *Psychiatric Annals*, *53*(3), 127–132. DOI: 10.3928/00485713-20230215-02 PMID: 37781171

Freimuth, V. S., & Quinn, S. C. (2004). The contributions of health communication to eliminating health disparities. *American Journal of Public Health*, *94*(12), 2053–2055. DOI: 10.2105/AJPH.94.12.2053 PMID: 15569949

Funk, C., & Lopez, M. H. (2022). *A brief statistical portrait of U.S. Hispanics.* Pew Research Center. https://www.pewresearch.org/science/2022/06/14/a-brief-statistical-portrait-of-u-s-hispanics/

Gadon, M., Balch, G. I., & Jacobs, E. A. (2007). Caring for patients with limited English proficiency: The perspectives of small group practitioners. *Journal of General Internal Medicine*, *22*(S2, Suppl 2), 341–346. DOI: 10.1007/s11606-007-0311-4 PMID: 17957422

Galemba, R., & Kuhn, R. (2021). "No place for old men": Immigrant duration, wage theft, and economic mobility among day laborers in Denver, Colorado. *The International Migration Review*, *55*(4), 1201–1230. DOI: 10.1177/01979183211001370 PMID: 36518637

Gallegos, A. M., Trabold, N., Cerulli, C., & Pigeon, W. R. (2021). Sleep and interpersonal violence: A systematic review. *Trauma, Violence & Abuse*, *22*(2), 359–369. DOI: 10.1177/1524838019852633 PMID: 31131736

Galvan, F. H., Wohl, A. R., Carlos, J.-A., & Chen, Y.-T. (2015). Chronic stress among Latino day laborers. *Hispanic Journal of Behavioral Sciences*, *37*(1), 75–89. DOI: 10.1177/0739986314568782

Gamez, A. M. (2024). *Overcoming Adversity*. Self-Publishing.

García-Sierra, R., Fernández-Cano, M. I., Manresa-Domínguez, J. M., Feijoo-Cid, M., Moreno Gabriel, E., Arreciado Marañón, A., Ramos-Roure, F., Segura-Bernal, J., & Torán-Monserrat, P. (2020). Psychological Distress and Somatization in Immigrants in Primary Health Care Practices. *Health Care*, *8*(4), 557. DOI: 10.3390/healthcare8040557 PMID: 33322209

Garcini, L. M., Daly, R., Chen, N., Mehl, J., Pham, T., Phan, T., Hansen, B., & Kothare, A. (2021). Undocumented immigrants and mental health: A systematic review of recent methodology and findings in the United States. *Journal of Migration and Health*, *4*, 100058. DOI: 10.1016/j.jmh.2021.100058 PMID: 34405198

Garcini, L. M., Domenech Rodríguez, M. M., Mercado, A., Silva, M., Cadenas, G., Galvan, T., & Paris, M. (2023). Anti-immigration policy and mental health: Risk of distress and trauma among deferred action for childhood arrivals recipients in the United States. *Psychological Trauma: Theory, Research, Practice, and Policy*, *15*(7), 1067–1075. DOI: 10.1037/tra0001228 PMID: 35482682

Gearing, R. E., Washburn, M., Brewer, K. B., Cabrera, A., Yu, M., & Torres, L. R. (2024). Pathways to mental health care: Latinos' help-seeking preferences. *Journal of Latina/o Psychology*, *12*(1), 1–17. DOI: 10.1037/lat0000237

Glick Schiller, N. (2003). The centrality of ethnography in the study of transnational migration: Seeing the wetlands instead of the swamp. In Foner, N. (Ed.), *American arrivals: Anthropology engages the new immigration* (pp. 99–128). School of American Research Press.

Goddard, C., & Bedi, G. (2010). Intimate partner violence and child abuse: A child-centred perspective. *Child Abuse Review*, *19*(1), 5–20. DOI: 10.1002/car.1084

Golash-Boza, T. (2009). The immigration industrial complex: Why we enforce immigration policies destined to fail. *Sociology Compass*, *3*(2), 295–309. DOI: 10.1111/j.1751-9020.2008.00193.x

Goldberg, M. (2000). Conflicting Principles in Multicultural Social Work. *Families in Society*, *81*(1), 12–21. DOI: 10.1606/1044-3894.1088

Gonsalves, C. J. (1992). Psychological stages of the refugee process: A model for therapeutic interventions. *Professional Psychology, Research and Practice*, *23*(5), 382–389. DOI: 10.1037/0735-7028.23.5.382

Gonzalez-Barrera, A. (2021). *Before COVID-19, more Mexicans came to the U.S. than left for Mexico for the first time in years.* Pew Research Center. https://www.pewresearch.org/short-reads/2021/07/09/before-covid-19-more-mexicans-came-to-the-u-s-than-left-for-mexico-for-the-first-time-in-years/

Gonzalez-Barrera, A., & Lopez, M. H. (2013). *Spanish is the most spoken non-English language in U.S. homes, even among non-Hispanics.* Pew Research Center. https://www.pewresearch.org/short-reads/2013/08/13/spanish-is-the-most-spoken-non-english-language-in-u-s-homes-even-among-non-hispanics/

Gonzalez-Barrera, A., Hamel, L., Artiga, S., & Presiado, M. (2024). *Language barriers in health care: findings from the KFF survey on racism, discrimination, and health.* KFF. https://www.kff.org/racial-equity-and-health-policy/poll-finding/language-barriers-in-health-care-findings-from-the-kff-survey-on-racism-discrimination-and-health/

Goodman-Bowling, J. (2018). *Labor, limits, and liberty: A study of day laborers at a grassroots collective in Southern California.* [Doctoral dissertation, University of Nevada, Reno]. Scholarworks. http://hdl.handle.net/11714/4849

Goodman-Bowling, J. (2024). Negotiating culture and educational expectations for Latin American migrants: Addressing challenges for parents, students, and educators. In Gamez, A. (Ed.), *Parental influence on educational success and wellbeing* (pp. 149–167). IGI Global., DOI: 10.4018/979-8-3693-1451-7.ch009

Gramlich, J., & Passel, J. (2024, September 27). U.S. immigrant population in 2023 saw largest increase in more than 20 years. *Pew Research Center.* https://www.pewresearch.org/short-reads/2024/09/27/u-s-immigrant-population-in-2023-saw-largest-increase-in-more-than-20-years/

Gray, T. (2023). Teaching and learning amid demographic change: A thematic review of school responses to newcomer students in the new Latinx diaspora. *Journal of Latinos and Education, 22*(2), 745–766. DOI: 10.1080/15348431.2020.1819284

Green, B. L. (2007). The role of trauma in forensic psychology: An overview. *Journal of Forensic Psychology Practice, 7*(1), 1–15. DOI: 10.1300/J158v07n01_01

Grieb, S. M., Platt, R., Vazquez, M. G., Alvarez, K., & Polk, S. (2023). Mental Health Stigma Among Spanish-Speaking Latinos in Baltimore, Maryland. *Journal of Immigrant and Minority Health, 25*(5), 999–1007. DOI: 10.1007/s10903-023-01488-z PMID: 37213041

Grove, C. L., & Torbiörn, I. (1985). A new conceptualization of intercultural adjustment and the goals of training. *International Journal of Intercultural Relations, 9*(2), 205–233. DOI: 10.1016/0147-1767(85)90008-2

Grubbs, V., Chen, A. H., Bindman, A. B., Vittinghoff, E., & Fernandez, A. (2006). Effect of awareness of language law on language access in the health care setting. *Journal of General Internal Medicine, 21*(7), 683–688. DOI: 10.1111/j.1525-1497.2006.00492.x PMID: 16808766

Guardia, D., Salleron, J., Roelandt, J.-L., & Vaiva, G. (2017). Prévalence des troubles psychiatriques et addictologiques auprès de trois générations successives de migrants: Résultats d'une étude menée en population générale. *L'Encéphale, 43*(5), 435–443. DOI: 10.1016/j.encep.2016.06.008 PMID: 27644920

Gutiérrez, R. (2019). *Mexican Immigration to the United States.* Oxford Research Encyclopedia of American History. https://oxfordre.com/americanhistory/view/10.1093/acrefore/9780199329175.001.0001/acrefore-9780199329175-e-146

H.R. (1990). *1048 - 101st Congress (1989-1990).* Hate Crime Statistics Act.

Haldar, S., Pillai, D., & Artiga, S. (2023). *Overview of health coverage and care for individuals with limited English proficiency (LEP)*. KFF. https://www.kff.org/racial-equity-and-health-policy/issue-brief/overview-of-health-coverage-and-care-for-individuals-with-limited-english-proficiency/

Han, A., Laranjo, H., & Friedman, S. M. (2009). The design and pilot of a translation aid to help ED clinicians enhance communication with Portuguese-speaking patients. *International Journal of Emergency Medicine*, *2*(1), 41–46. DOI: 10.1007/s12245-008-0081-8 PMID: 19390916

Harned, M. S., Korslund, K. E., & Linehan, M. M. (2014). A pilot randomized controlled trial of Dialectical Behavior Therapy with and without the Dialectical Behavior Therapy Prolonged Exposure protocol for suicidal and self-injuring women with borderline personality disorder and PTSD. *Behaviour Research and Therapy*, *55*, 7–17. DOI: 10.1016/j.brat.2014.01.008 PMID: 24562087

Haro, A., Kuhn, R., Rodriguez, M. A., Theodore, N., Melendez, E., & Valenzuela, A.Jr. (2020). Beyond occupational hazards: Abuse of day laborers and health. *Journal of Immigrant and Minority Health*, *22*(6), 1172–1183. DOI: 10.1007/s10903-020-01094-3 PMID: 32989653

Harrison, G., & Turner, R. (2011). Being a ‘Culturally Competent’ Social Worker: Making Sense of a Murky Concept in Practice. *British Journal of Social Work*, *41*(2), 333–350. DOI: 10.1093/bjsw/bcq101

Hartmann, M. (2019, November). *Human trafficking and immigrants*. The Exodus Road. https://theexodusroad.com/human-trafficking-and-u-s-immigration/?utm_term=&utm_campaign=&utm_source=adwords&utm_medium=ppc&hsa_tgt=dsa-19959388920&hsa_grp=123537986530&hsa_src=g&hsa_net

Hass, G., Yang, E., Monahan, K., Orloff, L., & Anver, B. (2014). Barriers and successes in U visas for immigrant victims: The experiences of legal assistance for victims grantees. *Arts Social Sci J S*, *1*, 2.

Hays, R.D., Ngo-Metzger, Q., Sorkin, D.H., Telfair, J., Weidmer, B.A., Weech-Maldonado, R., & Hurtado, M.P. (2006). Cultural Competency and Quality of Care: Obtaining the Patient's Perspective.

Hays, P. A. (2022). *Addressing cultural complexities in psychotherapy and clinical practice: An intersectional approach* (4th ed.). American Psychological Association.

Heath, M., Hvass, A. M. F., & Wejse, C. M. (2023). Interpreter services and effect on healthcare - a systematic review of the impact of different types of interpreters on patient outcome. *Journal of Migration and Health*, *7*, 100162. DOI: 10.1016/j.jmh.2023.100162 PMID: 36816444

Herman, J. L. (1992). *Trauma and recovery: The aftermath of violence—From domestic abuse to political terror*. Basic Books.

Herrenkohl, T. I., Jung, H., Lee, J. O., & Kim, M.-H. (2017). Effects of child maltreatment, cumulative victimization experiences, and proximal life stress on adult crime and antisocial behavior. Retrieved from https://www.ncjrs.gov/ pdffiles1/nij/grants/250506.pdf

Heyman, J. (2012). Capitalism and US policy at the Mexican border. *Dialectical Anthropology*, *36*(3), 263–277. DOI: 10.1007/s10624-012-9274-x

Hine, K. A., Porter, L. E., Westera, N. J., Alpert, G. P., & Allen, A. (2018). Exploring police use of force decision-making processes and impairments using a naturalistic decision-making approach. *Criminal Justice and Behavior*, *45*(11), 1782–1801. DOI: 10.1177/0093854818789726

Hodge, D. R., & Holtrop, C. R. (2002). Spiritual assessment: A review of complementary assessment models. *Social work and Christianity: Readings on the integration of Christian faith and social work practice, 2*, 167-192.

Holmes, S. M. (2013). *Fresh fruit, broken bodies: Migrant farmworkers in the United States*. University of California Press.

Homeland Security. (n.d.). *Immigration Options for Victims of Crime.* Retrieved October 18, 2024, from https://www.dhs.gov/immigration-options-victims-crime

Hope For Justice. (2024). Who is vulnerable to human trafficking. Retrieved from https://hopeforjustice.org/news/who-is-vulnerable-to-human-trafficking/#:~:text=Asylum%20seekers%2C%20displaced%20people%20and,be%20factors%20that%20create%20refugees

Hopper, E., & Hidalgo, J. (2006). Invisible chains: Psychological coercion of human trafficking victims. *Intercultural Human Rights Law Review*, *1*, 185–209.

Horton, S. B. (2016). *They leave their kidneys in the fields: Illness, injury, and illegality among U.S. farmworkers*. University of California Press. DOI: 10.1525/california/9780520283268.001.0001

House, T. W. (2022, March 16). *Fact Sheet: Reauthorization of the Violence Against Women Act (VAWA)*. The White House. https://www.whitehouse.gov/briefing-room/statements-releases/2022/03/16/fact-sheet-reauthorization-of-the-violence-against-women-act-vawa/

Hovens, J. G. F. M., Giltay, E. J., Spinhoven, P., Van Hemert, A. M., & Penninx, B. W. J. H. (2015). Impact of Childhood Life Events and Childhood Trauma on the Onset and Recurrence of Depressive and Anxiety Disorders. *The Journal of Clinical Psychiatry*, *76*(07), 931–938. DOI: 10.4088/JCP.14m09135 PMID: 25699690

Hunsinger, M., Christopher, M., & Schmidt, A. M. (2019). Mindfulness training, implicit bias, and force response decision-making. *Mindfulness*, *10*(12), 2555–2566. DOI: 10.1007/s12671-019-01213-8 PMID: 34413908

Hyland, P., Shevlin, M., Fyvie, C., & Karatzias, T. (2018). Posttraumatic Stress Disorder and Complex Posttraumatic Stress Disorder in *DSM-5* and *ICD-11*: Clinical and Behavioral Correlates. *Journal of Traumatic Stress*, *31*(2), 174–180. DOI: 10.1002/jts.22272 PMID: 29577450

Ikonte, C. O., Prigmore, H. L., Dawson, A. Z., & Egede, L. E. (2020). Trends in prevalence of depression and serious psychological distress in United States immigrant and non-immigrant populations, 2010—2016. *Journal of Affective Disorders*, *274*, 719–725. DOI: 10.1016/j.jad.2020.05.010 PMID: 32664007

İlimen, E. (2023). The Devil's Highway: The U.S. - Mexico border crossing, global influences and politics*. *Folklor / Edebiyat, 29*(113), 253–270. https://doi-org.libproxy.calbaptist.edu/10.22559/folklor.2277

Immigration and Customs Enforcement. (n.d.). *Human trafficking*. https://www.ice.gov/features/human-trafficking

Immigration and Nationality Act. (1952). 8 U.S.C. § 1182. Https://www.govinfo.gov/content/pkg/COMPS-1376/pdf/COMPS-1376.pdf

Immigration Policy. (2024). NNEDV. Retrieved October 18, 2024, from https://nnedv.org/content/immigration-policy/

Ingram, E. M. (2007). A Comparison of Help Seeking Between Latino and Non-Latino Victims of Intimate Partner Violence. *Violence Against Women*, *13*(2), 159–171. DOI: 10.1177/1077801206296981 PMID: 17251503

Ingram, M., McClelland, D. J., Martin, J., Caballero, M. F., Mayorga, M. T., & Gillespie, K. (2010). Experiences of immigrant women who self-petition under the Violence Against Women Act. *Violence Against Women*, *16*(8), 858–880. DOI: 10.1177/1077801210376889 PMID: 20679184

International Association of Chiefs of Police. (2019). *Enhance the response to hate crimes.*https://www.theiacp.org/sites/default/files/2019-04/IACP_Hate%20Crimes_Full%Report.pdf

Irizar, P., Gage, S. H., Field, M., Fallon, V., & Goodwin, L. (2021). The prevalence of hazardous and harmful drinking in the UK Police Service, and their co-occurrence with job strain and mental health problems. *Epidemiology and Psychiatric Sciences, 30*, e51. DOI: 10.1017/S2045796021000366 PMID: 34402422

Israel, E., & Batalova, J. (2020). Mexican Immigrants in the United States. *Migration Policy.*https://www.migrationpolicy.org/article/mexican-immigrants-united-states-2019

Jimenez, D. E., Bartels, S. J., Cardenas, V., & Alegría, M. (2013). Stigmatizing attitudes toward mental illness among racial/ethnic older adults in primary care. [PubMed: 23361866]. *International Journal of Geriatric Psychiatry, 28*(10), 1061–1068. DOI: 10.1002/gps.3928 PMID: 23361866

Jud, A., Pfeiffer, E., & Jarczok, M. (2020). Epidemiology of violence against children in migration: A systematic literature review. *Child Abuse & Neglect, 108*, 104634. DOI: 10.1016/j.chiabu.2020.104634 PMID: 32745801

Kaminer, D., Grimsrud, A., Myer, L., Stein, D. J., & Williams, D. R. (2008). Risk for post-traumatic stress disorder associated with different forms of interpersonal violence in South Africa. *Social Science & Medicine, 67*(10), 1589–1595. DOI: 10.1016/j.socscimed.2008.07.023 PMID: 18774211

Kandel, W. A. (2013). *Immigration provisions of the Violence Against Women Act.* VAWA.

Kapadia, F. (2024). Protecting immigrant children: A public health of consequence, March 2024. *American Journal of Public Health, 114*(3), 267–269. DOI: 10.2105/AJPH.2023.307569 PMID: 38382023

Karliner, L. S., Jacobs, E. A., Chen, A. H., & Mutha, S. (2007). Do professional interpreters improve clinical care for patients with limited English proficiency? A systematic review of the literature. *Health Services Research, 42*(2), 727–754. DOI: 10.1111/j.1475-6773.2006.00629.x PMID: 17362215

Kartarı, A. (2014). *Kültür, Farklılık, İletişim: Kültürlerarası İletişimin Kavramsal Dayanakları.* İletişim Yayınları.

Kenny, K. S., Merry, L., Brownbridge, D. A., & Urquia, M. L. (2020). Factors associated with cyber-victimization among immigrants and non-immigrants in Canada: A cross-sectional nationally-representative study. *BMC Public Health, 20*(1), 1–13. DOI: 10.1186/s12889-020-09492-w PMID: 33066741

Kenny, S., & Lobo, M. (2014). *Addressing Cultural Differences Whither Multiculturalism? F. Mansouri, & B. Ebanda de B'béri içinde, Global Perspectives on the Politics of Multiculturalism in the 21st Century: A Case Study Analysis*. Routledge.

KFF. (2025). *Key Facts on Health Coverage of Immigrants*. https://www.kff.org/racial-equity-and-health-policy/fact-sheet/key-facts-on-health-coverage-of-immigrants/

Kim, B. J. (2011). *Factors that Influence Quality of Life among Low-Income Elderly Korean Immigrants in Adult Day Health Care (ADHC)*. University of California.

Klika, J. B., Rosenzweig, J., & Merrick, M. (2020). Economic Burden of Known Cases of Child Maltreatment from 2018 in Each State. *Child & Adolescent Social Work Journal, 37*(3), 227–234. DOI: 10.1007/s10560-020-00665-5

Koff, M. D., & McGowan, J. J. (1999). MedSpanish: A language tool for the emergency department. In *Proceedings of the American Medical Informatics Association Symposium,* 565–569. https://pubmed.ncbi.nlm.nih.gov/10566422

Kolker, A. F., & Smith, H. R. (2024). *Immigration: Grounds of inadmissibility.*

Koocher, G. P., & Keith-Spiegel, P. (2016). *Ethics in psychology and the mental health professions: Standards and cases* (4th ed.). Oxford University Press.

Kop, N., Euwema, M., & Schaufeli, W. (1999). Burnout, job stress and violent behaviour among Dutch police officers. *Work and Stress, 13*(4), 326–340. DOI: 10.1080/02678379950019789

Kouyoumdjian, H., Zamboanga, B. L., & Hansen, D. J. (2003). Barriers to community mental health services for Latinos: Treatment considerations. *Clinical Psychology : a Publication of the Division of Clinical Psychology of the American Psychological Association, 10*(4), 394–422. DOI: 10.1093/clipsy.bpg041

Kroening, A. L. H., & Dawson-Hahn, E. (2019). Health Considerations for Immigrant and Refugee Children. *Advances in Pediatrics, 66*, 87–110. DOI: 10.1016/j.yapd.2019.04.003 PMID: 31230701

Kröger, C., Harbeck, S., Armbrust, M., & Kliem, S. (2013). Effectiveness, response, and dropout of dialectical behavior therapy for borderline personality disorder in an inpatient setting. *Behaviour Research and Therapy, 51*(8), 411–416. DOI: 10.1016/j.brat.2013.04.008 PMID: 23727659

Krogstad, J. M., Passel, J. S., Moslimani, M., & Noe-Bustamante, L. (2023). *Key facts about U.S. Latinos for National Hispanic Heritage Month.* Pew Research Center. https://www.pewresearch.org/short-reads/2023/09/22/key-facts-about-us-latinos-for-national-hispanic-heritage-month/

Krys, K., Vignoles, V. L., de Almeida, I., & Uchida, Y. (2022). Outside the "Cultural Binary": Understanding Why Latin American Collectivist Societies Foster Independent Selves. *Perspectives on Psychological Science, 17*(4), 1166-1187. (Original work published 2022)DOI: 10.1177/17456916211029632

Kurtz, D. L., Zavala, E., & Melander, L. A. (2015). The influence of early strain on later strain, stress responses, and aggression by police officers. *Criminal Justice Review*, *40*(2), 190–208. DOI: 10.1177/0734016814564696

Kutlu, Ö., & Sütlü, S. (2024). *Investigation of the Career Development Experiences of Women Managers: An Analysis From a Gender Perspective. M. Haoucha içinde, Empowering and Advancing Women Leaders and Entrepreneurs*. IGI Global. DOI: 10.4018/979-8-3693-7107-7.ch011

Kuusisto, T., & Kuusisto, R. (2015). Cyber world as a social system. In *Cyber security: Analytics, technology and automation* (pp. 31–43). Springer International Publishing. DOI: 10.1007/978-3-319-18302-2_2

Kymlicka, W. (1995). *Multicultural Citizenship: A Liberal Theory of Minority Rights*. Clarendon Press.

Kymlicka, W. (2007). *Multicultural Odysseys: Navigating the New International Politics of Diversity*. Oxford University Press. DOI: 10.1093/oso/9780199280407.001.0001

Lagdon, S., Armour, C., & Stringer, M. (2014). Adult experience of mental health outcomes as a result of intimate partner violence victimization: A systematic review. *European Journal of Psychotraumatology*, *5*(1), 24794. DOI: 10.3402/ejpt.v5.24794 PMID: 25279103

Lanesskog, D., Muñoz, J., & Castillo, K. (2020). Language is not enough: Institutional supports for Spanish speaking client-worker engagement in child welfare. *Journal of Public Child Welfare*, *14*(4), 435–457. https://doi-org.libproxy.calbaptist.edu/10.1080/15548732.2019.1621235. DOI: 10.1080/15548732.2019.1621235

Laub, J. H., & Vaillant, G. E. (2000). Delinquency and Mortality: A 50-Year Follow-Up Study of 1,000 Delinquent and Nondelinquent Boys. *The American Journal of Psychiatry*, *157*(1), 96–102. DOI: 10.1176/ajp.157.1.96 PMID: 10618019

League, A. D. (2018). *Mainstreaming hate: The anti-immigrant movement in the US*. Anti-Defamation League.

LeBrun, A., Hassan, G., Boivin, M., Fraser, S.-L., Dufour, S., & Lavergne, C. (2015). Review of child maltreatment in immigrant and refugee families. *Canadian Journal of Public Health = Revue Canadienne de Santé Publique, 106*(Suppl 7), eS45. https://doi.org/DOI: 10.17269/CJPH.106.4838

Lechner, E. (2007). Imigração e saúde mental. *Migrações*, 79–101. https://estudogeral.uc.pt/handle/10316/33297

Lechte, J., & Bottomley, G. (1993). *Difference, Postmodernity and Image in Multicultural Australia. G. Clark, D. Forbes, & R. Francis içinde, Multiculturalism, Difference and Postmodernism*. Longman Cheshire.

Lee, M., & Weber, P. (2023). *The Texas Shooter in a racist Walmart attack is going to prison. here's what to know about the case*. AP News. https://apnews.com/article/el-paso-walmart-texas-crusius-bf7d25f3567959ee8b121deabcf1d9a1

Leeb, R. T., Paulozzi, L., Melanson, C., Simon, T., & Arias, I. (2008) Child Maltreatment Surveillance: Uniform Definitions for Public Health and Recommended Data Elements, Version 1.0. Atlanta (GA): Centers for Disease Control and Prevention, National Center for Injury Prevention and Control.

Lee, H. Y., Rhee, T. G., Kim, N. K., & Ahluwalia, J. S. (2015). Health Literacy as a Social Determinant of Health in Asian American Immigrants: Findings from a Population-Based Survey in California. *Journal of General Internal Medicine, 30*(8), 1118–1124. DOI: 10.1007/s11606-015-3217-6 PMID: 25715993

Lee, J. S., Pérez-Stable, E. J., Gregorich, S. E., Crawford, M. H., Green, A., Livaudais-Toman, J., & Karliner, L. S. (2017). Increased Access to Professional Interpreters in the Hospital Improves Informed Consent for Patients with Limited English Proficiency. *Journal of General Internal Medicine*, *32*(8), 863–870. DOI: 10.1007/s11606-017-3983-4 PMID: 28185201

Lee, M., Bhimla, A., & Ma, G. X. (2020). Depressive Symptom Severity and Immigration-Related Characteristics in Asian American Immigrants. *Journal of Immigrant and Minority Health, 22*(5), 935–945. DOI: 10.1007/s10903-020-01004-7 PMID: 32221768

Leemis, R. W., Friar, N., Khatiwada, S., Chen, M. S., Kresnow, M., Smith, S. G., Caslin, S., & Basile, K. C. (2022). *The National Intimate Partner and Sexual Violence Survey: 2016/2017 report on intimate partner violence*. https://stacks.cdc.gov/view/cdc/124646#moretextPAmods.subject_name

LeMaster, J. W., Broadbridge, C. L., Lumley, M. A., Arnetz, J. E., Arfken, C., Fetters, M. D., Jamil, H., Pole, N., & Arnetz, B. B. (2018). Acculturation and post-migration psychological symptoms among Iraqi refugees: A path analysis. *The American Journal of Orthopsychiatry*, *88*(1), 38–47. DOI: 10.1037/ort0000240 PMID: 28253013

Levitt, P. (2001). *The transnational villagers*. University of California Press. DOI: 10.1525/9780520926707

Lewis, S. J., Koenen, K. C., Ambler, A., Arseneault, L., Caspi, A., Fisher, H. L., Moffitt, T. E., & Danese, A. (2021). Unravelling the contribution of complex trauma to psychopathology and cognitive deficits: A cohort study. *The British Journal of Psychiatry*, *219*(2), 448–455. DOI: 10.1192/bjp.2021.57 PMID: 34538875

Lightfoot, A. F., Thatcher, K., Eng, E., Merino, Y., Thomas, T., Simán, F. M., Coyne-Beasley, T., & Chapman, M. V. (2019). "What I wish my doctor knew about my life": Using photovoice with immigrant Latino adolescents to explore barriers to healthcare. *Qualitative Social Work: Research and Practice*, *18*(1), 60–80. https://doi-org.libproxy.calbaptist.edu/10.1177/1473325017704034. DOI: 10.1177/1473325017704034 PMID: 32973399

Linares, A. (2023). *Rise in hate crimes includes a "significant increase" against Latinos*. College of Social Sciences and Humanities. https://cssh.northeastern.edu/rise-in-hate-crimes-includes-a-significant-increase-against-latinos/

Lindert, J., Ehrenstein, O. S. V., Priebe, S., Mielck, A., & Brähler, E. (2009). Depression and anxiety in labor migrants and refugees – A systematic review and meta-analysis. *Social Science & Medicine*, *69*(2), 246–257. DOI: 10.1016/j.socscimed.2009.04.032 PMID: 19539414

Linehan, M. M., Korslund, K. E., Harned, M. S., Gallop, R. J., Lungu, A., Neacsiu, A. D., McDavid, J., Comtois, K. A., & Murray-Gregory, A. M. (2015). Dialectical behavior therapy for high suicide risk in individuals with borderline personality disorder: A randomized clinical trial and component analysis. *JAMA Psychiatry*, *72*(5), 475–482. DOI: 10.1001/jamapsychiatry.2014.3039 PMID: 25806661

Liu, C., Wang, D., Liu, C., Jiang, J., Wang, X., Chen, H., Ju, X., & Zhang, X. (2020). What is the meaning of health literacy? A systematic review and qualitative synthesis. *Family Medicine and Community Health*, *8*(2), e000351. DOI: 10.1136/fmch-2020-000351 PMID: 32414834

Lopes, L., Montero, A., Presiado, M., & Hamel, L. (2024). *Americans' Challenges with Health Care Costs*. KFF. https://www.kff.org/health-costs/issue-brief/americans-challenges-with-health-care-costs/

Lopez Vera, A., Thomas, K., Trinh, C., & Nausheen, F. (2023). A Case Study of the Impact of Language Concordance on Patient Care, Satisfaction, and Comfort with Sharing Sensitive Information During Medical Care. *Journal of Immigrant and Minority Health*, *25*(6), 1261–1269. DOI: 10.1007/s10903-023-01463-8 PMID: 36840903

Lou, C., Adams, G., Bernstein, H., Baird, C., Feng, A., Hagerman, L., & Lei, S. (2019). *Part of us: A data-driven look at children of immigrants*. Urban Institute.

Lugo, A. (2008). *Fragmented lives, assembled parts: Culture, capitalism, and conquest at the U.S.-Mexico border*. University of Texas Press.

Lum, D. (2003). *Culturally competent practice*. Thomson–Brooks/Cole.

Lustig, R. H. (2021). *Metabolical: The lure and the lies of processed food, nutrition, and modern medicine*. Harper Wave.

Luthar, S. S. (2006). Resilience in development: A synthesis of research across five decades. In Cicchetti, D., & Cohen, D. J. (Eds.), Developmental psychopathology: Vol. 3. *Risk, disorder, and adaptation* (pp. 739–795). Wiley.

Magaña, D. (2020). Local Voices on Health Care Communication Issues and Insights on Latino Cultural Constructs. *Hispanic Journal of Behavioral Sciences*, *42*(3), 300–323. DOI: 10.1177/0739986320927387

Maguire, J., Sizer, H., Mifsud, N., & O'Donoghue, B. (2020). Outcomes for migrants with a first episode of psychosis: A systematic review. *Schizophrenia Research*, *222*, 42–48. DOI: 10.1016/j.schres.2020.05.048 PMID: 32561236

Mahabir, D. F., O'Campo, P., Lofters, A., Shankardass, K., Salmon, C., & Muntaner, C. (2021). Classism and everyday racism as experienced by racialized health care users: A concept mapping study. *International Journal of Health Services*, *51*(3), 350–363. DOI: 10.1177/00207314211014782 PMID: 33949220

Marotta, V. (2014). *The multicultural, intercultural and transcultural subject. F. Mansouri, & B. Ebanda de B'béri içinde, Global Perspectives on the Politics of Multiculturalism in the 21st Century: A Case Study Analysis*. Routledge.

Martinez-Donate, A. P., Ejebe, I., Zhang, X., Guendelman, S., Lê-Scherban, F., Rangel, G., Gonzalez-Fagoaga, E., Hovell, M. F., & Amuedo-Dorantes, C. (2017). Access to Health Care among Mexican Migrants and Immigrants: A Comparison across Migration Phases. *Journal of Health Care for the Poor and Underserved*, *28*(4), 1314–1326. DOI: 10.1353/hpu.2017.0116 PMID: 29176097

Martin, N., Morales, S., & Theodore, N. (2007). Migrant worker centers: Contending with downgrading in the low-wage labor market. *GeoJournal*, *68*(2–3), 155–165. DOI: 10.1007/s10708-007-9083-y

Mason-Bish, H. (2015). Beyond the silo: Rethinking hate crime and intersectionality. In N. Hall, A. Corb, P. Giannasi, & J. G. D. Grieve (Eds.), *The Routledge International Handbook on Hate Crime* (pp. 24-33). essay, Routledge, Taylor & Francis Group.

Masten, A. S. (2001). Ordinary magic: Resilience processes in development. *The American Psychologist*, *56*(3), 227–238. DOI: 10.1037/0003-066X.56.3.227 PMID: 11315249

Maynard, B. R., Vaughn, M. G., Salas-Wright, C. P., & Vaughn, S. (2016). Bullying victimization among school-aged immigrant youth in the United States. *The Journal of Adolescent Health*, *58*(3), 337–344. DOI: 10.1016/j.jadohealth.2015.11.013 PMID: 26903431

Mazza, M., Marano, G., Del Castillo, A. G., Chieffo, D., Monti, L., Janiri, D., Moccia, L., & Sani, G. (2021). Intimate partner violence: A loop of abuse, depression and victimization. *World Journal of Psychiatry*, *11*(6), 215–221. DOI: 10.5498/wjp.v11.i6.215 PMID: 34168968

McAuliffe, M., & Triandafyllidou, A. (2021). *World Migration Report 2022*. International Organization for Migration. https://publications.iom.int/system/files/pdf/WMR-2022-EN_1.pdf

McGhee, D. (2008). *The End of Multiculturalism? Terrorism, Integration and Human Rights*. Open University Press.

McKenzie, K. C. (Ed.). (2022). *Asylum medicine: A clinician's guide*. Springer International Publishing., DOI: 10.1007/978-3-030-81580-6

McLaughlin, K. A., Koenen, K. C., Hill, E. D., Petukhova, M., Sampson, N. A., Zaslavsky, A. M., & Kessler, R. C. (2013). Trauma Exposure and Posttraumatic Stress Disorder in a National Sample of Adolescents. *Journal of the American Academy of Child and Adolescent Psychiatry*, *52*(8), 815–830.e14. DOI: 10.1016/j.jaac.2013.05.011 PMID: 23880492

Meffert, S. M., Musalo, K., McNiel, D. E., & Binder, R. L. (2010). The role of mental health professionals in political asylum processing. *The Journal of the American Academy of Psychiatry and the Law*, *38*(4), 479–489. PMID: 21156906

Mehta, C., Theodore, N., Mora, I., & Wade, J. (2002). *Chicago's undocumented immigrants: An analysis of wages, working conditions, and economic contributions*. https://www.semanticscholar.org/paper/Chicago%27s-undocumented-immigrants%3A-An-analysis-of-Mehta-Theodore/6457030c1296887962916ce526723bfb408e73a8

Melander, C., & Shmulyar Gréen, O. (2023). Language brokering as acts of care: Experiences of young migrants born in Poland and Romania living in Sweden. *Nordic Social Work Research*, *13*(4), 577–588. DOI: 10.1080/2156857X.2023.2199417

Melendres, M. (2020). Cultural competence in social work practice: Exploring the challenges of newly employed social work professionals. *Journal of Ethnic & Cultural Diversity in Social Work*, •••, 108–120.

Melikyan, Z. A., Agranovich, A. V., & Puente, A. E. (2019). 19—Fairness in psychological testing. In Goldstein, G., Allen, D. N., & DeLuca, J. (Eds.), *Handbook of Psychological Assessment* (4th ed., pp. 551–572). Academic Press., DOI: 10.1016/B978-0-12-802203-0.00018-3

Ménard, K. S., Arter, M. L., & Khan, C. (2016). Critical incidents, alcohol and trauma problems, and service utilization among police officers from five countries. *International Journal of Comparative and Applied Criminal Justice*, *40*(1), 25–42. DOI: 10.1080/01924036.2015.1028950

Mercado, A., Antuña, C., Bailey, C., Garcini, L., Hass, G., Henderson, C., Koslofsky, S., Morales, F., & Venta, A. (2022). Professional guidelines for psychological evaluations in immigration proceedings. *Journal of Latina/o Psychology*, *10*(4), 253–276. Advance online publication. DOI: 10.1037/lat0000209

Merriam-Webster. (n.d.). *Immigrant definition & meaning*. Merriam-Webster. Retrieved from https://www.merriam-webster.com/dictionary/immigrant#:~:text=im%C2%B7%E2%80%8Bmi%C2%B7%E2%80%8Bgrant,to%20take%20up%20permanent%20residence

Messing, J. T., Amanor-Boadu, Y., Cavanaugh, C. E., Glass, N. E., & Campbell, J. C. (2013). Culturally competent intimate partner violence risk assessment: Adapting the danger assessment for immigrant women. *Social Work Research*, *37*(3), 263–275. DOI: 10.1093/swr/svt019

Meyers, R. S. (2020). *Conducting psychological assessments for U.S. immigration cases*. Springer International Publishing., DOI: 10.1007/978-3-030-49868-9

Miao, X.-R., Chen, Q.-B., Wei, K., Tao, K.-M., & Lu, Z.-J. (2018). Posttraumatic stress disorder: From diagnosis to prevention. *Military Medical Research*, *5*(1), 32. DOI: 10.1186/s40779-018-0179-0 PMID: 30261912

Migration Policy Institute. (2024). *Children in U.S. Immigrant Families*. (2013, November 13). Retrieved from https://www.migrationpolicy.org/programs/data-hub/charts/children-immigrant-families

Miller, L. (2013). Psychological evaluations in the criminal justice system: Basic principles and best practices. *Aggression and Violent Behavior, 18*(1), Issue 1, p. 83-91. .DOI: 10.1016/j.avb.2012.10.005

Miller, K. K., Brown, C. R., Shramko, M., & Svetaz, M. V. (2019). Applying Trauma-Informed Practices to the Care of Refugee and Immigrant Youth: 10 Clinical Pearls. *Children (Basel, Switzerland)*, *6*(8), 94. DOI: 10.3390/children6080094 PMID: 31434278

Mitchell, K. (2004). Geographies of Identity: Multiculturalism Unplugged. *Progress in Human Geography*, *28*(5), 641–651. DOI: 10.1191/0309132504ph510pr

Mohammadifirouzeh, M., Oh, K. M., Basnyat, I., & Gimm, G. (2023). Factors Associated with Professional Mental Help-Seeking Among U.S. Immigrants: A Systematic Review. *Journal of Immigrant and Minority Health*, *25*(5), 1118–1136. DOI: 10.1007/s10903-023-01475-4 PMID: 37000385

Mölsä, M., Kuittinen, S., Tiilikainen, M., Honkasalo, M.-L., & Punamäki, R.-L. (2017). Mental health among older refugees: The role of trauma, discrimination, and religiousness. *Aging & Mental Health*, *21*(8), 829–837. DOI: 10.1080/13607863.2016.1165183 PMID: 27080403

Monnat, S. M., & Chandler, R. F. (2015). Long-term physical health consequences of adverse childhood experiences. *The Sociological Quarterly*, *56*(4), 723–752. DOI: 10.1111/tsq.12107 PMID: 26500379

Moore, R. (2023). *Man who killed 23 at El Paso Walmart pleads guilty to hate crimes*. The Texas Tribune. https://www.texastribune.org/2023/02/08/el-paso-walmart-shooting-pleads-guilty/

Morrison, A. M., Campbell, J. K., Sharpless, L., & Martin, S. L. (2024). Intimate Partner Violence and Immigration in the United States: A Systematic Review. *Trauma, Violence & Abuse*, *25*(1), 846–861. DOI: 10.1177/15248380231165690 PMID: 37078533

Moslimani, M., & Passel, J. (2024, September 27). *What the data says about immigrants in the U.S.* Pew Research Center. https://www.pewresearch.org/short-reads/2024/09/27/key-findings-about-us-immigrants/

Moslimani, M., & Passel, J. S. (2024). *What the data says about immigrants in the U.S.* Pew Research Center. https://www.pcwresearch.org/short-reads/2024/09/27/key-findings-about-us-immigrants/

Moslimani, M., & Passel, J. S. (2024). What the data says about immigrants in the U.S. Pew Research Center. Retrieved from https://www.pewresearch.org/short-reads/2024/09/27/key-findings-about-us-immigrants/#:~:text=Where%20do%20most%20U.S.%20immigrants,%25)%20and%20West%20(33%25).

Moslimani, M., Lopez, M. H., & Noe-Bustamante, L. (2023). *11 facts about Hispanic origin groups in the U.S.* Pew Research Center. https://www.pewresearch.org/short-reads/2023/08/16/11-facts-about-hispanic-origin-groups-in-the-us/

Munir, S., & Takov, V. (2024). Generalized Anxiety Disorder. In *StatPearls*. StatPearls Publishing., https://www.ncbi.nlm.nih.gov/books/NBK441870/

Murray, K. E., Davidson, G. R., & Schweitzer, R. D. (2010). Review of refugee mental health interventions following resettlement: Best practices and recommendations. *The American Journal of Orthopsychiatry*, *80*(4), 576–585. DOI: 10.1111/j.1939-0025.2010.01062.x PMID: 20950298

NASW. (2015). Standards and Indicators for Cultural Competence in Social Work Practice. https://www.socialworkers.org/Practice/NASW-Practice-Standards-Guidelines/Standards-and-Indicators-for-Cultural-Competence-in-Social-Work-Practice adresinden alındı

Nater, U. M., Skoluda, N., & Strahler, J. (2013). Biomarkers of stress in behavioural medicine. *Current Opinion in Psychiatry*, *26*(5), 440–445. DOI: 10.1097/YCO.0b013e328363b4ed PMID: 23867656

National Center on Domestic and Sexual Violence (NCDSV). (2024, October 18). *Immigrant Power and Control Wheel*. Retrieved from https://www.familyjusticecenter.org/wp-content/uploads/2017/10/Immigrant-Power-_-Control-Wheel-Domestic-Abuse-Intervention-Project.pdf

National Children's Alliance. (2024). *National Statistics on Child Abuse*. Retrieved October 20, 2024, from https://www.nationalchildrensalliance.org/media-room/national-statistics-on-child-abuse/

National Immigration Forum. (2019). Push or Pull Factors: What Drives Central American Migrants to the U.S.? https://immigrationforum.org/article/push-or-pull-factors-what-drives-central-american-migrants-to-the-u-s/

National Immigration Women's Advocacy Project. (2015). *Comparing forms of immigration relief for immigrant victims of crime.* Author. Retrieved from http://niwaplibrary.wcl.American.edu/pubs/imm-relief-forms-comparison

National Organization for Women (NOW). (2024, October 17). Intimate partner violence undocumented and immigrant women. https://now.org/wp-content/uploads/2017/06/Learn-More-IPV-and-Immigrant-Womenpdf.pdf

National Resource Center on Domestic Violence (NRCDV). (2021). *Public Policy & Advocacy* Retrieved August 6, 2021, from https://nrcdv.org/public-policy

Nazer, D., & Greenbaum, J. (2020). Human trafficking of children. *Pediatric Annals, 49*(5), e209–e214. DOI: 10.3928/19382359-20200417-01 PMID: 32413148

Neal, T. M. S., Slobogin, C., Saks, M. J., Faigman, D. L., & Geisinger, K. F. (2020). Psychological Assessments in Legal Contexts: Are Courts Keeping "Junk Science" Out of the Courtroom? *Psychological Science in the Public Interest, 20*(3), 135-164. (Original work published 2019)DOI: 10.1177/1529100619888860

Negele, A., Kaufhold, J., Kallenbach, L., & Leuzinger-Bohleber, M. (2015). Childhood Trauma and Its Relation to Chronic Depression in Adulthood. *Depression Research and Treatment, 2015*, 1–11. DOI: 10.1155/2015/650804 PMID: 26693349

Negi, N. J. (2013). Battling discrimination and social isolation: Psychological distress among Latino day laborers. *American Journal of Community Psychology, 51*(1–2), 164–174. DOI: 10.1007/s10464-012-9548-0 PMID: 22864958

NeMoyer, A., Rodriguez, T., & Alvarez, K. (2019). Psychological Practice with Unaccompanied Immigrant Minors: Clinical and Legal Considerations. *Translational Issues in Psychological Science, 5*(1), 4–16. DOI: 10.1037/tps0000175 PMID: 30882017

Nielsen, D. S., Abdulkadir, L. S., Lynnerup, C., & Sodemann, M. (2020). 'I had to stifle my feelings' – Bilingual health professionals translating for family members in a healthcare setting. A qualitative study. *Scandinavian Journal of Caring Sciences, 34*(4), 929–937. DOI: 10.1111/scs.12800 PMID: 31830311

NIJC. (2022). *NIJC procedural manual for asylum representation*. National Immigrant Justice Center. https://immigrantjustice.org/for-attorneys/legal-resources/file/nijc-procedural-manual-asylum-representation-pdf

Nipperess, S., & Williams, C. (2019). *Introduction. S. Nipperess, & C. Williams içinde, Critical Multicultural Pratice in Social Work New Perspectives and Practices*. Routledge.

Njie-Carr, V. P., Sabri, B., Messing, J. T., Suarez, C., Ward-Lasher, A., Wachter, K., Marea, C. X., & Campbell, J. (2020). Understanding Intimate Partner Violence among Immigrant and Refugee Women: A Grounded Theory Analysis. *Journal of Aggression, Maltreatment & Trauma, 30*(6), 792–810. DOI: 10.1080/10926771.2020.1796870 PMID: 34483645

Norman, R. E., Byambaa, M., De, R., Butchart, A., Scott, J., & Vos, T. (2012). The Long-Term Health Consequences of Child Physical Abuse, Emotional Abuse, and Neglect: A Systematic Review and Meta-Analysis. *PLoS Medicine, 9*(11), e1001349. DOI: 10.1371/journal.pmed.1001349 PMID: 23209385

Novak, E. A., Kulig, T. C., & Doña-Reveco, C. (2021). *Human trafficking and the T visa process: Insights from legal representatives working with victims from Latin America*. OLLAS Reports., DOI: 10.32873/uno.dc.ollas.1016

NPS. (n.d.) Statue of Liberty: The New Colossus. Retrieved from https://www.nps.gov/stli/learn/historyculture/colossus.htm#:~:text=%22Give%20me%20your%20tired%2C%20your,refuse%20of%20your%20teeming%20shore

O'Hara, A. F., Violanti, J. M., Levenson, R. L.Jr, & Clark, R. G.Sr. (2013). National police suicide estimates: Web surveillance study III. *International Journal of Emergency Mental Health, 15*(1), 31–38. PMID: 24187885

Öçal, M., & Korkmaz, A. (2021). Neo-Liberalizmin Gölgesinde Sosyal Devlet: Emek ve Emeğin Örgütlenmesi Nereye Gidiyor? Sosyoloji Divanı, 27-49.

Öçal, M., & Kutlu, Ö. (2023). A Study on Welfare and Living Conditions of Disadvantaged Groups: The Case of Burdur Province. Journal of Management and Economics Research, 410-425.

Öçal, M., & Kutlu, Ö. (2024). İstihdamın Karanlık Yüzü: Ter Atölyelerine (Sweatshop) İnsani Bir Bakış ve Ter İndeksi ile Bir Kıyaslama. Çalışma ve Toplum, 1391-1424.

Öçal, M. (2023a). *Çalışma Yaşamında Göçmenler. M. Zubaroğlu Yanardağ, & B. Erkoç içinde, Göç ve Sosyal Hizmet*. Akademisyen Kitabevi.

Öçal, M. (2023b). *Bir Sosyal Devlet Ödevi Olarak Sosyal Gelişim ve Sosyal Kalkınmanın Teşviki. M. Öçal içinde, Sosyal Gelişimin Teşvikinde Kuramlar, Politikalar ve Eylemler*. Detay Yayıncılık.

Öçal, M., & Korkmaz, A. (2020). *Sosyal Dışlanma ve Sosyal Dışlanmanın Toplumsal Refah Üzerine Etkisi. M. Kasapoğlu, M. Öztürk, & M. Öçal içinde, Spor Yoluyla Sosyal Uyum*. Detay Yayıncılık.

Oehme, K., Donnelly, E. A., & Martin, A. (2012). Alcohol abuse, PTSD, and officer-committed domestic violence. *Policing. Journal of Policy Practice*, *6*(4), 418–430. DOI: 10.1093/police/pas030

Oh, H., Trinh, M. P., Vang, C., & Becerra, D. (2020). Addressing Barriers to Primary Care Access for Latinos in the U.S.: An Agent-Based Model. *Journal of the Society for Social Work and Research*, *11*(2), 165–184. https://www.journals.uchicago.edu/doi/full/10.1086/708616. DOI: 10.1086/708616

Ojeda, L., Flores, L. Y., Meza, R. R., & Morales, A. (2011). Culturally competent qualitative research with Latino immigrants. *Hispanic Journal of Behavioral Sciences*, *33*(2), 184–203. DOI: 10.1177/0739986311402626

Ojito, M. A. (2014). *Hunting season: Immigration and murder in an All-American town*. Beacon Press.

Oladipo, G. (2024). Racism is embedded in our society': how attacks on immigrants in Ohio highlight US disinformation crisis. The Guardian. Retrieved from https://www.theguardian.com/us-news/2024/sep/18/trump-republicans-springfield-aurora-political-disinformation

Ordóñez, J. T. (2015). *Jornalero: Being a day laborer in the USA*. University of California Press.

Organista, K. C. (2008). Mexican migration for dummies: What social workers and the public need to know. *Journal of Ethnic & Cultural Diversity in Social Work*, *16*(3–4), 189–198. DOI: 10.1300/J051v16n03_16

Organista, K. C., & Kubo, A. (2005). Pilot survey of HIV risk and contextual problems and issues in Mexican/Latino migrant day laborers. *Journal of Immigrant Health*, *7*(4), 269–281. DOI: 10.1007/s10903-005-5124-0 PMID: 19813293

Organista, K. C., & Ngo, S. (2019). Cultural and community resources protect Latino migrant day laborers from discrimination-related distress. *Cultural Diversity & Ethnic Minority Psychology*, *25*(2), 232–241. DOI: 10.1037/cdp0000211 PMID: 30010347

Organista, K. C., Worby, P., Quesada, J., Arreola, S. G., Kral, A. H., & Khoury, S. (2013). Sexual health of Latino migrant day labourers under conditions of structural vulnerability. *Culture, Health & Sexuality*, *15*(1), 58–72. DOI: 10.1080/13691058.2012.740075 PMID: 23140484

Orloff, L., Angel, C., & Robinson, S. (2013). *Empowering survivors: Legal rights of immigrant victims of sexual assault.*

Ornelas, I. J., Yamanis, T. J., & Ruiz, R. A. (2020). The Health of Undocumented Latinx Immigrants: What We Know and Future Directions. *Annual review of public health, 41*, 2 89–308. https://doi.org/DOI: 10.1146/annurev-publhealth-040119-094211

Ortega, A. N., Rodriguez, H. P., & Bustamante, A. V. (2015). Policy dilemmas in Latino health care and implementation of the Affordable Care Act. *Annual Review of Public Health*, *36*(1), 525–544. https://doi-org.libproxy.calbaptist.edu/10.1146/annurev-publhealth-031914-122421. DOI: 10.1146/annurev-publhealth-031914-122421 PMID: 25581154

Osborn, P., & Karandikar, S. (2022). Practice-based knowledge perspectives of cultural competence in social work. ournal of Ethnic & Cultural Diversity in Social Work, 285-297.

Osooli, M., Ohlsson, H., Sundquist, J., & Sundquist, K. (2023). Major depressive disorders in young immigrants: A cohort study from primary healthcare settings in Sweden. *Scandinavian Journal of Public Health*, *51*(3), 315–322. DOI: 10.1177/14034948211019796 PMID: 34120516

Öztürk, A. (2020). *Mülteci Çocukların Sorunları ve Kültürel Yetkinlik Çerçevesinde Mülteci Çocuklarla Çalışma. F. Paslı, & H. Aslantürk içinde, Çocuklarla Çalışma: Temel Alanlar, Uygulamalar, Güncel Tartışmalar*. Nobel.

Pandey, M., Maina, R. G., Amoyaw, J., Li, Y., Kamrul, R., Michaels, C. R., & Maroof, R. (2021). Impacts of English language proficiency on healthcare access, use, and outcomes among immigrants: A qualitative study. *BMC Health Services Research*, *21*(1), 741. DOI: 10.1186/s12913-021-06750-4 PMID: 34311712

Parekh, B. (2004). *Dialogue between cultures*. Routledge.

Park, T., Mullins, A., Zahir, N., Salami, B., Lasiuk, G., & Hegadoren, K. (2021). Domestic Violence and Immigrant Women: A Glimpse Behind a Veiled Door. *Violence Against Women*, *27*(15–16), 2910–2926. DOI: 10.1177/1077801220984174 PMID: 33506739

Parreñas, R. S. (2002). The care crisis in the Philippines: Children and transnational families in the new global economy. In Ehrenreich, B., & Hochschild, A. R. (Eds.), *Global woman: Nannies, maids, and sex workers in the new economy* (pp. 39–54). Metropolitan Books.

Parreñas, R. S. (2005). *Children of global migration: Transnational families and gendered woes*. Stanford University Press. DOI: 10.1515/9781503624627

Pascual-Leone, A., Kim, J., & Morrison, O.-P. (2017). Working with Victims of human trafficking. *Journal of Contemporary Psychotherapy*, *47*(1), 51–59. DOI: 10.1007/s10879-016-9338-3

Passel, J. S., & Krogstad, J. M. (2024). *What we know about unauthorized immigrants living in the U.S.* Pew Research Center. https://www.pewresearch.org/short-reads/2024/07/22/what-we-know-about-unauthorized-immigrants-living-in-the-us/

Pearson, A., Srivastava, R., Craig, D., Tucker, D., Grinspun, D., Bajnok, I., Griffin, P., Long, L., Porritt, K., Han, T., & Gi, A. A. (2007). Systematic review on embracing cultural diversity for developing and sustaining a healthy work environment in healthcare. *International Journal of Evidence-Based Healthcare*, *5*(1), 54–91. DOI: 10.1111/j.1479-6988.2007.00058.x PMID: 21631782

Pearson, L. B. (1957). *The Four Faces of Peace. The Nobel Peace Prize 1957.* The University of Oslo.

Pedron, S. M., & da Cruz, J. D. A. (2021). US Immigration and Human Traffifficking Overlap. International Social Science Review (Online), 97(4), 0_1-19.

Penninx, B. W., Pine, D. S., Holmes, E. A., & Reif, A. (2021). Anxiety disorders. *Lancet*, *397*(10277), 914–927. DOI: 10.1016/S0140-6736(21)00359-7 PMID: 33581801

Peréz-Torres, R. (1993). Nomads and Migrants: Negotiating a Multicultural Postmodernism. *Cultural Critique*, •••(26), 161–189. DOI: 10.2307/1354459

Perreira, K. M., & Ornelas, I. (2013). Painful Passages: Traumatic Experiences and Post-Traumatic Stress among U.S. Immigrant Latino Adolescents and their Primary Caregivers. *The International Migration Review*, *47*(4), 976–1005. DOI: 10.1111/imre.12050 PMID: 24385676

Petereit-Haack, G., Bolm-Audorff, U., Romero Starke, K., & Seidler, A. (2020). Occupational Risk for Post-Traumatic Stress Disorder and Trauma-Related Depression: A Systematic Review with Meta-Analysis. *International Journal of Environmental Research and Public Health*, *17*(24), 9369. DOI: 10.3390/ijerph17249369 PMID: 33327657

Pham, A. T., van Dijk, B. A. C., van der Valk, E. S., van der Vegt, B., van Rossum, E. F. C., & de Bock, G. H. (2024). Chronic stress related to cancer incidence, including the role of metabolic syndrome components. *Cancers (Basel)*, *16*(11), 2044. Advance online publication. DOI: 10.3390/cancers16112044 PMID: 38893162

Pignon, B., Amad, A., Pelissolo, A., Fovet, T., Thomas, P., Vaiva, G., Roelandt, J.-L., Benradia, I., Rolland, B., & Geoffroy, P. A. (2018). Increased prevalence of anxiety disorders in third-generation migrants in comparison to natives and to first-generation migrants. *Journal of Psychiatric Research*, *102*, 38–43. DOI: 10.1016/j.jpsychires.2018.03.007 PMID: 29597072

Pillai, D., & Artiga, S. (2023). *Overview of Health Coverage and Care for Individuals with Limited English Proficiency (LEP)*. KFF. https://www.kff.org/racial-equity-and-health-policy/issue-brief/overview-of-health-coverage-and-care-for-individuals-with-limited-english-proficiency/

Pinedo-Turnovsky, C. (2006). *Doing the corner: A study of immigrant day laborers in Brooklyn, New York* (Doctoral dissertation, City University of New York).

Pinedo-Turnovsky, C. (2019). *Daily labors: Marketing identity and bodies on a New York City street corner*. Temple University Press.

Polat, S. (2020). *Multicultural Structure of Schools and Intercultural Education. S. Polat içinde, Empowering Multiculturalism and Peacebuilding in Schools*. IGI Global.

Popal, F. (2021). *Surviving or thriving? what it takes for immigrants to succeed*. Bush Presidential Center., https://www.bushcenter.org/catalyst/state-of-the-american-dream/popal-what-it-takes-to-make-it-in-america

Portes, A. (2001). Introduction: The debates and significance of immigrant transnationalism. *Global Networks*, *1*(3), 181–194. DOI: 10.1111/1471-0374.00012

Prabhu, M., & Baranoski, M. (2012). Forensic mental health professionals in the immigration process. *The Psychiatric Clinics of North America*, *35*(4), 929–946. DOI: 10.1016/j.psc.2012.08.012 PMID: 23107571

Pumariega, A., Rogers, K., & Rothe, E. (2005). Culturallycompetentsystemsofcare for children's mental health: Advances and challenges. *Community Mental Health Journal*, *41*(5), 539–555. DOI: 10.1007/s10597-005-6360-4 PMID: 16142537

Quesada, J., Arreola, S., Kral, A., Khoury, S., Organista, K. C., & Worby, P. (2014). "As good as it gets": Undocumented Latino day laborers negotiating discrimination in San Francisco and Berkeley, California, USA. *City & Society*, *26*(1), 29–50. DOI: 10.1111/ciso.12033 PMID: 24910501

Quiroz, A. D., Boothe, R., Cruz, H., Palnati, S. R., & Bhakta, S. (2024). Primary Care Perceptions Among Spanish-Speaking Populations: A Comprehensive Review. *Cureus*, *16*(9), e68736. DOI: 10.7759/cureus.68736 PMID: 39371846

Qureshi, A., & Eiroa-Orosa, F. (2013). *Training for overcoming health disparities in mental health care: Interpretive-relational cultural competence*. Hogrefe Publishing. https://repository.uel.ac.uk/download/ffe867cdf7cf37eb40320e3a4b7f3a159f97b4f100cfc503a8c1b5d4dd739f5c/280351/Qureshi%2C%20Eiroa-Orosa%20-%202012%20-%20Cultural%20Variations%20in%20Psychopathology.%20From%20Research%20to%20Practice.pdf

Ragsdale, S. (2013). Immigrants in the United States of America. *Advances in Historical Studies*, *2*(03), 167–174. DOI: 10.4236/ahs.2013.23021

Raj, A., & Silverman, J. (2002). Violence against immigrant women: The roles of culture, context, and legal immigrant status on intimate partner violence. *Violence Against Women*, *8*(3), 367–398. DOI: 10.1177/10778010222183107

Ramirez, A. S., Willis, G., & Rutten, L. F. (2017). Understanding Spanish-Language response in a national health communication survey: *Implications for health communication research.Journal of Health Communication*, *22*(5), 442–450. DOI: 10.1080/10810730.2017.1304470 PMID: 28414618

Rana, K., Kent, J. L., & Page, A. (2025). Housing inequalities and health outcomes among migrant and refugee populations in high-income countries: A mixed-methods systematic review. *BMC Public Health*, *25*(1), 1098. DOI: 10.1186/s12889-025-22186-5 PMID: 40121396

Rao, A., Pillai, D., Artiga, S., Hamel, L., Schumacher, S., Kearney, A., & Presiado, M. (2024). *Five key facts about immigrants with limited English proficiency.* KFF. https://www.kff.org/racial-equity-and-health-policy/issue-brief/five-key-facts-about-immigrants-with-limited-english-proficiency/

Rasmussen, A., Crager, M., Baser, R. E., Chu, T., & Gany, F. (2012). Onset of Posttraumatic Stress Disorder and Major Depression Among Refugees and Voluntary Migrants to the United States. *Journal of Traumatic Stress*, *25*(6), 705–712. DOI: 10.1002/jts.21763 PMID: 23184423

Rathod, J. M. (2016). Danger and dignity: Immigrant day laborers and occupational risk. *Seton Hall Law Review*, *46*(3), 813–882. PMID: 27066611

Reavell, J., & Fazil, Q. (2017). The epidemiology of PTSD and depression in refugee minors who have resettled in developed countries. *Journal of Mental Health (Abingdon, England)*, *26*(1), 74–83. DOI: 10.1080/09638237.2016.1222065 PMID: 27684305

Revens, K. E., Gutierrez, D., Paul, R., Reynolds, A. D., Price, R., & DeHaven, M. J. (2021). Social support and religiosity as contributing factors to resilience and mental wellbeing in Latino immigrants: A community-based participatory research study. *Journal of Immigrant and Minority Health*, *23*(5), 904–916. DOI: 10.1007/s10903-021-01179-7 PMID: 33715112

Richter-Levin, G., & Xu, L. (2018). How could stress lead to major depressive disorder? *IBRO Reports*, *4*, 38–43. DOI: 10.1016/j.ibror.2018.04.001 PMID: 30155523

Rintell, L. S., Buchholz, K. R., & Gladstone, T. R. G. (2021). Depression. In W. O'Donohue & M. Zimmermann (Eds.), *Handbook of Evidence-Based Prevention of Behavioral Disorders in Integrated Care* (pp. 101–137). Springer International Publishing. DOI: 10.1007/978-3-030-83469-2_6

Rivera, T. (2023). A social-ecological approach to Latino immigrant trauma and intervention: An integrative review. *Journal of Immigrant and Minority Health*, *25*(4), 916–924. https://doi-org.libproxy.calbaptist.edu/10.1007/s10903-023-01474-5. DOI: 10.1007/s10903-023-01474-5 PMID: 37004677

Rodriguez, C. (2019). Latino/a citizen children of undocumented parents negotiating illegality. *Journal of Marriage and Family*, *81*(3), 713–728. https://doi-org.libproxy.calbaptist.edu/10.1111/jomf.12551. DOI: 10.1111/jomf.12551

Rogers, R. G. (2025). *The Dire Mental Health Effects of Restrictive Immigration Policies*. U.S. Committee for Refugees and Immigrants. https://refugees.org/the-dire-mental-health-effects-of-restrictive-immigration-policies/

Rosenberg, J. (2019). Why are you seeking refuge? Conducting evaluations of Central American asylum seekers. *Journal of Human Rights and Social Work*, *4*(4), 229–237. DOI: 10.1007/s41134-019-00097-x

Rutter, M. (2012). Resilience as a dynamic concept. *Development and Psychopathology*, *24*(2), 335–344. DOI: 10.1017/S0954579412000028 PMID: 22559117

Sabri, B., Campbell, J. C., & Messing, J. T. (2018). Intimate partner homicides in the United States, 2003-2013: A comparison of immigrants and nonimmigrant victims. *Journal of Interpersonal Violence*, *36*(9–10), 4735–4757. DOI: 10.1177/0886260518792249 PMID: 30095027

Sabri, B., Nnawulezi, N., Njie-Carr, V. P. S., Messing, J., Ward-Lasher, A., Alvarez, C., & Campbell, J. C. (2018). Multilevel risk and protective factors for intimate partner violence among African, Asian, and Latina immigrant and refugee women: Perceptions of effective safety planning interventions. *Race and Social Problems*, *10*(4), 348–365. DOI: 10.1007/s12552-018-9247-z PMID: 31289602

Sacco, L. N. (2019). *The Violence Against Women Act (VAWA): Historical overview, funding, and reauthorization.*

Saechao, F., Sharrock, S., Reicherter, D., Livingston, J. D., Aylward, A., Whisnant, J., Koopman, C., & Kohli, S. (2012). Stressors and barriers to using mental health services among diverse groups of first-generation immigrants to the United States. *Community Mental Health Journal, 48*(1), 98–106. DOI: 10.1007/s10597-011-9419-4 PMID: 21655942

Salami, B., Salma, J., & Hegadoren, K. (2019). Access and utilization of mental health services for immigrants and refugees: Perspectives of immigrant service providers. *International Journal of Mental Health Nursing, 28*(1), 152–161. DOI: 10.1111/inm.12512 PMID: 29984880

Salas-Wright, C. P., Kagotho, N., & Vaughn, M. G. (2014). Mood, anxiety, and personality disorders among first and second-generation immigrants to the United States. *Psychiatry Research, 220*(3), 1028–1036. DOI: 10.1016/j.psychres.2014.08.045 PMID: 25223256

Sanchez, T. F. (2013). Californian strawberries: Mexican immigrant women sharecroppers, labor, and discipline. *Anthropology of Work Review, 34*(1), 15–22. DOI: 10.1111/awr.12003

Sangalang, C. C., Becerra, D., Mitchell, F. M., Lechuga-Peña, S., Lopez, K., & Kim, I. (2019). Trauma, Post-Migration Stress, and Mental Health: A Comparative Analysis of Refugees and Immigrants in the United States. *Journal of Immigrant and Minority Health, 21*(5), 909–919. DOI: 10.1007/s10903-018-0826-2 PMID: 30244330

Santambrogio, J., Cimminiello, N., Wisidagamage Don, P., Leon, E., Miragliotta, E., Capuzzi, E., Colmegna, F., & Clerici, M. (2024). Influence of post-migration living difficulties on mental health among refugees and asylum seekers: A scoping review on clinical tools. *The International Journal of Social Psychiatry, 70*(7), 1191–1201. DOI: 10.1177/00207640241251748 PMID: 39049583

Santisteban, D. A., Mena, M. P., & Abalo, C. (2012). Bridging Diversity and Family Systems: Culturally Informed and Flexible Family Based Treatment for Hispanic Adolescents. *Couple & Family Psychology, 2*(4), 246–263. DOI: 10.1037/cfp0000013 PMID: 24772378

Schouler-Ocak, M. (Ed.). (2015). *Trauma and Migration: Cultural Factors in the Diagnosis and Treatment of Traumatised Immigrants*. Springer International Publishing., DOI: 10.1007/978-3-319-17335-1

Schultze-Krumbholz, A., Pfetsch, J. S., & Lietz, K. (2022). Cyberbullying in a multicultural context—Forms, strain, and coping related to Ethnicity-Based Cybervictimization. *Frontiers in Communication, 7*, 846794. DOI: 10.3389/fcomm.2022.846794

Schumacher, S., Hamel, L., Artiga, S., Pillai, D., Kearney, A., & Presaido, M. (2024). Most Hispanic Immigrants Say Their Lives Are Better In The US But Face Financial And Health Care Challenges: The 2023 KFF/LA Times Survey of Immigrants. KFF January 2024.

Scott, M., Weaver, S., & Kamimura, A. (2018). Experiences of immigrant women who applied for Violence Against Women Act (VAWA) Self- petition in the United States: Analysis of legal affidavits. *Diversity and Equality in Health and Care, 15*(4). Advance online publication. DOI: 10.21767/2049-5471.100168

Segal, U. A., & Mayadas, N. S. (2005). Assessment of issues facing immigrant and refugee families. *Child Welfare, 84*(5), 563–583. PMID: 16435651

Sege, R. D., Amaya-Jackson, L., Flaherty, E. G., Idzerda, S. M., Legano, L. A., Leventhal, J. M., & Sege, R. D. (2017). Clinical considerations related to the behavioral manifestations of child maltreatment. *Pediatrics, 139*(4), e20170100.

Seghetti, L. M., & Bjelopera, J. P. (2012). The Violence Against Women Act: Overview, legislation, and federal funding. *Congressional Research Service, 10*, 1–35.

Selten, J.-P., Van Der Ven, E., & Termorshuizen, F. (2020). Migration and psychosis: A meta-analysis of incidence studies. *Psychological Medicine, 50*(2), 303–313. DOI: 10.1017/S0033291719000035 PMID: 30722795

Sentell, T., Shumway, M., & Snowden, L. (2007). Access to mental health treatment by English language proficiency and race/ethnicity. *Journal of General Internal Medicine, 22*(S2, Suppl 2), 289–293. DOI: 10.1007/s11606-007-0345-7 PMID: 17957413

Shelley, L. (2013). Human trafficking as a form of transnational crime. In *Human trafficking* (pp. 116–137). Willan.

Shelton, D., Kesten, K., Zhang, W., & Trestman, R. (2011). Impact of a dialectic behavior therapy—Corrections Modified (DBT-CM) upon behaviorally challenged incarcerated male adolescents. *Journal of Child and Adolescent Psychiatric Nursing, 24*(2), 105–113. DOI: 10.1111/j.1744-6171.2011.00275.x PMID: 21501287

Shen, A. (2017). *What we know (and don't know) about immigrants and violent crime*. The Trace. https://www.thetrace.org/2017/02/immigrants-violent-crime-facts-donald-trump/?gad_source=1&gclid=Cj0KCQjwhb60BhClARIsABGGtw8XHP94atHLfCqxKeRuIdlG2m2jLQKo5p5yVm_dz7pUdFFYrpDaaBgaAuvOEALw_wcB

Sherwood, L., Hegarty, S., Vallières, F., Hyland, P., Murphy, J., Fitzgerald, G., & Reid, T. (2019). Identifying the key risk factors for adverse psychological outcomes among police officers: A systematic literature review. *Journal of Traumatic Stress*, *32*(5), 688–700. DOI: 10.1002/jts.22431 PMID: 31553502

Shibley, M. G., & Holt, M. (2022). *Conducting immigration evaluations: A practical guide for mental health professionals*. Routledge. https://api.taylorfrancis.com/content/books/mono/download?identifierName=doi&identifierValue=10.4324/9781003139973&type=googlepdf

Simich, L. (2006). Hidden Meanings of Health Security: Migration Experiences and Systemic Barriers to Mental Well-Being among Non-status Migrants in Canada. *International Journal of Migration, Health and Social Care*, *2*(3/4), 16–27. DOI: 10.1108/17479894200600024

Singer, E., Eswarappa, M., Kaur, K., & Baranowski, K. A. (2020). Addressing the need for forensic psychological evaluations of asylum seekers: The potential role of the general practitioner. *Psychiatry Research*, *284*(112752), 112752. Advance online publication. DOI: 10.1016/j.psychres.2020.112752 PMID: 32000095

Sliwinski, K., Kutney-Lee, A., McHugh, M. D., & Lasater, K. B. (2024). A Review of Disparities in Outcomes of Hospitalized Patients with Limited English Proficiency: The Importance of Nursing Resources. *Journal of Health Care for the Poor and Underserved*, *35*(1), 359–374. https://pmc.ncbi.nlm.nih.gov/articles/PMC11047028/ . DOI: 10.1353/hpu.2024.a919823 PMID: 38661875

Sloan, M. (2018). *T visas protect victims of human trafficking and strengthen community relationships*.

Smith, A. K., Sudore, R. L., Pérez-Stable, E. J., Smith, A. K., Sudore, R. L., & Pérez-Stable, E. J. (2009). Palliative care for Latino patients and their families: Whenever we prayed, she wept. *Journal of the American Medical Association*, *301*(10), 1047–E1. https://doi-org.libproxy.calbaptist.edu/10.1001/jama.2009.308. DOI: 10.1001/jama.2009.308 PMID: 19278947

Smith, B. L. (2018). Spanish-speaking psychologists in demand. *Monitor on Psychology*, *49*(6). https://www.apa.org/monitor/2018/06/spanish-speaking

Smith, S. G., Zhang, X., Basile, K. C., Merrick, M. T., Wang, J., Kresnow, M., & Chen, J. (2018). *The National Intimate Partner and Sexual Violence Survey (NISVS): 2015 Data Brief*. National Center for Injury Prevention and Control, Centers for Disease Control and Prevention.

Soto Mas, F., & Jacobson, H. E. (2018). Advancing Health Literacy Among Hispanic Immigrants: The Intersection Between Education and Health. *Health Promotion Practice*, *20*(2), 251–257. https://www.doi.org/10.1177/1524839918761865. DOI: 10.1177/1524839918761865 PMID: 29564920

Southern Poverty Law Center. (2009). *Climate of fear: Latino immigrants in Suffolk County, N.Y.*https://www.splcenter.org/20090831/climate-fear-latino-immigrants-suffolk-county-ny

Southern Poverty Law Center. (2019). *Terror from the right.* https://www.splcenter.org/terror-from-the-right

Spencer, C. M., Stith, S. M., & Cafferky, B. (2022). What Puts Individuals at Risk for Physical Intimate Partner Violence Perpetration? A Meta-Analysis Examining Risk Markers for Men and Women. *Trauma, Violence & Abuse*, *23*(1), 36–51. DOI: 10.1177/1524838020925776 PMID: 32431231

Squires, A. (2018). Strategies for overcoming language barriers in healthcare. *Nursing Management*, *49*(4), 20–27. DOI: 10.1097/01.NUMA.0000531166.24481.15 PMID: 29528894

Stanley, E. A., & Larsen, K. L. (2022). Stressed out: The missing influence of stress arousal in emotion's role in political decision-making. *Political Psychology*, *43*(4), 798–808. DOI: 10.1111/pops.12793

Stavenhagen, R. (2002). The Return of the Native. Occasional Papers No. 27: University of London Institute of Latin American Studies.

Steel, C., Haddock, G., Tarrier, N., Picken, A., & Barrowclough, C. (2011). Auditory Hallucinations and Posttraumatic Stress Disorder Within Schizophrenia and Substance Abuse. *The Journal of Nervous and Mental Disease*, *199*(9), 709–711. DOI: 10.1097/NMD.0b013e318229d6e8 PMID: 21878787

Sternberg, R. M., Nápoles, A. M., Gregorich, S., Paul, S., Lee, K. A., & Stewart, A. L. (2016). Development of the Stress of Immigration Survey: A Field Test Among Mexican Immigrant Women. *Family & Community Health*, *39*(1), 40–52. DOI: 10.1097/FCH.0000000000000088 PMID: 26605954

Stevelink, S. A. M., Opie, E., Pernet, D., Gao, H., Elliott, P., Wessely, S., Fear, N. T., Hotopf, M., & Greenberg, N. (2020). Probable PTSD, depression and anxiety in 40,299 UK police officers and staff: Prevalence, risk factors and associations with blood pressure. *PLoS One*, *15*(11), e0240902. DOI: 10.1371/journal.pone.0240902 PMID: 33180769

Stonbraker, S., Schnall, R., & Larson, E. (2015). Tools to measure health literacy among Spanish speakers: An integrative review of the literature. *Patient Education and Counseling, S0738-3991(*15)30020-3 . Advance online publication. https://doi.org/DOI: 10.1016/j.pec.2015.07.012

Stone, J., & Moskowitz, G. B. (2011). Non-conscious bias in medical decision making: What can be done to reduce it? *Medical Education*, *45*(8), 768–776. DOI: 10.1111/j.1365-2923.2011.04026.x PMID: 21752073

Straiton, M. L., Aambø, A. K., & Johansen, R. (2019). Perceived discrimination, health and mental health among immigrants in Norway: The role of moderating factors. *BMC Public Health*, *19*(1), 1–13. DOI: 10.1186/s12889-019-6649-9 PMID: 30894173

Striffler, S. (2005). *Chicken: The dangerous transformation of America's favorite food*. Yale University Press.

Stubbe, D. E. (2020). Practicing Cultural Competence and Cultural Humility in the Care of Diverse Patients. *Focus - American Psychiatric Publishing*, *18*(1), 49–51. DOI: 10.1176/appi.focus.20190041 PMID: 32047398

Subudhi, C. (2014). Culture and mental illness. *Social Work Practice in Mental Health: Cross-Cultural Perspectives, 141*, 132–140. https://www.researchgate.net/profile/Chittaranjan-Subudhi-2/publication/270762975_Culture_and_Mental_Illness/links/54b4adac0cf28ebe92e4818f/Culture-and-Mental-Illness.pdf

Subu, M. A., Holmes, D., Arumugam, A., Al-Yateem, N., Maria Dias, J., Rahman, S. A., Waluyo, I., Ahmed, F. R., & Abraham, M. S. (2022). Traditional, religious, and cultural perspectives on mental illness: A qualitative study on causal beliefs and treatment use. *International Journal of Qualitative Studies on Health and Well-being*, *17*(1), 2123090. DOI: 10.1080/17482631.2022.2123090 PMID: 36097886

Sue, D. W., Capodilupo, C. M., Torino, G. C., Bucceri, J. M., Holder, A., Nadal, K. L., & Esquilin, M. (2007). Racial microaggressions in everyday life: Implications for clinical practice. *The American Psychologist*, *62*(4), 271–286. DOI: 10.1037/0003-066X.62.4.271 PMID: 17516773

Sullivan, K., & Orloff, L. (2013). *BREAKING BARRIERS: A COMPLETE GUIDE TO LEGAL RIGHTS AND RESOURCES FOR BATTERED IMMIGRANTS*.

Sundvall, M., Tidemalm, D. H., Titelman, D. E., Runeson, B., & Bäärnhielm, S. (2015). Assessment and treatment of asylum seekers after a suicide attempt: A comparative study of people registered at mental health services in a Swedish location. *BMC Psychiatry*, *15*(1), 235. DOI: 10.1186/s12888-015-0613-8 PMID: 26446409

Sütlü, S. (2022). *Policies on Gender Equality. S. Sütlü, & D. Say Şahin içinde, Disadvantaged Groups: A Social Policy Perspective*. Eğitim Yayınevi.

Syed, S., Ashwick, R., Schlosser, M., Jones, R., Rowe, S., & Billings, J. (2020). Global prevalence and risk factors for mental health problems in police personnel: A systematic review and meta-analysis. *Occupational and Environmental Medicine*, *77*(11), 737–747. DOI: 10.1136/oemed-2020-106498 PMID: 32439827

Szaflarski, M., Cubbins, L. A., & Meganathan, K. (2017). Anxiety Disorders among US Immigrants: The Role of Immigrant Background and Social-Psychological Factors. *Issues in Mental Health Nursing*, *38*(4), 317–326. DOI: 10.1080/01612840.2017.1287790 PMID: 28379742

Tazi, K. Y., Rogers, R., & Chang, Y.-T. (2023). Forensic evaluations for immigration courts: A critical commentary on legal and ethical considerations. *Psychological Injury and Law*, *16*(4), 303–319. DOI: 10.1007/s12207-023-09489-x

Theodore, N. (2020). Regulating informality: Worker centers and collective action in day-labor markets. *Growth and Change*, *51*(1), 144–160. DOI: 10.1111/grow.12343

Theodore, N. (2023). Day-Labor Worker Centers: Advancing New Models of Equity and Inclusion in the Informal Economy. *Economic Development Quarterly*, *37*(4), 363–374. DOI: 10.1177/08912424231165004

Theodore, N., Valenzuela, A.Jr, & Meléndez, E. (2009). Worker centers: Defending labor standards for migrant workers in the informal economy. *International Journal of Manpower*, *30*(5), 422–436. DOI: 10.1108/01437720910977634

Timshel, I., Montgomery, E., & Dalgaard, N. T. (2017). A systematic review of risk and protective factors associated with family related violence in refugee families. *Child Abuse & Neglect*, *70*, 315–330. DOI: 10.1016/j.chiabu.2017.06.023 PMID: 28683372

Torres, S. A., Santiago, C. D., Walts, K. K., & Richards, M. H. (2018). Immigration policy, practices, and procedures: The impact on the mental health of Mexican and Central American youth and families. *The American Psychologist*, *73*(7), 843–854. https://doi-org.libproxy.calbaptist.edu/10.1037/amp0000184. DOI: 10.1037/amp0000184 PMID: 29504782

Trabsa, A., Redolar-Ripoll, D., Vargas, L., Llimona, A., Hogg, B., Valiente-Gómez, A., Pérez, V., Moreno-Alcázar, A., & Amann, B. L. (2023). A comparison of PTSD and traumatic event rates in a clinical sample of non-refugee immigrants and native-born individuals with a psychotic disorder: A case-control study. *European Journal of Psychotraumatology, 14*(2), 2263151. DOI: 10.1080/20008066.2023.2263151 PMID: 37846737

Trevillion, K., Oram, S., Feder, G., & Howard, L. M. (2012). Experiences of domestic violence and mental disorders: A systematic review and meta-analysis. *PLoS One, 7*(12), e51740. DOI: 10.1371/journal.pone.0051740 PMID: 23300562

Tulli, M., Salami, B., Begashaw, L., Meherali, S., Yohani, S., & Hegadoren, K. (2020). Immigrant mothers' perspectives of barriers and facilitators in accessing mental health care for their children. *Journal of Transcultural Nursing, 31*(6), 598–605. DOI: 10.1177/1043659620902812 PMID: 32013750

Turner, M. (2023). *Red and blue, who's hating who: An Examination of differences in hate crimes within traditional red and blue states*. ProQuest. https://www.proquest.com/openview/9ab583d83f6d5b8b1b22c708dacbb8ee/1?pq-origsite=gscholar&cbl=18750&diss=y

Tuttle, C. (2012). *Mexican women in American factories: Free trade and exploitation on the border*. University of Texas Press.

Twersky, S. E., Jefferson, R., Garcia-Ortiz, L., Williams, E., & Pina, C. (2024). The Impact of Limited English Proficiency on Healthcare Access and Outcomes in the U.S.: A Scoping Review. *Healthcare (Basel), 12*(3), 364. DOI: 10.3390/healthcare12030364 PMID: 38338249

U.S. Citizenship and Immigration Services (USCIS, 2014). Immigration relief for abused children, Special Immigrant Juvenile Status. Retrieved from Immigration_Relief_for_Abused_Children-FINAL.pdf (uscis.gov)

U.S. Citizenship and Immigration Services. (2024). *DHS implements keeping families together*. https://www.uscis.gov/newsroom/news-releases/dhs-implements-keeping-families-together

U.S. Department of Homeland Security. (2017). *Deferred action for parents of Americans and lawful permanent residents recession memo ("Dapa"): Homeland Security*. https://www.dhs.gov/publication/deferred-action-parents-americans-and-lawful--residents-recession-memo-dapa

U.S. Department of Homeland Security. (2024). *Application for waiver of grounds of inadmissibility*. USCIS. https://www.uscis.gov/i-601

U.S. Department of Justice. (2023). *Texas man sentenced to 90 consecutive life sentences for 2019 mass shooting at Walmart in El Paso, Texas, killing 23 people and injuring 22 others*. https://www.justice.gov/opa/pr/texas-man-sentenced-90-consecutive-life-sentences-2019-mass-shooting-walmart-el-paso-texas

U.S. Department of Justice. (2024). *Adjudication statistics: Total asylum applications*. U.S. Department of Justice, Executive Office for Immigration Review. https://www.justice.gov/eoir/media/1344871/dl?inline

U.S. N.A.R.A. (2021). *Alien victims of certain qualifying criminal activity. 8 C.F.R. §214.14*. United States: National Archives and Records Administration (US NARA): Office of the Federal Register. https://www.govinfo.gov/app/details/CFR-2021-title8-vol1/CFR-2021-title8-vol1-sec214-14

Ungar, M. (2011). *The social ecology of resilience: A handbook of theory and practice*. Springer.

United Nations. (2020). International migrant stock. https://www.un.org/development/desa/pd/content/international-migrant-stock

United Nations. (n.d.). *Migrant smuggling*. https://www.unodc.org/unodc/en/human-trafficking/migrant-smuggling/migrant-smuggling.html

United States Census Bureau. (2020). *People that speak English less than very well in the United States*. Public Tableau. https://public.tableau.com/app/profile/us.census.bureau/viz/shared/TSN7T2CMX

United States Census Bureau. (2024). *How do Hispanic or Latino Groups in the United States Compare?* Census.Gov. https://www.census.gov/library/visualizations/interactive/population-pyramid-hispanic-origin.html

United States Citizenship and Immigration Services. (2024). *USCIS policy manual*. U.S. Citizenship and Immigration Services. Https://www.uscis.gov/policy-manual

United States Department of Health and Human Services. (1996) Health Insurance Portability and Accountability Act of 1996. https://aspe.hhs.gov/reports/health-insurance-portability-accountability-act-1996

United States Department of Justice. (2022). *Human trafficking*. United States Department of Justice. https://www.justice.gov/humantrafficking

Urzúa, Á., Caqueo-Urízar, A., & Aragón, D. (2020). Prevalencia de sintomatología ansiosa y depresiva en migrantes colombianos en Chile. *Revista Medica de Chile*, *148*(9), 1271–1278. DOI: 10.4067/S0034-98872020000901271 PMID: 33399702

Valdés, G. (2020). (Mis)educating the children of Mexican-origin people in the United States: The challenge of internal language borders. *Intercultural Education, 31*(5), 548–561. DOI: 10.1080/14675986.2020.1794122

Valdez, Z., Plankey-Videla, N., Murga, A. L., Menchaca, A. C., & Barahona, C. (2019). Precarious entrepreneurship: Day laborers in the U.S. Southwest. *The American Behavioral Scientist, 63*(2), 225–243. DOI: 10.1177/0002764218794232

Valdivieso-Mora, E., Peet, C. L., Garnier-Villarreal, M., Salazar-Villanea, M., & Johnson, D. K. (2016). A Systematic Review of the Relationship between Familism and Mental Health Outcomes in Latino Population. *Frontiers in Psychology, 7*, 1632. DOI: 10.3389/fpsyg.2016.01632 PMID: 27826269

Valenzuela, A.Jr, Theodore, N., Meléndez, E., & Gonzalez, A. L. (2006). *On the corner: Day labor in the United States*. UCLA Center for the Study of Urban Poverty.

van der Kolk, B. A. (2014). *The body keeps the score: Brain, mind, and body in the healing of trauma*. Viking.

Vargas-Willis, G., & Cervantes, R. C. (1987). Consideration of Psychosocial Stress in the Treatment of the Latina Immigrant. *Hispanic Journal of Behavioral Sciences, 9*(3), 315–329. DOI: 10.1177/07399863870093007

Vélez-Coto, M., Rute-Pérez, S., Pérez-García, M., & Caracuel, A. (2021). Unemployment and general cognitive ability: A review and meta-analysis. *Journal of Economic Psychology, 87*, 102430. DOI: 10.1016/j.joep.2021.102430

Verhage, A., Noppe, J., Feys, Y., & Ledegen, E. (2018). Force, stress, and decision-making within the Belgian police: The impact of stressful situations on police decision-making. *Journal of Police and Criminal Psychology, 33*(4), 345–357. DOI: 10.1007/s11896-018-9262-4

Vesti. (2023). *Immigration and refugees: Understanding the challenges and opportunities*. LinkedIn. https://www.linkedin.com/pulse/immigration-refugees-understanding-challenges-opportunities/

Victims of Trafficking and Violence Protection Act of 2000, 22 U.S.C. § 7101 (2000). https://www.govinfo.gov/content/pkg/PLAW-106publ386/pdf/PLAW-106publ386.pdf

Violanti, J. M. (2018). *Police officer suicide*. Oxford University Press.

Violanti, J. M., Fekedulegn, D., Andrew, M. E., Charles, L. E., Hartley, T. A., & Burchfield, C. M. (2011). Adiposity in policing: Mental health consequences. *International Journal of Emergency Mental Health, 13*(4), 257–266. PMID: 22900459

Violanti, J. M., Gu, J. K., Charles, L. E., Fekedulegn, D., & Andrew, M. E. (2021). Dying for the job: Police mortality, 1950–2018. *Policing. Journal of Policy Practice*, *44*(6), 1168–1187. DOI: 10.1093/police/paaa066 PMID: 37200948

Violanti, J. M., Owens, S. L., McCanlies, E., Fekedulegn, D., & Andrew, M. E. (2019). Law enforcement suicide: A review. *Policing. Journal of Policy Practice*, *42*(2), 141–164. DOI: 10.1093/police/pay057

Vukcevic, M., Momirovic, J., & Puric, D. (2016). Adaptation of Harvard Trauma Questionnaire for working with refugees and asylum seekers in Serbia. *Psihologija (Beograd)*, *49*(3), 277–299. DOI: 10.2298/PSI1603277V

Wahass, S. H. (2005). The role of psychologists in health care delivery. *Journal of Family & Community Medicine*, *12*(2), 63–70. PMID: 23012077

Walker, L. (1984). *The battered women syndrome*. Springer.

Walker, L. E., Shapiro, D., & Akl, S. (2020). *Introduction to forensic psychology: Clinical and social psychological perspectives*. Springer International Publishing., DOI: 10.1007/978-3-030-44470-9

Walker, R., & Staton, M. (2000). Multiculturalism in Social Work Ethics. *Journal of Social Work Education*, *36*(3), 449–462. DOI: 10.1080/10437797.2000.10779021

Wallace, L. S., DeVoe, J. E., Heintzman, J. D., & Fryer, G. E. (2009). Language Preference and Perceptions of Healthcare Providers' Communication and Autonomy Making Behaviors among Hispanics. *Journal of Immigrant and Minority Health*, *11*(6), 453–459. DOI: 10.1007/s10903-008-9192-9 PMID: 18814028

Walter, N., Bourgois, P., & Loinaz, H. M. (2004). Masculinity and undocumented labor migration: Injured Latino day laborers in San Francisco. *Social Science & Medicine*, *59*(6), 1159–1168. DOI: 10.1016/j.socscimed.2003.12.013 PMID: 15210088

Wand, A. P. F., Pourmand, D., & Draper, B. (2020). Working with interpreters in the psychiatric assessment of older adults from culturally and linguistically diverse backgrounds. *International Psychogeriatrics, 32(*1), p.11-16. DOI: 10.1017/S1041610219000280

Wang, S.-K., Feng, M., Fang, Y., Lv, L., Sun, G.-L., Yang, S.-L., Guo, P., Cheng, S.-F., Qian, M.-C., & Chen, H.-X. (2023). Psychological trauma, posttraumatic stress disorder and trauma-related depression: A mini-review. *World Journal of Psychiatry*, *13*(6), 331–339. DOI: 10.5498/wjp.v13.i6.331 PMID: 37383283

Warsi, Z. (2023). Hundreds of immigrants have reported sexual abuse at Ice facilities. Most cases aren't investigated. PBS News. Retrieved from https://www.pbs.org/newshour/nation/hundreds-of-immigrants-have-reported-sexual-abuse-at-ice-facilities-most-cases-arent-investigated

Waters, A. R., Zamora, E. R., Fluchel, M., Warner, E. L., Rosen, S., Gwilliam, V., Tavor, G. E., Morales, J. P., & Kirchhoff, A. C. (2021). A qualitative inquiry of communication based barriers to the diagnosis of pediatric cancer: Perceptions of primarily Spanish-speaking caregiver. *Patient Education and Counseling*, *504*(6), 1503–1509. DOI: 10.1016/j.pec.2021.09.028 PMID: 34598802

Weber, O., Klemp, J., Chmetz, F., Daliani, A., Diserens, E. A., & Faucherre, F. (2023). Interpreter-mediated psychiatric assessments: Metacommunication as key. *Transcultural Psychiatry*, *60*(4), 626–636. DOI: 10.1177/13634615221119383 PMID: 36083232

Weiss, R. A., & Rosenfeld, B. (2012). Navigating cross-cultural issues in forensic assessment: Recommendations for practice. *Professional Psychology, Research and Practice*, *43*(3), 234–240. DOI: 10.1037/a0025850

Wells, A., Lagomasino, I., Palinkas, L., Green, J., & Gonzalez, D. (2013). Barriers to depression treatment among low-income, Latino emergency department patients. *Community Mental Health Journal*, *49*(4), 412–418. https://doi-org.libproxy.calbaptist.edu/10.1007/s10597-012-9547-5. DOI: 10.1007/s10597-012-9547-5 PMID: 23054150

Widom, C. S., Czaja, S. J., Bentley, T., & Johnson, M. S. (2012). A prospective investigation of physical health outcomes in abused and neglected children: New findings from a 30-year follow-up. *American Journal of Public Health*, *102*(6), 1135–1144. DOI: 10.2105/AJPH.2011.300636 PMID: 22515854

Widom, C. S., & Maxfield, M. G. (2001). *An update on the "cycle of violence."*. National Institute of Justice Research Brief., DOI: 10.1037/e528142006-001

Wiggins, K. (2024). What Congress should do about hate crime statistics. https://www.lawfaremedia.org/article/what-congress-should-do-about-hate-crime-statistics#:~:text=To%20improve%20hate%20crime%20statistics,impose%20hate%20crime%20reporting%20mandates

Williams, M. T., Peña, A., & Mier-Chairez, J. (2017). Tools for assessing racism-related stress and trauma among Latinos. In Benuto, L. T. (Ed.), *Toolkit for counseling Spanish-speaking clients*. Springer., DOI: 10.1007/978-3-319-64880-4_4

Williams, M. T., Printz, D., & DeLapp, R. C. (2018). Assessing racial trauma with the Trauma Symptoms of Discrimination Scale. *Psychology of Violence*, *8*(6), 735–747. DOI: 10.1037/vio0000212

Wilson, E., Chen, A. H., Grumbach, K., Wang, F., & Fernandez, A. (2005). Effects of limited English proficiency and physician language on health care comprehension. *Journal of General Internal Medicine*, *20*(9), 800–806. DOI: 10.1111/j.1525-1497.2005.0174.x PMID: 16117746

Wilson, F. E., Hennessy, E., Dooley, B., Kelly, B. D., & Ryan, D. A. (2013). Trauma and PTSD rates in an irish psychiatric population: A comparison of native and immigrant samples. *Disaster Health*, *1*(2), 74–83. DOI: 10.4161/dish.27366 PMID: 28228990

Worby, P. A., & Organista, K. C. (2013). Contextual influences on the drinking of male Latino immigrant day laborers. *Substance Use & Misuse*, *48*(5), 391–403. DOI: 10.3109/10826084.2013.765481 PMID: 23461665

Wylie, L., Van Meyel, R., Harder, H., Sukhera, J., Luc, C., Ganjavi, H., Elfakhani, M., & Wardrop, N. (2018). Assessing trauma in a transcultural context: Challenges in mental health care with immigrants and refugees. *Public Health Reviews*, *39*(1), 22. DOI: 10.1186/s40985-018-0102-y PMID: 30151315

Wynia, M. K., & Osborn, C. Y. (2010). Health literacy and communication quality in health care organizations. *Journal of Health Communication*, *15*(2), 102–115. DOI: 10.1080/10810730.2010.499981 PMID: 20845197

Xie, M., & Baumer, E. P. (2021). Immigrant status, citizenship, and victimization risk in the United States: New findings from the National Crime Victimization Survey (NCVS). *Criminology*, *59*(4), 610–644. DOI: 10.1111/1745-9125.12278 PMID: 35177865

Yllö, K., & Torres, M. G. (2016). *Marital rape: Consent, marriage, and social change in global context (Eds).* Oxford University Press.

Young, J., Binford, W., Bochenek, M. G., & Greenbaum, J. (2024). Health Risks of Unaccompanied Immigrant Children in Federal Custody and in US Communities. *American Journal of Public Health*, *114*(3), 340–346. DOI: 10.2105/AJPH.2023.307570 PMID: 38330256

Zaidi, R., & Sah, P. K. (2025). "Just make them feel welcomed": Examining newcomer ESL students' intersectional racism in Canadian schools. *International Multilingual Research Journal*, *19*(2), 1–18. DOI: 10.1080/19313152.2025.2476838

Zangeneh, M., & Al-Krenawi, A. (Eds.). (2019). *Culture, Diversity and Mental Health—Enhancing Clinical Practice*. Springer International Publishing., DOI: 10.1007/978-3-030-26437-6

Zghal, A., El-Masri, M., McMurphy, S., & Pfaff, K. (2021). Exploring the impact of health care provider cultural competence on new immigrant health-related quality of life: A cross-sectional study of Canadian newcomers. *Journal of Transcultural Nursing*, *32*(5), 508–517. DOI: 10.1177/1043659620967441 PMID: 33095098

Zhou, A. Q., Lee, H. Y., & Lee, R. M. (2019). Who has low health literacy and does it matter for depression? Findings from aggregated and disaggregated racial/ethnic groups. *Cultural Diversity & Ethnic Minority Psychology*, *25*(1), 73–81. DOI: 10.1037/cdp0000210 PMID: 30714769

About The Contributors

Ana M. Gamez, Ph.D., MBA, serves as a Professor of Psychology with tenure at California Baptist University, with over 20 years of teaching experience. She also serves as the Program Director and Practicum Director for the graduate program in Forensic Psychology. Dr. Gamez is a licensed clinical psychologist and the President and Chief Psychologist of Bee Haven Psychological & Behavioral Health Wellness, Inc., a psychological clinic that provides comprehensive psychological evaluations for immigration cases throughout California—T-Visa, U-Visa, Asylum, Hardship, Extreme Hardship, N-648, criminality, and substance abuse evaluations. She authored the book titled "Overcoming Adversity: An Immigrant's Perspective." She is also a retired Police Psychologist with the Los Angeles County Sheriff's Department, where she provided organizational consultations to department executives, program development, training, employee wellness, curriculum development, emergency response, and clinical services. Dr. Gamez offers nonprofit leadership to community organizations to help them fulfill their mission and vision. Her passion for assisting first responders led her to serve as the Chief Executive Officer for Badge of Life, 501 (C)(3), an agency that provides comprehensive services to first responders, promoting their physical and psychological well-being through awareness, support, evidence-based training, and education. Dr. Gamez has served as a national grant reviewer, published author, and researcher. Her research interests include forensic and police psychology, trauma, ethics, police misconduct and corruption, substance abuse, immigration, diversity, inclusion, and leadership. She has authored multiple books and articles and is a journal reviewer. She earned a Ph.D. in clinical psychology (LLU), an MBA in general business (WTAMU), an M.S. in forensic psychology (CSULA), a B.A. in psychology (CSULA), and a graduate certificate in diversity and inclusion from Cornell University.

***

Usharani Bhimavarapu is working as an Assistant Professor in the Computer Science and Engineering Department at Koneru Lakshmaiah Education Foundation at Vaddeswaram, Andhra Pradesh, India. She has been teaching from last 14 years with emphasis on Data Mining, Machine Learning, and Data Structure. She communicated more than 40 research papers in SCI, SCIE, Scopus indexed Journals. She has authored 12 books in programming languages like CPP, Java, Python, HTML, CSS and so on. Dr. Jude D. Hemanth received his B.E degree in ECE from Bharathiar University in 2002, M.E degree in communication systems from Anna University in 2006 and Ph.D. from Karunya University in 2013. His research areas include Computational Intelligence and Image processing. He has authored more than 230 research papers in reputed SCIE indexed International Journals and Scopus indexed International Conferences. His Cumulative Impact Factor is more than 350. He has published 37 edited books with reputed publishers such as Elsevier, Springer and IET.

Daniel Abdala earned a Bachelor of Arts in Sociology with a concentration in Criminology and a minor in Psychology from the University of Portland. He also holds an Associate Degree in Kinesiology Wellness from Mt. San Antonio College. Currently, he is pursuing a graduate degree in Forensic Psychology at California Baptist University, where he is also a student-athlete competing on the Men's Cross Country and Track and field teams.

Jerrondralyn K. Beltran holds a Master of Arts in Forensic Psychology from California Baptist University and a Bachelor of Arts in Psychology from the University of California - Riverside. Before beginning her graduate education, she served the courts and the community as a probation officer for 10 years, primarily supervising adult offenders. Jerrondralyn has remained closely connected to the criminal justice system through an internship with the district attorney's office.

Lizbeth Gaona is an assistant professor at California Baptist University in Riverside, California. She has extensive experience working as clinical consultant and clinical supervisor in community mental health programs. She received her B.A. in psychology from University of California, Los Angeles, her Master's in Social Work at California State University, Los Angeles and her doctorate at the USC Suzanne Dworak-Peck School of Social Work. Before returning to academia to pursue a doctorate, as a licensed clinical social worker, Dr. Gaona received rigorous clinical training with the Los Angeles County Department of Mental Health at Harbor UCLA Medical Center. Dr. Gaona was intensively trained in DBT in 2010 and has received training in DBT for Substance Abuse, DBT+PE (Prolonged Exposure), and DBT-ACES (Accepting the Challenges of Exiting the System).

From 2014-2015 Dr. Gaona served as the Director of the DBT-ACES program at Harbor UCLA Adult Outpatient Psychiatry Clinic. Along with her colleagues Dr. Gaona founded the first DBT Spanish adherent program within Los Angeles County in 2007. Dr. Gaona also participated in dissemination and implementation efforts of adherent cognitive behavior therapy in a collaborative project between the Los Angeles County Department of Mental Health and the Association of Cognitive and Behavior Therapy (A-CBT) and continues to serve as a DBT program consultant for Los Angeles County Department of Mental Health. In addition, Dr. Gaona serves a board member for th Association of Cognitive and Behavior Therapy (A-CBT). Some of Dr. Gaona's research interests include, community mental health outcomes, serious mental illness, culturally adapted evidenced based intervention research, evidenced based treatment outcomes across cultures, religion and trauma.

LizGomez is a bilingual licensed clinical social worker with years of practice with ethnic minority populations diagnosed with serious mental illnesses. Liz is also a clinical supervisor who has provided supervision for associate social workers seeking licensure. Liz provides evidence-based therapy in a collaborative, supportive, and affirming environment. Liz respects and incorporates a person's personal values, experiences and culture and utilizes an unconditional positive regard approach, allowing the client to feel fully accepted as they are without judgment.

Julie Goodman-Bowling serves as Professor of Anthropology and Chair of the Division of Family and Culture at California Baptist University. An applied, cultural anthropologist, her expertise centers on labor and migration, transnationalism and globalization, and the dynamics of identity formation. With over sixteen years of teaching experience, Dr. Goodman-Bowling brings a contagious passion for anthropology, inspiring students through the transformative journey of learning from and about others.

Özge Kutlu graduated from Social Work and Social Policy Master's Program in 2022. She is a doctoral student in the Social Work program at Hacettepe University. Kutlu, who worked as a Social Worker at Burdur Provincial Health Directorate between 2019-2023, has been working as a lecturer in Burdur Mehmet Akif Ersoy University Elderly Care program since February 2023. She works on the provision of rights-based social work practices for the elderly and their families.

Dylan Lacson holds a Master of Arts in Forensic Psychology at California Baptist University. Originally from the Philippines, he completed his undergraduate studies at Ateneo de Manila University, earning a Bachelor of Science in Psychology with a concentration in pre-medicine. He later obtained a certificate in Forensic Psychology from Washington University in St. Louis before relocating to the United

States for his graduate education. While completing his studies at California Baptist University, he was a graduate research assistant in the Forensic Research Lab and a teaching assistant for graduate classes. In addition, he undertook additional research experience as a graduate research assistant for the Maternal Health Network of San Bernardino, contributing to quantitative research focused on the quality and accessibility of maternal and mental health services for vulnerable populations.

Kelsey A. Michaels holds a Master of Arts in Forensic Psychology from California Baptist University, and a Bachelor of Arts in Psychology from the University of California, Riverside. Passionate about research, she is dedicated to advancing the field of forensic psychology through both academic and practical contributions. Her research spans a variety of fields, including forensic psychology, public health, and neurodevelopment. While at California Baptist University, her work focused on psychological evaluations in U.S. immigration proceedings and police psychology. In addition, she served as an intern at the Office of Violence Prevention, Los Angeles County Department of Public Health, where she analyzed organizations supporting victims of gender-based violence and assisted with gun violence prevention efforts. Previously, Kelsey worked as a research assistant at the Riverside University Health System's Comparative Effectiveness and Clinical Outcomes Research Center, helping develop a survey on vaccine hesitancy. She also supported suicide prevention research at the Community Translational Research Institute. While studying at UC Riverside, Kelsey led an undergraduate project on infant attentional selection at the Perception-Action Development Lab and contributed to neurodevelopmental research at the Kids Interaction and Neurodevelopment Lab. She has published research in Vaccines, exploring COVID-19 vaccine acceptance, hesitancy, and refusal among healthcare workers. As an undergraduate researcher, she was awarded the Undergraduate Research Mini-Grant at UC Riverside in 2020 for her project on infant attention. She also presented her research at the 2020 R'PSYC Conference, where she received the Best Novel Research Question and Highlighted Presentation awards. With a strong academic foundation and a commitment to both scholarly excellence and community impact, Kelsey is dedicated to advancing the field of forensic psychology while making valuable contributions to public health and safety.

Jasmine Morando is a fourth-year doctoral candidate in clinical psychology at California Baptist University, with a Master of Arts in Clinical Psychology and a Master of Science in Counseling Psychology from California Baptist University. Her clinical experience includes practicum training at the Department of State Hospitals - Patton, where she conducts forensic evaluations and assessments; Brea Olinda Unified School District, where she performed psychoeducational evaluations and provided school-based psychotherapy; and Psychological Services of Riverside, where she provided psychotherapy to adults and children. Furthermore, Jasmine has served as a bilingual registered associate marriage and family therapist at Trinity Youth Services, where she provided mental health services to underserved populations. She had the opportunity to collaborate with the Office of Refugee Resettlement, providing services to unaccompanied immigrant minors residing in the United States. Jasmine has served as a guest lecturer at California Baptist University and is currently working on a doctoral dissertation exploring mental health services in faith-based organizations. Her research experience also includes co-authoring a manuscript on the use of a Spanish primer in interventional radiology. Jasmine is bilingual in Spanish and English and has conducted assessments and therapy in both languages. Her commitment to working with underserved populations is a driving force behind her professional development.

Garrett P. Murrieta, M.A., is an adjunct professor at California Baptist University in the Masters in Forensic Psychology program. He also works at Hodson Private Investigations as an insurance investigator. He served five years in the United States Marine Corps as a security forces team leader, CQB team member, marksmanship coach, and infantry team leader. His interests include cult indoctrination, theology, philosophy, forensic psychology, personality psychology, and constitutional law. He earned an M.A. in Forensic Psychology (CBU) and a dual B.A. in Psychological Science and Criminology, Law, and Society (UCI).

AbbieNelson is an Assistant Professor at Southeast Missouri State University in the Department of Criminal Justice, Social Work and Sociology. She is a Licensed Clinical Social Worker with 18 years of experience working in the areas of trauma, domestic violence, sexual assault, and immigration. She has practiced in the United States, Mexico, and Guatemala. Her research interests include holistic interventions for survivors of intimate partner violence, the connection between nutrition and mental health, matricentric feminism, and global practice. She teaches a variety of clinical, practice, and policy social work classes.

John Park, Ph.D. is an associate professor of psychology at California Baptist University. He completed his doctoral studies at Loma Linda University in clinical psychology. He has also completed his postdoctoral fellowship at Dartmouth Medical Center in the department of psychiatry with a specialization in the treatment of anxiety and mood disorders, and behavioral medicine.

Joshua T. Shadwick is an Assistant Professor at Southeast Missouri State University in the Department of Criminal Justice, Social Work and Sociology. He teaches both undergraduate and graduate courses on topics ranging from research methods to gangs. His research interests include the justice system's response to social problems, police investigations, and wildlife crime. Dr. Shadwick's research has been published in peer-reviewed journals such as, Policing: An International Journal, Deviant Behavior, and Criminal Justice Policy Review.

Sneha Shenoy is a BSc Psychology student at PES University, Bangalore, with interests in community, forensic, and neuropsychology. She has contributed to academic literature on trauma, neuroscience, and mental health interventions. Sneha holds a Harvard Medical School certificate in autistic adults' care and is pursuing an online neuropsychology course from the University of Chicago. Her work focuses on chronic health, resilience, and well-being.

Mikaylin Turner holds a Master of Science in Criminal Justice. Her research interests focus on the study of hate crimes, exploring the sociological and legal implications of bias-motivated offenses, focusing on prevention strategies, victim advocacy, and policy reform. She is passionate about contributing to scholarship that advances understanding marginalized communities' experiences within the criminal justice system.

Index

L

M

P

R

S

T

U

V

www.ingramcontent.com/pod-product-compliance
Ingram Content Group UK Ltd.
Pitfield, Milton Keynes, MK11 3LW, UK
UKHW050947290926
15470UKWH00005B/1682

9 798369 379448